500

OF THE MOST IMPORTANT HEALTH TIPS YOU'LL EVER NEED

An A–Z of alternative health hints to help over 200 conditions

Hazel Courteney

With Stephen Langley and Gareth Zeal

D1392249

This edition published 2008 for Index Books Ltd

First published in Great Britain by
CICO Books
20-21 Jockey's Fields
London WC1R 4BW
020 7025 2280

Copyright © CICO Books 2001, 2006, 2008

First edition published 2001

Revised editions printed 2006, 2008

Text copyright © Hazel Courteney 2001, 2006, 2008

The right of Hazel Courteney to be identified as the author of this work has been asserted by her in accordance with the Copyright, Designs and Patents Act 1988.

All rights reserved. No part of this publication may be reproduced, stored in or introduced into a retrieval system, or transmitted in any form or by any means, electronic, mechanical, photocopying, recording or otherwise, without the prior written permission of the copyright holder and publisher.

10 9 8 7 6 5 4 3

A CIP catalogue record for this book is available from the British Library

ISBN-13: 978 1 904991 37 3

ISBN-10: 1 904991 37 8

Jacket design by Jerry Goldie

Designed by Jerry Goldie

Printed in Singapore by Tien Wah Press

PUBLISHERS' NOTE:
Always consult a doctor before undertaking any of the advice, exercise plans, or supplements suggested in this book. While every attempt has been made to ensure the medical information in this book is entirely safe and correct and up to date at the time of publication, the Publishers accept no responsibility for consequences of the advice given herein. If in any doubt as to the nature of your condition, consult a qualified medical practitioner.

The Publishers also accept no responsibility for changes in prices, stockist arrangements and locations mentioned herein.

Hazel Courteney is an award-winning, respected health and spiritual writer and speaker based in the UK. In 1997 she was voted Health Journalist of the Year for her column in *The Sunday Times*. Today Hazel writes regular features and columns for various publications. During her eight years as a weekly health columnist, Hazel answered more than 50,000 readers' health queries. This is her fourth health book. Hazel has also written two highly acclaimed spiritual/science books, and is currently working on her third. For more information on Hazel's work, log on to her website at www.hazelcourteney.com

Other books by Hazel Courteney:

500 of the Most Important Ways to Stay Younger Longer
Divine Intervention
The Evidence for the Sixth Sense
Mind and Mood Foods
Body and Beauty Foods

Gareth Zeal BSc is a nutritionist and health writer with 20 years' experience. He runs a busy health practice in London and regularly lectures around the UK. You can reach him via his office, on 020 7924 0970.

Stephen Langley ND, DipHom, DBM, DipAc, OMD is a registered Naturopath, Homeopath, Acupuncturist, Doctor of Chinese Medicine, and Medical Herbalist. He lectures in Naturopathic Medicine at the College of Naturopathic Medicine (CNM) in London, Bristol, Manchester, Dublin, Galway and Belfast, as well as running a busy health practice in London and lecturing globally. Stephen has studied Holistic Medicine in China, India, America, Australia, Tibet and Japan. He can be reached via the Hale Clinic. See page 361 for contact details.

Emma Wells Dip ION is a nutritional therapist based in Brighton, who runs a busy nutritional practice as well as lecturing at the Institute for Optimum Nutrition in London and Raworth. You can contact her by logging on to her website www.smartnutrition.co.uk, or at her office on 01273 775480.

AUTHOR'S NOTE

Throughout the book, we have in many instances suggested specific amounts of nutrients. This is to ensure that sufficient amounts of the nutrient are taken to benefit a specific condition. In places where no specific amounts are suggested, take the supplements daily, according to the instructions on the label or from your health professional.

I have mentioned only those books that I have found particularly useful, but whatever you are suffering from, believe me, there is a specialist book on it. Remember, you will fail only if you give up.

This book is not intended as a substitute for conventional medical counselling. Never stop taking prescribed medicine without first consulting your doctor. Always inform your doctor of any supplements or herbs you are taking in case these are contraindicated with your drugs.

During the last 20 years I have read hundreds of books and many phrases and facts have remained in my mind. Wherever possible, I have acknowledged the source of these phrases and facts, and to those whose names I have forgotten, my apologies for any unintentional oversights.

For the latest update on EC rulings regarding which supplements may or may not be available in the future, see page 8.

Acknowledgements

Revising this book has been a five-month labour of love. Several wonderful people have contributed to make this updated version truly special. To my original co-author Gareth Zeal, thanks for all our lengthy Sunday morning phone calls. My dear friend Stephen Langley – thanks for spending several days with me keeping me up-to-date on the latest news in naturopathy, and for your patience during the final read-through. To nutritionist, Emma Wells, thanks for writing several sections and contributing some of your knowledge to a host of others. A special thank you goes both to homeopathic pharmacist Margo Marrone, and to herbalist Malcolm Simmonds – for your time and patience and for sharing your knowledge.

Also my gratitude to Ali Hadi at Kudos Vitamins for having such great integrity and for allowing his nutritionists Shazia and Dana to check many of the conditions. Thank you ladies. Dear Sue Croft, at Consumers for Health Choice, thank you for keeping me up-to-date on the latest information on European legislation and for being a very special lady.

This section would not be complete without also sending a big hug to Lindsay Ross-Jarrett – who checked dozens of phone numbers and figures.

Finally, thanks as always to my wonderful husband Stuart – who has eaten a fair amount of baked beans whilst I have completed this update – I owe you a fabulous dinner!

For Victoria

I Love You

Mum

INTRODUCTION

WHY THERE IS STILL AN URGENT NEED FOR THIS BOOK ...

When I first wrote this book back in 2000, one in four people were developing cancer at some point in their lives – that figure is now one in three. Certain cancer charities state this will shortly become one in every two people. Furthermore, more than eight million men and women in the UK are obese, that's one in five adults. Among six- to 15-year-olds obesity has trebled from 5% in 1990 to 16% in 2004. This in turn has triggered an explosion of late-onset diabetes which affects more than two million people in the UK alone and costs the NHS five and a half billion pounds a year to treat. That's £165 a second.

The 'good' news is that in 2000 heart disease killed 140,000 people, and last year it killed *only* 110,000. Nevertheless the UK still has one of the highest death rates from heart disease in the world.

The continuing tragedy is that virtually all these conditions, are, in the majority of cases, totally preventable. The average adult eats 60 pounds of sugar a year – and people wonder why late-onset diabetes is now becoming common even in teenagers! Twenty years ago the average age for late-onset diabetes to occur was 50.

Yes, thousands of people have changed their diets and lifestyles, and thanks to excellent columnists, such as Dr John Briffa and naturopath Stephen Langley, plus great TV shows, such as "You Are What You Eat" with Dr Gillian McKeith, the message about what constitutes a healthy diet and healthy lifestyle is getting through.

However, we still have some way to go: binge drinking among young people is on the rise; 15 million people in the UK still smoke and, in 2004, they smoked more than 55 million cigarettes. Four-hundred-and-fifty children start smoking every day.

Human nature is perverse. Everyone knows that smoking, and passive smoking, can kill; but not all youngsters or their parents realize that binge drinking can severely damage the liver. Specialists are seeing youngsters in their twenties with liver damage usually associated with unhealthy 50-year-olds. Why? Because most youngsters – and many adults – think that it's never going to happen to them ... until it does.

How much better it would be if we could take not only a lot more responsibility for our own health, but also learn more about our bodies with the aim of preventing them becoming sick in the first place. Unfortunately, too many people still hand total responsibility for their health to their overworked doctor. Most GPs are caring, hard-working people, but during their six years at medical school they are lucky to receive four hours' training in how diet, taking the right supplements, and lifestyle can greatly improve and prevent many illnesses. Most of their courses are sponsored by drugs companies, which is why prescribing a pill for our illnesses remains their usual response. But this practice rarely addresses the root cause of the condition.

Almost everyone is looking for a single magic bullet to help alleviate their health problems. Most of us are in a hurry and yet happy to react to misleading health information which appears in the media with alarming regularity. But help is at hand. Certified organic food has really taken off and virtually all supermarkets now offer excellent ranges of organic produce. Prices have come down – and most people definitely prefer organic.

The more we eat organic the less hormone-disrupting chemicals we swallow. Unfortunately, each year, more than 31 tonnes of 50 of the mostly extensively used pesticides are still sprayed over our fruits, vegetables and grains. But at long last this may soon change. In September 2005 The Royal Commission on Environmental Pollution stated that fears linking cancers, miscarriages and numerous diseases to overuse of pesticides may be justified. It's taken a long time. Antibiotic residues are in our water, too, along with hormone residues from the pill and HRT.

In 2000 I also wrote about how the 31 million mobile phones in use were linked with depression and various cancers. There are now more than 52 million mobiles in use in the UK – many by children – even though the Government has issued warnings that young children should not use mobile phones. If you add the negative affects of mobile phones to the microwaves, computers, and all electrical equipment which pulse us with harmful electromagnetic radiation, and again to the affects of our diets and lifestyles, you soon realize that it's the cumulative effects of these factors that is triggering the tidal wave of illness we experience today. Our bodies were never designed to eat so much rubbish and ingest so many chemicals and they are telling us that they have simply had enough. We have caused most of the problems we face today – but the good news is that we can change or reverse many of them.

MRSA has been triggered by our overuse of antibiotics – but many doctors don't know that Manuka honey and bee propolis, as well as herbs such as pau d'arco and St John's wort have been scientifically proven to destroy MRSA and many other superbugs.

We also know that if hyperactive and violent children and adults are given a healthier diet along with the right supplements, they become calmer and easier to live with. Trial after trial – including a brilliant TV series with nutritionist Patrick Holford – has shown just how diet can affect one's mood.

In the meantime, I'll bet most of you have never heard of Thieves Essential Oil. Made with a blend of cloves, lemon, eucalyptus and rosemary, Thieves has been scientifically tested and found to have a 99.996% kill-rate against all airborne bacteria. Its name derives from the days when 15th-century thieves rubbed these oils on themselves to avoid contracting bubonic plague while they robbed the bodies of the dead and dying. Find details of this amazing therapeutic oil in the new MRSA section. With so many diseases on the increase, and with various bacteria mutating into deadlier strains faster than doctors can kill them, the time has come to discover new ways to protect ourselves.

For this reason I have completely revised and updated this book to give you access to the latest developments in the alternative health field. I have included many new headings, including Hepatitis and Food Poisoning, both of which are on the increase. You will also discover why taking liquid hyaluronic acid – a naturally occurring protein in the body – can help to keep your joints and skin younger.

Throughout this book I and my colleagues have given numerous, often little-known but well-researched solutions to many health problems plus a host of proven remedies, nutrients and ideas to improve your health on a day-to-day basis. We also offer alternative answers to many common symptoms that even your doctor may not recognize – to help you become your own health detective. Remember: the body is perfectly capable of healing itself when it is given the right tools for the job.

May our work give you good health – today and all days.

Hazel Courteney

IS OUR RIGHT TO TAKE SUPPLEMENTS UNDER THREAT?

Sue Croft, a director of CHC Consumers for Health Choice, spends her life lobbying MPs and regulators (the people who make claims on how we live our lives), both in the UK and in Brussels, to help us retain our freedom to choose. She says that "As things stand [November 2005] we are still set to lose many of our nutritional supplements, the biggest threat is to specific specialist sources of nutrients such as the chelated- and yeast-based types of minerals. The dose levels of vitamins and minerals they will allow us to take may not be set for another two years, although work has already started on examining safety issues. Also, most of the people in the Member States of the EU are not used to taking higher-dose nutrients – and unfortunately the majority view that wants low dosages could prevail. For instance the current RDI (Recommended Daily Intake) for vitamin C, needed for more than 40 functions in the body, is 60mg, but this is only just sufficient to prevent scurvy. Yet this is the dose that is mostly available in Europe – and those countries with the largest number of votes, France and Germany, want to keep it that way. Even though there are thousands of published and verified scientific studies showing that appropriate higher dosages are both safe and beneficial, we still have a fight on our hands. This is why we are using all our influence to push the British Government to wade in to this argument on our behalf.

The signs so far are positive, but time is of the essence. What most people don't understand is that our nutritional products are sold under Food Law: they have to be 100% safe – as safe as a loaf of bread or a tomato. And just because a medicine has a product licence (which allows the makers to make specific beneficial claims, and can cost millions of pounds that vitamin companies just don't have) it doesn't make it safe. Vioxx, the arthritis drug, was granted a medicinal licence and has been taken by 20 million people. Unfortunately, many are now dead and others are bringing massive law suits against the makers of this drug. There has been only one recorded incidence of death from anyone taking supplements, and that was a small child who swallowed a whole bottle of his mother's high-dose prescription iron tablets. In the past 11 years there have been only eleven reported cases of people claiming symptoms such as tingling fingers and toes from taking certain nutrients to excess, which rapidly recede once those supplements are stopped. Yet more than 40,000 people die annually thanks to prescription drugs."

Like Sue, I feel very strongly about this subject and I hope you will write to your MP and MEP to tell them of the health benefits you have experienced thanks to taking supplements. For the latest news regarding this unwelcome legislation log onto CHC's website: www.healthchoice.org.uk

WHY YOU NEED NUTRITIONAL SUPPLEMENTS

How many times have you heard people say "Surely if I eat a healthy balanced diet, I will not need to take vitamins and minerals."

"Expensive pee!" others exclaim.

When I started writing about health almost 15 years ago, I thought "Oh, it won't take long for people to change once they know the facts." I was wrong. The Government's campaign encouraging everyone to eat five portions of fruit and vegetables a day has fallen mainly on deaf ears. A few people have changed but the fact remains that as little as 5% of the Western population eats a truly healthy, balanced diet. The majority talk about healthy eating, but in reality continue to eat far too much pre-packaged, refined junk foods that are often packed with salt, sugar, additives and saturated fats. A few people still do not comprehend that the human body is literally made of food molecules, so your body is largely made up from what you have eaten during the last year.

Also, during the past five years, most commercial growers – especially from overseas – are harvesting more and more of their fruit and vegetables long before they are ripe. Research in Spain and at Oregon State University in America have found that when, for example, cherries are picked before being ripe the vitamin C content is halved. When blackberries were picked early, the green ones contained 74mg of anthocyanins (the blue pigment that is great for your eyes and immune system) compared with 317mg in the naturally ripened fruits. Add to this the fact that most fresh produce is flown halfway round the world – and then stored for long periods which itself hugely depletes nutrient levels – the message is obvious: as much as possible buy more fresh, ripe, locally grown foods.

To survive, the human body needs 50 factors, these are 13 vitamins, 21 minerals, 9 amino acids, 2 essential fatty acids, plus carbohydrate, fibre, air, water and light. As our bodies cannot manufacture these substances, we must take them in from external sources – through our diet and by taking the right supplements. If the body becomes deficient in nutrients, negative symptoms will eventually result.

We can all have treats and really enjoy them – but we must stop living on them. Many times I have watched people fill their supermarket trolleys with white bread, prepackaged meals, cakes, chocolate bars and fizzy drinks. Almost all this refined, prepackaged and processed food contains virtually no vitamins, essential fats, minerals or fibre. We are bombarded with food advertisements claiming that products are 'packed with added vitamins'. Have you ever asked yourself why the manufacturers need to add vitamins, if the food is supposed to be nutritious in the first place?

Dr Richard Passwater, who has worked as a research scientist in Maryland, USA, for 40 years, states that refined sugars have had 99.9% of all their natural nutrients removed, and the only reason that there is 0.1% nutritional value left is because the manufacturing companies cannot figure out how to remove the last 0.1%. White flour and mass-produced oils are the same. Tinned foods are sterilised at high temperatures to kill any bacteria. How many nutrients do you think are left after these processes?

Without doubt I advocate organic farming and the more farmers who switch to organic methods, the fewer pesticides and herbicides (known to deplete even more nutrients from our food) will be in our food, water and air. And organic food has been proven to contain more nutrients than non-organic produce. Fewer chemicals means less acid rain, less pollution and less sickness. GM foods to my mind are another BSE/CJD-scenario waiting to happen – I would never knowingly eat GM foods. Intensive farming methods still use far too many antibiotics for their livestock – which definitely add to our health problems.

Natural mineral levels in soil in many countries, including the UK, are dropping, and if vital nutrients such as selenium, known to reduce the incidence of cancer and heart disease, are not in our soil they are never going to make it into our fruits and vegetables. This is why, in countries such as Finland, selenium has been added to all fertilisers since 1984. As a result sperm counts have risen and incidence of heart disease is falling.

Unfortunately, some people still compare vitamins, minerals and essential fats in capsule forms, to prescription drugs – but remember that essential nutrients are essential to life.

All these nutrients work synergistically, or together, inside the body. In a perfect world it is always preferable to ingest all the nutrients we need from a varied diet. But most people do not.

Our eating habits have changed drastically during recent years. As little as 50 years ago, it was routine for the family to sit and eat home-cooked meals with freshly picked vegetables and fruits from a local farm or allotment. Today, this tradition seems to have all but disappeared. The longer fresh food is stored and cooked, the more nutrients are lost. If you leave an orange in a fridge for more than three days, up to 50% of the vitamin C content disappears. And, because the modern diet is less than perfect, we need to come to a compromise – hence I take nutritional supplements and recommend specific nutrients in this book.

Many governments suggest minimum amounts of nutrients, called RDIs – Recommended Daily Intakes. In Europe there are RDIs for 19 nutrients and yet there are 45 essential nutrients required for health. Confusion is rife as RDIs vary from country to country, so whom do we believe? Initially, the idea of RDIs was to prevent obvious signs of deficiency, such as scurvy (vitamin-C deficiency) in soldiers in the trenches in 1941. However, they do not represent the quantities of nutrients we require for optimum health. Nor do they represent the levels of vitamins and minerals we need to protect our bodies from the pollutants and toxins in our modern environment. What is more, RDIs take no account of individual requirements such as age, gender or the health status of the person. For example, the current RDI for vitamin C is 60mg – but to ingest this amount from your diet you would need to eat 10 apples, 3 kiwi fruits or 2 large freshly picked oranges. In the US, the RDI for the mineral chromium, which has been proven to halve the incidence of late-onset diabetes, is 120mcg; yet in the UK or Europe no RDI exists. And to add insult to injury this is one of the minerals that the EU has excluded from its guidance list. This is lunacy. But there is hope. A few years ago, I met a man aged 73 who had been refused heart surgery as his arteries were so blocked. He was deemed a lost cause, totally breathless, he could not even walk across the room. A nutritional physician friend took him on. First, she completely changed his diet, then gave him supplements proven to thin blood naturally, lower cholesterol levels and to help clear some of the plaque that had built up in his arteries. Under medical supervision he was also taught yoga. After several months he slowly but surely regained his health. Today he climbs Alpine slopes as a hobby. It's never too late to change. And as Western doctors are now seeing plaque in the arteries of children as young as 10, change is imperative.

We all need to start eating food that is as unprocessed and unrefined as possible. Natural, locally grown organic food, without pesticides and additives, plus taking the right supplements is the way forward. There are now more than half a million clinical research papers showing that taken in the right amounts nutritional supplements can, and do, work.

IMPORTANT HINTS TO NOTE BEFORE TAKING SUPPLEMENTS

If you are taking any prescription drugs you must advise your doctor of any supplements or herbs you wish to take in case of complications. For example, the drug warfarin thins the blood, but so does vitamin E and the herb *Ginkgo biloba*. If you decide to begin taking supplements you must check with your GP so that you can have regular blood tests. Then, in time and with your doctor's permission, hopefully you can reduce your intake of drugs.

- It is important to note that vitamins, minerals and essential fatty acids are nutrients essential to life – but herbs are powerful medicines. Many prescription drugs are based on herbs. Herbs themselves are not essential to life, but, when taken in the appropriate amounts and for the appropriate time, have proven to be of great benefit for many conditions. Generally, take herbs for no more than 3 months at a time, have a month or so without them and then, if you feel the need, begin taking them again. Generally look for whole herbal preparations in powder form, rather than herbal extracts that have been standardised for one particular 'active' ingredient. 'Whole herb' preparations can also be safer. For example, nearly every recorded adverse health reaction, which resulted in the problems with Kava Kava were caused by Kava-standardised extracts. For help with any herbs suggested in this book, call a qualified herbalist or health professional, or contact *The Specialist Herbal Supplies* on 0870 774 4494 Website: www.shs100.com

- Supplements taken regularly in the long term almost always produce beneficial effects, but don't expect miracles in a week. Supplements are not magic bullets, but stimulate the body's natural healing processes, giving long-term health benefits. Generally speaking, supplementation with nutrients produces improvements in health more slowly than prescription medication, which normally just suppresses symptoms. If you start a course of vitamins, minerals or any supplements, take them regularly for at least two months in order to see the benefits. Any changes in your health may be very subtle.

- Some supplements currently on the market have less than optimum quantities of beneficial ingredients. In general you get what you pay for. Some low-priced supplements contain relatively small amounts of nutrients or forms of nutrients. The better quality and usually more expensive supplements generally provide better value for money in the long term.

- Most vitamins have a good shelf life but cease to be effective if you keep them for too long. Be aware of sell-by dates and always keep your vitamins in a cool, dry place – never expose them to direct sunlight.

- If you find that vitamin C irritates your gut, try Esther C, or vitamin C in an ascorbate form. There is also Crystal C which is based on sodium ascorbate. It is pH neutral and even in higher doses should not cause any irritation. Visit www.crystalc.co.uk. Vitamin C is more effective when taken in repeated small doses throughout the day with food.

- Take supplements with food, which ensures better absorption, unless otherwise stated on the label.

- Avoid taking any supplements with tea, coffee or alcohol as these can block absorption of certain nutrients, especially iron.

- Some people have reactions to certain supplements but this is quite rare. This is usually caused not by the nutrients themselves but by a reaction to one or more of the other ingredients contained in the supplement. In general, better quality supplements containing hypoallergenic ingredients are less likely to give rise to adverse reactions. If you suffer a negative reaction to any supplement or herb, stop taking it immediately. For example, most glucosamine supplements are mainly derived from crushed crab shells – so, if you are highly sensitive to shellfish, ask for the vegetarian version derived from corn which is now available from health shops.

- Products derived from bees, in extremely rare cases, may cause a reaction in anyone who suffers a severe sensitivity to bee stings. Obviously if you know this is a problem avoid products related to bees! In the case of bee propolis, this would also apply to tree resins.
- The supplements suggested in this book can be taken by anyone over the age of 16. For children's dosages, seek professional guidance.
- Probiotics (friendly bacteria), more commonly known as acidophilus, should also contain bifidus strain bacteria. All probiotic preparations keep better in glass bottles and should be kept either in a fridge or freezer. There are now various probiotics available that do not need to be kept refrigerated and can survive stomach acid – but these should be taken immediately after food unless otherwise directed.
- Natural source, full-spectrum vitamin E is better absorbed and retained by the body than synthetic forms.
- If you are pregnant, or planning a pregnancy, do not take any supplement containing more than 3000iu of vitamin A per day. Most manufacturers state whether supplements are unsuitable to be taken during pregnancy. The UK Government warns that pregnant women should consume no more than one portion of liver a week, as liver is high in Vitamin A – and too much vitamin A is linked to calcium loss. One portion of liver may contain 30,000 to 40,000iu of vitamin A, but such a risk would occur only at about 85,000iu a day. In fact too much of *any* animal protein will deplete calcium from the body. We need to realize that vitamin A is vital for a healthy immune system, for healthy skin, eyes and a healthy pregnancy at modest levels. To overdose on vitamin A you would need to take more than 30,000iu daily for a month or more. If in doubt take natural-source beta carotenes, which naturally convert to vitamin A in the body and have not been linked to reducing bone mass.
- Do not take separate iron supplements if you are over 50 unless you have been diagnosed with a medical condition that requires extra supplementation as iron accumulates in the body, and too high a level is linked with heart disease and strokes. **Never leave iron tablets near children.**
- Keep all supplements away from young children. Any substance taken in excess can cause harm – even water. Follow the manufacturer's instructions unless your health professional advises otherwise.
- If you have any problem taking pills and cannot find liquid formulas at your health shop use an inexpensive tablet crusher. To order call **Health Plus** on 01323 872277 or visit their website: www.healthplus.co.uk; or call Orange Burst on 01273 558112 or visit their website: www.lemonburst.net
- The supplements we suggest should be taken in most instances until the condition is alleviated. For maintenance nutrients see under *General Supplements* on page 160.
- If you are in any doubt about the amount of supplements you or your children should be taking, always consult a qualified health practitioner.

HOW TO USE THIS BOOK
AND KEY TO CODES

Throughout this book we have suggested numerous formulas – and given the names of the companies that make them. All their details are here if you wish to contact them. If we have mentioned no company, shop or brand name, then the listed supplements should be readily available from good health food stores worldwide.

No one is more aware than myself of the thousands of alternative supplements now available. In this book we have suggested many specific brands, which we have used, and/or come to trust over many years. If we tried to mention every brand by name, this book would not be an easy-to-read book of hints, but a lengthy encyclopaedia. Our choices of specific brands in no way infers that they are better or more beneficial than others on the market. If you have specific brands that you know and trust, check with your own suppliers or health shop who, I am sure, will stock similar supplements to those recommended. It is well worth noting that virtually every reputable supplement company has its own in-house qualified nutritionists who are happy to help you. Don't be afraid to call them. Most of these suppliers are happy to post orders anywhere worldwide.

BC
BioCare Ltd
Lakeside, 180 Lifford Lane, Kings Norton, Birmingham, B30 3NU
Tel: 0121 433 3727
Fax: 0121 433 8705
Email: customerservices@biocare.co.uk
Website: www.biocare.co.uk

BLK
Blackmores are now called Naturopathic Health and Wellness
Tel (general-public mail order): 0870 770 0980
Email: info@apotheke20-20.co.uk
If you need to speak to a nutritionist who knows the Blackmores' range call: 0208 995 2293
Any practitioners wanting to order the Blackmores range should call G&G on 0870 770 0976

FSC
FSC vitamins are now called BHM Healthgroup
Lancaster Road, Carnaby Industrial Estate, Bridlington, East Yorkshire YO15 3QY
Tel: 01262 607890
Fax: 01262 424012
Email: sales@beehealth.com
Website: www.bhmhealthgroup.com

HN
Higher Nature Ltd
The Nutrition Centre, Burwash Common, East Sussex, TN19 7LX
Tel: 01435 883484
Fax: 0870 066 4010
Orders: 0800 458 4747

Helpline: 0800 458 4747
Email: info@higher-nature.co.uk
Website: www.highernature.co.uk

KVH
Kudos Vitamins and Herbals Ltd
Units 2 & 2A, Quidhampton Business Units, Polhampton Lane, Overton, Hampshire RG25 3EA
Tel: 01256 773299; Freephone: 0800 389 5476; Fax: 01256 771631
Email: info@kudosvitamins.com
Website: www.kudosvitamins.com

NP
Nature's Plus (they make a great range for children)
Nutrigroup Ltd, Waterloo House, 1 Waterloo Road, Epsom, Surrey, KT19 8AY
Tel: 01372 724216
Email: sales@nutriglow.com
Website: www.nutriglow.com

NC
The Nutri Centre
The Hale Clinic, 7 Park Crescent, London, W1N 3HE
Tel: 020 7436 5122; or Freephone: 0800 587 2290
Fax: 020 7436 5171
Bookshop tel: 020 7323 2382; fax: 020 7636 0276
Email: enq@NutriCentre.com
Website: www.NutriCentre.com

OP
The Organic Pharmacy
396 Kings Road, London SW10 OLN
Tel: 020 7351 2232
Email: organp@dircon.co.uk
Website: www.theorganicpharmacy.com

PN
Pharma Nord (UK) Ltd
Telford Court, Morpeth, NE61 2DB
Tel: 01670 519989
Fax: 01670 534903
Email: info@pharmanord.co.uk
Website: www.multivits.co.uk

PW
Pharm West Inc.
4640 Admiralty Way # 423, Marina Del Rey, California 90292, USA
Tel. UK and Ireland: 00 353 46 943 7317
Fax UK and Ireland: 00 353 46 943 7310
Tel. US: 001 310 301 4015

Fax US: 001 310 577 0296
Email: infodesk@pharmwest.com
Website: www.pharmwest.com

SL
Sloane Health Shop
27 Kings Road, London SW3 4RT
Tel: 020 7730 7046
Or: 50 High Street, Esher, Surrey, KT10 9QY
Tel: 01372 465864

SVHC
Solgar Vitamin and Herb Company
Aldbury, Tring, Herts HP23 5PT
Tel: 01442 890 355
Fax: 01442 890 366
For technical support or to speak to a nutritionist tel: 01442 890355
Email: solgarinfo@solgar.com
Website: www.solgar-vitamins.co.uk
Solgar Vitamin and Herb Company
500 Willow Tree Road, Leonia, New Jersey 07605, USA
Consumers' tel: 001 877 765 4274
For retail stores call: 001 800 645 2246
Website: www.solgar.com

SHS
Specialist Herbal Supplies
This company uses 'whole herbs' and is run by Malcolm Simmonds BAc, MH, MBRI
Portslade Hall, 18 Station Road, Portslade, Brighton, BN41 1GB
Tel: 0870 774 4494
Fax: 01273 424345
Email: sales@shs100.com
Website: www.shs100.com

Therapeutic Grade Essential Oils
By Young Living in the USA, these are some of the finest and most healing bio-dynamic oils I have found. In the UK for help as to which oil you need for your specific condition call Susie Anthony on 01749 679900 or log on to her website: www.psalifemastery.com and look for the **Resources** pages.

ABSORPTION <small>(see also *Coeliac Disease, Indigestion, Low Stomach Acid* and *Stress*)</small>

We are not only what we eat, but also what our bodies are able to absorb and eliminate. Many people presume that every item of food they swallow is automatically absorbed into their system, but there is a vital intermediate stage. You swallow food, and if chewed thoroughly, then a form of amylase, an enzyme in your saliva, begins breaking down your food. But if you are stressed, and as we age, levels of amylase fall causing more absorption problems. Amylase is 30 times more abundant in the average 25-year-old than the average 80-year-old.

The chewing process also alerts the stomach that food is on its way, which triggers stomach-acid production, ready to begin the digestion process. Chewing is the first and very important stage of digestion. Your stomach does not have any teeth! With ageing, and problems like gastritis, stomach-acid production is also reduced. Without these natural digestive aids, absorption of nutrients through our gut walls and into the bloodstream is greatly diminished. Therefore vital nutrients needed for tissue repair and cellular regeneration can sometimes pass through the body and out the other end undigested.

Absorption mostly takes place in the small intestine, but as we age enzymes produced by the pancreas (which helps to further break down sugars, proteins and fats) are also reduced. As the pace of modern life is increasing, more and more people, even young people, suffer varying degrees of absorption problems. Stress also has a negative effect on the digestive process as it reduces absorption by shutting down enzyme production.

Symptoms of malabsorption include hair loss, low energy levels, chronic fatigue, weight loss or gain, poor bone density, dry and wrinkled skin, and dry hair and nails. Naturopath, Steve Langley says, "Almost all disease is linked to deficiency of nutrients and toxicity within the body, therefore if you get your digestive system in good working order, a huge amount of health problems could be avoided."

Foods to Avoid

- Reduce your intake of red meats and heavy, rich meals. Concentrated proteins and fats, such as red meat and cheese, are harder to digest as they require more work as well as oxygen to break them down completely. We need to maintain a high oxygen level in our tissues to keep our bodies healthy. And all junk foods reduce oxygen levels and accelerate loss of enzyme reserves in the body.
- Avoid croissants, burgers, fried foods, excessive high-sugar foods and full-fat dairy produce. The more unnatural your diet, the more the body has to produce enzymes to digest your food, and over time negative symptoms can arise.
- Cooked cheese is really hard on your digestive system.
- Modern refined wheat and related products are often hard to digest as we lack the necessary enzymes.
- Avoid drinking too much fluid with meals, which dilutes the stomach acid – the very substance you need for digesting your meal.

Friendly Foods

- Raw, steamed or lightly cooked foods retain more enzymes, which aid digestion. Papaya is rich in papain, which aids in the breakdown of foods in the stomach and small intestine. It is best eaten before a main meal.
- Pineapple is rich in the enzyme bromelain, which again aids digestion. Eat a small amount before main meals.
- Generally increase your intake of fresh raw foods. Eat a salad at least once daily in summer. Light stir-fries and steamed vegetables are also fine.
- If you have a problem with wheat, try spelt, millet, buckwheat, amaranth or quinoa-based breads, which are available in most supermarkets and health stores.
- Try rice, corn, buckwheat or millet-based pastas, which are also easier to digest.
- If you have a problem with cow's milk, try rice, almond, oat or goat's milk, which are gentler on the stomach.
- A glass of red wine can help to stimulate stomach-acid production.

Useful Remedies

- Take a digestive enzyme capsule with all main meals. Available from health stores.
- You can also take hydrochloric acid (HCl) with pepsin capsule with main meals, but only if you have been diagnosed as suffering from low stomach acid (see under *Low Stomach Acid*).
- Bitter herbs such as gentian, in tincture form, can be taken 15 minutes before each meal to stimulate production of stomach acid and digestive enzymes.
- A teaspoon of apple cider vinegar in a little water taken before main meals can also help increase stomach-acid production.

Helpful Hints

- Try not to eat late at night as this places an extra burden on the digestive system.
- Chew thoroughly, and as much as possible eat sitting down in a relaxed frame of mind. Not always easy, but this simple act really aids digestion.
- Avoid eating for about an hour after rigorous exercise.
- Don't eat large meals when you are under stress. Keep them small and light.
- If your digestive system is playing up, try 'food combining'. Basically this means separating concentrated proteins, such as meat, fish, eggs and cheese, from concentrated carbohydrates, such as potatoes, rice, bread and pasta. So, if for example you are eating fish, eat it with vegetables rather than potatoes. And if you have pasta, then also eat this with vegetables but not meat or fish. Eat fruit in-between or 15–20 minutes before a meal rather than after a main meal. Fruit likes a quick passage through the gut and if it gets 'stuck' behind a main meal, gas and bloating can result. This is especially true of melon. Some nutritionists now state that food combining is old fashioned but naturopath Stephen Langley says, "There is no doubt that anyone with digestion and absorption problems would find lets say pasta and meat together pretty hard to digest. I have seen thousands of patients who have been helped by this method of eating – especially those who want to lose weight." For this reason eat melon on its own as a starter, and don't combine with other fruits, as melon has an even quicker transit time than other fruits, which again can trigger fermentation and bloating in the gut.

ACID–ALKALINE BALANCE

(see also *Arthritis, Indigestion and Low Stomach Acid*)

Nutritionists and health professionals have long understood the importance of maintaining a healthy acid/alkaline balance. At last this subject is receiving wider attention. For good health the body needs to maintain a certain acid–alkaline balance and keeping this balance is one of the crucial keys to remaining healthy and also slowing the ageing process. Every cell functions more efficiently when it is predominantly alkaline.

In general the body needs to be around 70% alkaline and 30% acid. But in the West the average person is 80% acid and 20% alkaline, hence why we are suffering so many acid conditions such as arthritis. Many people confuse the term acid-forming with the term acidic, but they are entirely different. Everything we swallow, once metabolised within the body, breaks down into either an alkaline or acid mineral based ash or residue. Whether a substance is alkaline or acid is determined by its pH (potential Hydrogen). Stomach acid can be as low as pH 1.5, very acid, whereas saliva after eating could be as high as pH 8, which is very alkaline. Your blood has a pH which is slightly alkaline – between 7.35 and 7.45 – and this level needs to be maintained at all costs. If it becomes too acid, the blood (via the kidneys) withdraws alkalising minerals from anywhere it can find them; beginning with the hair, skin and nails and then moving on through the body until it begins drawing minerals from the bones, which in time contributes to conditions such as osteoporosis.

Unfortunately most modern lifestyles and diets are almost all acid-forming and if the body remains in an acid state for too long, this acidity triggers degenerative diseases. A high acid-forming diet also has a negative effect on tooth enamel – especially pre-packaged concentrated fruit juices. Acid-forming foods deplete calcium from the body, while alkaline foods increase the body's ability to absorb calcium from the diet.

Emotions greatly affect this balance: stress and anger trigger more acidity within the body, whereas feelings of being in control, in love and breathing deeply through the nose re-alkalises the body. Basically harmony alkalises and disharmony acidifies.

Practically every major degenerative disease, including some cancers, is triggered by an over-acid system. When the pH is out of balance, your skin and hair become dull, the nervous system is affected and you may suffer insomnia, arthritis, rheumatism, aching joints, skin conditions, candida, fungal infections, muscle pain and gout, which are all common symptoms of an over-acid system.

Foods to Avoid

- It's important to realise that just because a food is acid-forming it is not necessarily unhealthy. Proteins are acid-forming, but they are also essential for good health. Therefore, if you tend to eat two large meat-based meals daily, reduce it to one. Make the other a fish-based meal, or eat pulses such as soya, aduki or pinto beans.
- Basically all animal produce and egg yolks are acid-forming. Duck, venison, grouse and pheasant, lamb, beef and pork are all acid-forming. Fish, turkey and chicken are also acid-forming, but do not contain such high levels of uric acid as red meat.
- Milk and yoghurt are alkaline before digestion but become acid-forming once digested. This is why milk products are calming to an over-acid oesophagus if you suffer from an acid-type reflux after food. But in the long term this would exacerbate arthritic type conditions. It's just a case of getting a balance.
- All nuts are acid-forming except almonds, fresh coconut, and chestnuts.
- All grains are also acid-forming with the exception of millet, buckwheat, amaranth and quinoa. Whole grains are a healthy food and remember: these foods are not to be eliminated *per se*, you just need to be aware of what is acid-forming.
- All refined sugars found in cakes, biscuits, pre-packaged desserts, whips and so on are acid-forming. Chocolate is a truly acid-forming treat, it's high in oxalic acid which is linked to kidney stones – so, don't overdo it!

- Wine, beer, spirits, coffee, tea, fizzy drinks and sweetened fruit juices are all highly acid-forming.
- All drugs, prescription and social, such as cannabis, are also acidic.
- Cranberries, plums, prunes and rhubarb are highly acid-forming. But again I reiterate, these foods are healthy – in fact prunes (dried plums) are very anti-ageing. Everything in moderation.
- Mass-produced malt vinegar, a waste product of the brewing industry, is also acid-forming in the body.

Friendly Foods
- Honey and brown-rice syrup are alkalising. But don't overdo these foods – as they are sugar! If you eat too much of them, the sugar converts to fat and lives on your hips. Again just get a balance.
- All vegetables are alkaline but the best are wheat grass, alfalfa, kelp, seaweed, parsley, watercress, carrots, endives and celery. All green foods are high in chlorophyll, which is rich in magnesium, a major alkalising mineral.
- Cabbage, kale, broccoli, spring greens, green beans and asparagus are all great alkaline foods. Spinach contains oxalic acid, but it breaks down into an alkaline residue.
- All fruits are healthy, and you should eat them freely, but be aware that cranberries, plums, prunes and rhubarb are highly acid-forming and to a lesser degree so are blueberries, blackberries, raspberries and strawberries.
- The most alkalising fruits are cantaloupe melons (and all melons), papaya, dates, especially dried dates, mangoes, lemons, limes and figs. In case you are wondering, it's the alkaline mineral content and not the sugar content that determines whether a food is acid or alkaline forming in the body.
- Oranges, grapefruit, pineapple, cherries, kiwi and tomatoes contain acids, but they make an alkaline ash within the body after they are digested. People who suffer indigestion immediately after a meal, and may have an over acid stomach, often say these types of foods make their problem worse, this is because they are acid on contact and until digested. However, they make an alkaline residue once they reach the small intestine. This is why apple cider vinegar or lemon juice, with a little honey and warm water, help to re-alkalise the body and reduce symptoms of arthritis and inflammatory conditions. Take 1tsp of each twice daily.
- Use a little organic sea salt, which is rich in alkalising minerals.
- Drink more green tea, especially Bancha tea, with a little added honey.
- Apple cider vinegar, preferably organic, has an alkalising effect within the body. It also helps increase stomach-acid production as it is acid on contact, but alkalising after digestion.

Useful Remedies
- Ask at your health shop for powdered organic formulas that contain wheat grass, spirulina, chlorella, alfalfa, broccoli and green foods and take daily.
- Dr Gillian McKeith makes a Living Food Energy Powder, available from all health stores.
- Take a multi-mineral formula that contains 600mg of calcium, 300–500mg of magnesium, 25mg of zinc, 90mg of potassium, in a colloidal or chelated form, which are more easily absorbed.
- Sodiphos – sodium phosphate – helps to reduce lactic acid (and uric acid) build-up and re-alkalises an over acid system. Take 600mg daily for 3 months. BLK

Helpful Hints
- Stress, anger and smoking contribute to an over-acid system.
- Breathing deeply and regularly helps to re-alkalise the body. This is because when you breathe more oxygen into the body, it has an alkaline effect. When we are under stress, we tend to shallow-breathe, which leaves more carbon dioxide, more acidity, in the tissues.

- Do not brush your teeth immediately after eating or drinking high acid-forming foods and drinks, as you can lose more tooth enamel. Simply drink a little water and swill it around the mouth to help neutralise the acids.
- Meditation also re-alkalises the body (see *Meditation*).
- When you first wake, the body is very acid, so having fruit for breakfast helps to re-alkalise the system. A great diet for summer breakfasts – but in winter you need to keep warmer and fruit won't do the job, so try porridge sweetened with a freshly grated apple or any chopped fruit. Breakfast is also a great time to drink freshly made juices. But too much orange juice can over stimulate production of stomach acid, so go for diluted apple or pear juice as an alternative. Also, apple, carrot or celery juice with a little added fresh root ginger is also highly alkalising.
- For more information read *Alkalize or Die* by Theodore A Barody (Holographic Health).

ACID STOMACH   (see also *Indigestion* and *Low Stomach Acid*)

Many people complain about having an acid stomach, often mistakenly presuming that they produce too much stomach acid – hydrochloric acid, which is known as HCl. In fact, sufferers from acid stomach regularly produce too much stomach acid at the wrong times – usually in response to stress, or overindulgence in caffeine, alcohol or sugar – which all leave the stomach with too little stomach acid for digesting foods. And as the average person eats approximately 50+ tons of food in their lifetime, which requires 300 litres of digestive juices to break it down, it's no wonder that we are suffering more and more digestive disorders. Typical symptoms are feelings of heartburn, acid reflux, indigestion, bloating and general discomfort. When you are under prolonged stress or are exhausted, your digestive system is greatly weakened. Never underestimate how long-term, negative stress and chronic exhaustion can affect the body (see also *Stress*).

Foods to Avoid
- Reduce your intake of coffee, colas, black tea, alcohol and sugar.
- Full-fat cheeses and rich, creamy foods.
- Fried and very fatty foods.
- Oily, spicy foods (such as an Indian take-away with lots of sauce), which are usually packed with refined vegetable oils. These types of meals – if high in fat – are hard to digest.
- Concentrated fruit juices, especially orange, lemon and grapefruit, and raw tomato juice, which can make the problem worse. Buy non-concentrates and dilute with water.
- Reduce your intake of wheat-based foods, which can be a problem for people with acid stomach (especially croissants, white bread and pre-packaged, mass-produced pies and cakes).

Friendly Foods
- Eat more whole grains such as brown rice, quinoa, kamut or amaranth, and try lentil, corn, buckwheat, millet- or spelt-based pastas, breads and cereals. Rice cakes, amaranth and spelt crackers are often easier to digest than wheat. If you adore bread, try small amounts of wholemeal varieties.
- Include plenty of lightly cooked vegetables and fruits in your diet, which are easier on the digestive system.
- Try making more fruit compotes or lightly grilled fruit kebabs without sugar. Use a little honey or chopped organic dried fruits to sweeten.
- Choose low-fat meats such as venison, turkey, duck and chicken without the skin, and include

plenty of fresh fish in your diet.
- Replace full-fat cows' milk with organic rice, soya or goats' milk.
- Experiment with caffeine-free herbal teas, such as fennel and liquorice, which reduce acidity. Camomile, meadowsweet and fresh mint teas soothe the gut.
- Fresh root ginger is very calming to the gut, as is lightly cooked cabbage, or cabbage juice made from raw cabbage.
- Eat more live, low-fat yoghurts.

Useful Remedies
- De-glycyrrhized liquorice helps to protect and heal the lining of the oesophagus and stomach. Chew 1–2 tablets 20 minutes before a meal. It can also be used as an alternative to antacids after meals. Available from health shops.
- Ask at your local health shop or pharmacy for a *Peppermint Formula* containing ingredients such as peppermint, gentian, fennel or camomile, which can be taken after foods.
- Slippery Elm Plus is a supplement containing slippery elm, marsh mallow and gamma oryzanol which all help to soothe the stomach lining. **BC**
- The mineral salt sodium phosphate helps to balance excess acidity. Take 100mg 3 times daily. **BLK**

Helpful Hints
- Chew all foods thoroughly and avoid drinking too much with meals, as this dilutes the stomach acid, which you need to digest your meal.
- Eat little and often, avoiding large, heavy meals. The larger the meal, the greater the burden on your digestive system. Small meals are especially important if you are stressed, as stress increases stomach acid at inappropriate times.
- Take time out to eat your meals calmly – do not eat on the run. Avoid large meals if you are feeling upset.
- If you are prone to nervous conditions, join a yoga, meditation or T'ai chi class and learn to relax. Get plenty of exercise, but no strenuous exercise immediately after eating. Walking for 10–15 minutes after a meal greatly aids digestion.
- Drink peppermint, fennel, camomile or green teas after a meal.
- Food combining helps an acid stomach: this means separating proteins and starches to aid digestion. Basically if you are eating a protein such as meat or fish, eat this with salad or vegetables but not potatoes, pasta or bread; conversely, when you eat bread, pasta or potatoes, eat them with vegetables or salad, not protein. Read *The Complete Book of Food Combining* by Kathryn Marsden, Piatkus. Many people become reliant on antacids to control their symptoms, when making a few simple changes to the diet and eating pattern can produce very significant relief in most cases. Antacids can harm the body if used excessively and many contain aluminium, which has been implicated in Alzheimer's disease.

ACNE
(see also *Liver Problems* and *Rosacea)*

Many adolescents experience acne owing to the massive increase in hormone production, which often leads to overproduction of sebum, or naturally produced oils in the skin that cause blockages in the skin's sebaceous glands. Teenagers are also notorious for eating a poor nutrient deficient diet – and taking too many fizzy drinks and too much alcohol – which will exacerbate this problem. Sugar and fat are the biggest offenders. For adults, acne often results from internal toxicity, which can be caused by many factors. Constipation, candida (a yeast fungal overgrowth; see *Candida*) or food intolerances can all trigger this problem. Pre-menstrual women can also experience acne. The key factor in controlling and preventing acne is to look after your liver and ensure that toxins can be eliminated. Once the system becomes overloaded it begins dumping toxins into the skin, hence constipation and poor skin often go hand in hand.

Foods to Avoid

- Many teenagers ingest up to 60 tsp of sugar daily in refined snacks, cola-type drinks, croissants, cakes, sweets and so on. Therefore these types of foods have to be greatly reduced, if the acne is to be healed.
- Most mass-produced, pre-packed meals, cakes, biscuits and pies, which are high in sugar, salt and saturated fats, which place a great strain on the liver.
- Full-fat cheeses and dairy produce, fried foods and greasy burger-type foods.

Friendly Foods

- Eat more beetroot, kale, celeriac and artichoke, which help to cleanse the liver.
- Chickpeas, soya, black-eyed, haricot and cannellini beans as well as pulses help the body to excrete excess hormones.
- Eat Japanese and Thai foods, such as miso and tempeh, which help to regulate hormones.
- Include more fresh vegetables and fruits such as figs in your diet – this is especially true of teenagers who tend to eat a very poor diet. We can all do this for a certain time but symptoms will arise once the body becomes very toxic.
- Drink 8 glasses of water daily.
- Add a tablespoonful of linseeds and sunflower seeds to high-fibre, low-sugar breakfast cereal.
- Snack on unsulphured dried apricots and dates as well as raw, unsalted nuts and seeds.
- Raw wheat germ and avocados are rich in vitamin E, which nourishes the skin.
- See also *General Health Hints*.

Useful Remedies

- Zinc has been shown to be as successful as taking certain antibiotics for this condition – take 30mg of zinc up to 3 times daily until the condition improves. For every 15mg of zinc, you should also take 1mg of copper to maintain a healthy balance within the body.
- Take a good quality B-complex vitamin plus a multi-vitamin and mineral daily.
- With acne, hormones are often an important factor. Herbs that should help include blessed thistle, squaw vine, cramp bark, and raspberry leaf. These are available as a liquid or capsules. **SHS**
- To help support the liver, try a formula based on barberry, wild yam and dandelion. Take this for 3 months. **SHS**
- Saw palmetto, red clover, agnus castus, calendula, echinacea and dandelion formula is a very useful formula for balancing testosterone levels in women – take 15 drops twice daily in liquids. **OP**
- Vitamin A is essential for healthy skin; if you are not pregnant or planning a pregnancy take up to 30,000iu taken daily for up to two months and then reduce to 3000iu daily.
- Natural source, full-spectrum vitamin E 200–400iu daily reduces the tendency to scarring and helps maintain healthy skin.
- Essential fats are also important because saturated, trans and hydrogenated fats displace EFAs in the body – take 1g of Omega 3 fish oil daily.

Helpful Hints

- *The Sher System* is a skin regime especially formulated for problem skin. Contact The Sher System, 30 New Bond Street, London, W1S 2RN Tel: 020 7499 4022. Website: www.sher.co.uk
- *Rosa Mosqueta*, a Latin American plant-based oil, can be used topically to heal scars, but don't use on active acne. Use once the acne is no longer active. **OP**

■ Taking liquid hyaluronic acid (a natural component of skin) daily in water helps to heal any scarring on the skin. For details call Modern Herbals on 01274 889047. Website: www.modern-herbals.com

■ Tea tree oil is highly antiseptic. Add a few drops to bath water or use cream, soap or lotion on the affected areas.

■ Kali Brom 6c is a homeopathic remedy that helps if the acne is on the face, chest and shoulders. Homeopathic Silica 6c is also useful twice daily. This may trigger symptoms to increase for a short time as toxins are released – but this will balance out after a couple of weeks.

■ Exercise encourages free flow of sebum and detoxification of the body through sweating.

■ Many readers have benefited from taking aloe vera juice internally and using the gel externally.

■ A thorough detox is useful for clearing acne (see *Liver*).

ADHD – Attention Deficit Hyperactivity Disorder (see *Hyperactivity*)

ADRENAL EXHAUSTION (see *ME* and *Stress*)

AGEING

Today there are approximately 390 million people aged over 65 in the world – by 2030 over 20% of the world's 6 billion people will be over 65. Governments worry about the health-cost burden of the so-called 'pensioners' and yet if you begin taking more responsibility for your health from today by eating sensibly, reducing stress and taking more exercise, then you could have the capability to live a healthy, productive life until at least 100. In fact, a woman born today has a 40% chance of living to 150. Keep in mind that 60 is the new 40!

An example of good nutrition and its effects on health and the ageing process is found in the Hunza population of northern Pakistan. The Hunzas are renowned for their average lifespan of between 100 and 120 years. These simple people live a long life with virtually no illness. Dr Jay F. Hoffman, who was sent to study the Hunzas by the American Geriatrics Society, wrote "Here is a land where people do not have our common diseases, such as heart ailments, cancer, arthritis, high blood pressure, diabetes, tuberculosis, hayfever, asthma, liver and gall bladder trouble, constipation or many other ailments that plague the rest of the world" – in other words all the modern-day Western illnesses that tend to accompany the process of ageing.

As we age biological changes take place throughout our bodies. Our heart muscle becomes thinner, the capacity of our kidneys reduces and all of our organs go through some physiological change. However, these changes are not necessarily associated with illness or disease. And none of these changes cause ill health or disease on their own. The process of ageing is the breakdown of key biological functions of our mind and body and is directly related to our environment, diet, lifestyle and outlook on life.

The single most common result of the process of ageing and the leading cause of death worldwide is cardiovascular disease. Dr Michael Colgan, a renowned nutritional research scientist in the US, says that if people could eat more of the right foods and change their lifestyles, then 98% of cardiovascular disease cases and 80% of cancers would be preventable. Also that late-onset diabetes, which is reaching epidemic proportions in Western countries, is a direct consequence of over-consumption of sugar, plus stress and overuse of stimulants. It is both avoidable and manageable by good nutrition (see also *Diabetes*).

And if you eat the right foods, and take the right supplements and hormones, then a 60-year-old can have the Biological Ageing Markers – such as blood pressure, cholesterol count, lean body mass, bone density, skin thickness and so on – of a 40-year-old.

So, what causes the deterioration of our body that we call ageing? It is now accepted that the ageing process and virtually all disease is the result of free radical damage to the cells in one form or another. Hence why antioxidants such as vitamins A, C and E, plus minerals such as selenium hold one of the major keys to slowing down the ageing process. Free radicals are produced by our bodies when oxygen is used to create energy and during everyday processes such as breathing and eating. There is much misinformation on free radicals, which are also vital to life. They are created by the billion daily – they help to neutralize viruses and bacteria and help to kill cancer cells, so there are positive purposes for a certain amount of free radicals (also known as oxidants) in the body. But over time, as the body begins to accumulate *excess* free radicals, which proliferate when insufficient antioxidants are present, the system becomes overwhelmed by these unstable molecules that then break down our DNA, trigger deterioration in our blood vessels and brain, and cause damage to virtually every cell of our body. You can reduce free-radical accumulation by cutting down on burned or smoked foods, exposure to air pollution, pesticides, overuse of mobile phones, and excessive sunbathing, additives and stress; and by taking more potent antioxidants, which are listed below.

Inflammation is another major contributor to ageing. Degenerative diseases that are associated with inflammation in the tissues are; arteriosclerosis, Alzheimer's, Parkinson's, diabetes, arthritis, ME, cancer, and allergies. Sources of inflammation are chronic low-level infections, and toxicity from ingesting too many foods containing additives, a deficiency in essential nutrients, foods to which we have an intolerance, and heavy metals such as mercury and aluminium.

Physical activity is crucial in helping to slow down the ageing process but severe exertion generates large amounts of free radicals and inflammation in the body. This may explain why people who spend so much time in the gym do not always survive longer than those who don't, and why some marathon runners and aerobics instructors age more quickly. As always, we need everything in a balance and this is the secret to slowing the ageing process.

Also, how often do you here people say, "It's all in my genes"? And if their parents died young, many people presume they have inherited the likelihood that they might do the same. Yes our genes do play a huge part in the dice of life and how well or otherwise you age, but if your genes stay healthy then your body stays healthy. If you live a healthy lifestyle you can change which genes are expressed. In other words if your parents and grandparents died of heart attacks you may well have a pre-disposition for heart problems at some point. But if you live a different lifestyle and eat healthier foods, you can change the chemistry within the body and tip the scales in your favour. Genes are repairable and alterable, they adjust to our environment and state of mind. Generally, people who live to a great age are positive, adaptable and hard-working; they eat a good breakfast and consume plenty of freshly, locally grown fruits and vegetables.

Jeanne Calment, a French lady, lived to 122; she gave up smoking at the age of 120 in 1995 saying "it had become a habit" and died two years later. She was one in six billion, which shows that there are always exceptions to every rule.

Don't underestimate the extent to which your thoughts and stress levels can affect both your general health and the rate at which you age. If you repeatedly say "It's to be expected at my age", don't be surprised if you age faster.

In my twenties and thirties I was obsessed with ageing and spent too much time rushing around having the latest anti-ageing therapies instead of simply enjoying being young. Learn to enjoy the moment, know that you can only do your best, and have some fun.

Foods to Avoid

- Sugar triggers an inflammatory response in the body and ages the skin as much as smoking or regular sunbathing. And if you don't burn up sugar during exercise, it converts to fat in the body.
- Cut down on foods with a high sugar content, such as refined carbohydrates – breads, cakes, biscuits, pastries, pasta – and sweets and concentrated fruit juice. A diet of more than 40% carbohydrate intake can cause insulin resistance (see *Insulin Resistance*). Also, the body has a limited capacity to store carbohydrate in the liver and muscles and will turn excess carbohydrate into fat tissue.
- Artificial sweeteners including Aspartame (Nutrasweet and Canderel), saccharin, and Sucralose are synthetic forms of sugar that the body does not utilise well.
- Fried foods and all refined hydrogenated/trans fats (see *Fats You Need To Eat*).
- Artificial preservatives and chemicals, including MSG.
- Municipal tap water is known to contain many chemicals, hormone and antibiotic residues and in some areas fluoride – which can accumulate in the body causing many health problems. Fit a good water filter under your sink and make sure it's serviced regularly. Otherwise I drink Fiji, Volvic or Spa waters.
- Cut down on stimulants such as caffeine, fizzy drinks and alcohol.
- Reduce your intake of full-fat dairy products.
- Avoid shellfish, which tend to feed in polluted coastal waters.
- Non-organic, preserved, smoked and cured meats (deli-type meats and bacon), as the chemicals used are carcinogenic.
- Avoid tinned, microwaved and pre-packaged foods.
- Avoid industrially produced battery eggs and chickens.
- Cut down on non-organic red meats.
- Cut down on sodium-based table salts. Use mineral rich sea salts in moderation. I use Himalayan Crystal Salt, which is rich in organic source minerals. For your nearest stockists contact Best Care Products on 01342 410303, or log on to www.bestcare-UK.com

Friendly Foods

- Oily fish, linseeds, fresh fruit, vegetables, salads, nuts and oatmeal will all help to reduce inflammation in the body. As much as possible eat locally grown fresh foods.
- Sip water throughout the day; try to drink 6–8 glasses daily.
- Eat organic foods as much as you can as they contain far lower levels of potentially dangerous pesticides and chemicals. Also, organic veggies contain more nutrients than non-organic ones.
- A good anti-ageing diet should be composed of 50% vegetables (non-starchy, such as sweet potatoes), 20% protein (meat, cheese, fish etc), and 20% fruits, and 10% grains (brown rice, quinoa, buckwheat, millet or spelt). The vegetables should be raw or lightly cooked to preserve the nutrient content, the protein should include vegetable proteins like organic soya beans, mung beans, aduki beans and so on, as well as some animal protein. Fruits should be uncooked and whole as opposed to juiced. The grains are best as whole grains such as brown rice rather than flour-based foods.
- Eat more thyme, which has powerful antioxidant properties. Otherwise use therapeutic grade oils on your spine and the soles of your feet for optimum anti-ageing effects. For more details call Susie Anthony on 01749 679900 for details of some of the finest oils I have ever come across.

Anti-ageing Nutrients

■ For years I have taken up to 30 nutrients a day to help boost my immune system, nourish my skin, protect my bones, eyes, heart, circulation, brain and so on, which in turn helps slow down the ageing process. Eventually I became so fed up with taking so many pills, with the help of Kudos Vitamins and Herbals based in the UK, I helped develop a multi-nutrient formula, containing food-state, GM-free, highly absorbable vitamins, minerals, antioxidants, amino acids, brain nutrients, essential fats, isoflavones, green foods, and specific anti-ageing nutrients such as carnosine and CoQ10 (see below) that both men and women of all ages can take once daily. It offers protection to help slow ageing at every level. It is called Kudos 24 Multi-Active Age Management Complex – for full details and a list of the ingredients, see *General Supplements*.

■ If you prefer your own supplements, then take a good-quality multi-vitamin/mineral plus an antioxidant formula. Always include an extra gram of vitamin C.

Below are listed some of the most anti-ageing nutrients currently known:

ALPHA-LIPOIC ACID is an important antioxidant that has the unique ability to pass into the brain, where it helps recycling of other antioxidants, such as vitamins C and E, plus glutathione. It also removes heavy metals like aluminium, mercury and lead from the brain, which helps to protect against Alzheimer's, Parkinson's and senile dementia. Because it is both water- and fat-soluble, it is easily absorbed in the gut. ALA also helps prevent and treat some of the complications of diabetes. Take 200mg daily with food.

ACETYL L-CARNITINE (ALC) is a natural substance present in the human body, especially the muscles and brain. It helps to combat 2 major factors involved with brain ageing, diminished brain-cell metabolism and reduced circulation in the brain. ALC easily crosses the blood-brain barrier and its role in protecting neurological function has been well established. The use of acetyl L-carnitine with alpha lipoic acid is now being considered a major breakthrough for preventing the process of ageing. Take 1000mg daily on an empty stomach. Most companies now sell ALC and ALA in a combination formula. **HN**

CARNOSINE is a naturally occurring antioxidant made within the body and as we age the levels fall. High concentrations of carnosine are present in long-lived cells such as in nerve tissues and people who live longer have higher levels of this nutrient. Carnosine has been shown to help reverse age related damage especially in the skin. It also blocks amyloid production, the substance found in the brains of Alzheimer's patients. Other emerging benefits are its apparent anti-cancer effects, the removal of toxic metals from the body and it is a great immune booster. It is found in lean red meat and chicken. For optimum anti-ageing results take 50–100mg daily. Take on an empty stomach in between meals.

Co-enzyme Q10 is an essential factor in energy production within the cells. CoQ10 is a vitamin-like substance that is manufactured in the liver. As we age production slows down. CoQ10 facilitates and regulates the oxidation of fats and sugars into energy. CoQ10 has profound anti-ageing effects on the brain; it also helps protect the heart. Parkinson's patients tend to be low in CoQ10, which has also been shown to inhibit cancer-cell growth and protect breast tissue, be excellent for allergy-management, boost energy levels, protect from gum disease, and act as an antioxidant. If you want to stay younger longer, take 100mg daily. If you are taking Statin drugs to lower your cholesterol levels, it is important to replenish CoQ10, which is greatly depleted by Statins (see *Cholesterol*).

OMEGA-3 ESSENTIAL FATS More than 2,000 scientific studies have demonstrated the wide range of problems associated with omega-3 fatty acid deficiencies. The modern diet is almost devoid of omega-3s. In fact, researchers believe that at least 60% of people are deficient in omega-3 fats. Essential fats keep the skin hydrated and supple, and are essential for hormone production, weight loss and controlling blood pressure. The brain cannot function properly without essential fatty acids. Fish oils are high in EPA and DHA – omega-3 fats that are not generally found in vegetable and nut sources that are vital for the brain and nervous system. The best sources are sardines, tuna, wild salmon, mullet, herring, trout, mackerel and anchovies. Excellent non-fish sources of omega-3 fats include flaxseeds (linseeds), walnuts, hemp and pumpkin seeds and to a lesser extent soybeans. Include these seeds and unrefined oils in your diet and for lots more information see *Fats You Need To Eat*.

Omega-6 essential fats are found in sunflower, sesame and pumpkin seeds, linseeds and their unrefined oils, and evening primrose oil. Most people have plenty of omega-6 EFAs in their diet from vegetable spreads and oils.

If you want to help keep your skin and joints more supple – begin taking liquid hyaluronic acid (HA) daily in water. HA is a naturally occurring protein in the body. HA is what makes young skin look plump and supple. Unfortunately as we age levels of HA in the body decline, resulting in wrinkles and joint problems. HA is used in thousands of beauty salons as an injectable to plump up lines. But it can also be taken internally in a liquid formula. Take 1ml daily in water on an empty stomach; very effective. For more details ask at your health store or call Modern Herbals on 01274 889047. Website: www.modernherbals.com

Helpful Hints

- People who are adaptable and have a positive outlook on life tend to live the longest.
- Never under estimate just how much your thoughts and stress levels can affect not only your health but also the speed at which you age. If you keep saying over and over "it's to be expected at my age", do not be surprised if you become sicker and age faster.
- Learn to say yes to what you do want in your life and no to what you don't.
- Have fun – laugh a lot. No one ever had engraved on their tombstone "I wish I had spent more time at the office." Find a balance.
- Stop worrying – as Dale Carnegie once said, "85% of things you worry about never happen" so stop worrying about the things you cannot change – concentrate on what you can change. And if you really want to change things in your own life and environment then take the steps necessary to begin the changes that you require. Be willing to *act* positively for the good of all, rather than just talking about it.
- Stop smoking, every cigarette you smoke can take 15 minutes off your life. Smoking ages your skin and depletes vital nutrients such as vitamin C, which are needed for healthy skin and bones, energy-production, and an active immune system.
- Take regular exercise, but not to excess.
- Being overweight can shorten your life by up to 10 years (see *Weight Problems*).
- Supplementing the hormone DHEA (see *Menopause*) can help reduce inflammation and ageing in the body. Don't take extra hormones unless you need them.
- Learn to meditate (see *Meditation*) for it has many proven anti-ageing benefits.
- Reduce your exposure to mobile phones and excessive electrical equipment.
- Reduce exposure to pesticides, herbicides and toxic chemicals. Eat and drink organic foods and drinks as much as possible.
- Too much sun will age your skin, but we do need some sunshine to produce vitamin D, which helps to keep bones healthy. Sunshine makes you feel good – everything in moderation. Wear a PABA-free UVA/UVB sunscreen to protect the skin.
- Don't overeat. Generally in the West, we tend to eat 40% more food than the body needs. Having said that, there are some people on calorie-restricted diets (proven to slow ageing) living on 1,200 calories a day, but some of them look awful! And food is meant to be a pleasure. We

can all enjoy treats and not feel guilty but we must stop living on treats.

■ Get sufficient sleep – it's the easiest way to look younger.

■ Cut down your stress-load as prolonged stress ages you (see *Stress*).

■ If you want to know how well or otherwise you are ageing, have your BioMarkers (this is your lean body mass, muscle strength, cholesterol, blood pressure, bone density, basal metabolic rate and so on) analysed at an anti-ageing clinic. HB Health (at 12 Beauchamp Place, London SW3 1NZ) offers this type of service. They have state-of-the-art equipment and a panel of longevity experts/doctors who can test your biological markers and offer you a complete and individual prescription (including chelation, hormones, supplements and therapies) for a longer life. For details call 020 7838 0765 or Email clinic@hbbeauchamp.com

■ Another great website for anti-ageing research is the Life Extension Foundation at www.lef.org. They run a very efficient postal service from the US and sell supplements that can be difficult to source in the UK. You can also order hormones such as DHEA and melatonin from the Foundation.

■ Dr Nick Delgardo is a member of the American Academy of Anti-ageing and his website www.growyoungandslim.com is well worth a look.

■ An ioniser helps clean the air in the room; negative ions have a relaxing effect on the body and nervous system.

■ For further reading on ageing read *500 of the Most Important Ways to Stay Younger Longer* by me (Cico Books).

■ Always use a body lotion after bathing – there are many fabulous organic vitamin creams now widely available from health stores. My favourites are from the Organic Pharmacy in London. **OP**

■ Laser therapy can help remove the visible signs of ageing, such as liver/ age spots (see *Age Spots*). Contact Laser Care Clinics who have 17 clinics in the UK. To arrange a free nurse consultation call them on 0800 028 7222. Website: www.lasercare-clinics.co.uk

AGE SPOTS

(see also *Liver Problems* and *Sunburn*)

If you look at young skin, it's almost always clear with an even tone, and age spots don't normally appear until the early 40s and onwards. If you look at the buttocks of an average 60-year-old woman, they will still look young and blemish-free. The best ways to reduce and avoid age spots is to take less sun, look after your liver and to ingest more antioxidants. Melanocytes are your melanin, or colour-producing cells, and over time, thanks to exposure to the sun, these fatty pigments or lipids begin to 'clump' together causing age spots (also known as liver spots), or uneven pigmentation of varying sizes and shapes, which begin to appear all over the body. They commonly appear on the backs of the hands, the face, the forearms, and eventually anywhere that is exposed regularly to the sun.

Foods to Avoid

■ Fried and barbecued foods, saturated fats found in full fat dairy products, meat pies, cakes, fatty meats and chocolates.

■ Alcohol and too many fats, which place a strain on your liver.

■ Mass-produced refined foods and meals, which are often packed with hydrogenated and trans fats, plus sugar, which all age the skin (see *Fats You Need To Eat*).

■ Reduce non-organic foods, which are often high in additives and pesticides.

Friendly Foods

- To help avoid age spots it is important that the body is eliminating unwanted fatty deposits properly. Lecithin granules, available from all health stores, help emulsify and break down fats. Take 1 tbsp daily over cereals, fruits and yoghurts. Lecithin is also found in soya products and eggs.
- Eat more antioxidant-rich foods, organic fruit and vegetables, especially red, orange or dark-green fruits and vegetables, such as carrots, apricots, pumpkin, broccoli, Chinese broccoli, pak choy, red peppers, red and purple berries and tomatoes.
- Use tahini or olive oil as a spread instead of hydrogenated margarines and spreads.

Useful Remedies

- Antioxidants help to mop up or neutralise the free-radical reactions that are triggered by sunbathing. Therefore, take a high-strength antioxidant formula. The antioxidant Astaxanthin has been shown to support sun-damaged skin. This antioxidant is found in marine algae that pink-coloured birds like flamingoes feed on. Higher Nature makes a high-strength Astaxanthin complex. **HN**
- Beta-carotene helps to encourage melanin production; make sure it's a natural source carotene complex that contains all the carotenoids.
- Potassium chloride is important also for removing congestion and fatty deposits in the tissues. You need 50mg potassium chloride per tablet x 3 a day. **BLK**
- Active H is a powerful antioxidant and many people taking this supplement have reported that after a few months of taking 2 x 250mg tablets daily, their age spots have disappeared. **NC**
- 1g of vitamin C daily.
- Essential fatty acids, known as EFAs, help to reduce the sun's negative effects. If taken regularly they help keep your skin looking younger for longer (see *Fats You Need To Eat*).

Helpful Hints

- Use a factor 15 sun screen on the backs of your hands and on your face, and take more care in the sun – you really will reap the benefits in later life.
- If you have young children keep in mind that a huge amount of skin damage can be done before a child reaches 16. If children are allowed to burn then they are more likely to suffer skin cancers in later life. Some sun is healthy, but all things in moderation. Over and over I see young children and teenagers on beaches in the midday sun with red, blistered skin and no hat! (See *Sunburn*)
- The secret is not to let the skin burn and turn bright red. We all know the sensible precautions – to cover up between 11am and 3pm and to always wear a hat in hot midday sun – but a huge majority of us are simply not doing it. Start protecting the skin from an early age. If you do want to tan, do it slowly – don't burn.
- Ask at your health store for an antioxidant-rich cream, there are now dozens of creams containing grape-seed extract, and vitamins C, E and so on. Use this on the age spots daily.
- Cigarettes age your skin. Stop smoking.
- Glycolic acid based creams are fairly successful especially when combined with Kojic acid. Dr Daniello makes excellent products – for details of stockists in the UK call 00 35 31 67 77 911.
- Modern lasers are highly successful at removing age spots, but make sure you see a dermatologist or doctor who has experience of this work. I had mine done at a Lasercare Clinic, 144 Harley Street by Dr Thomas Bozek. Tel: 020 7224 0988. They have 12 clinics around the UK with qualified personnel. For further details and to find your nearest clinic call 0800 028 7222 or log on to: www.lasercare-clinics.co.uk.

ALCOHOL

(see also *Liver Problems*)

Alcohol consumption at home has risen 48% in the last 10 years – and many young people are drinking excess amounts of cheap supermarket alcohol before going out for the evening. There has been an enormous rise in the number of young people who are bingeing on alcohol. It is a dangerous fashion. Specialists are now seeing 26-year-olds with liver problems usually associated with people over 50. In fact around 37% of young men and 23% of young women regularly binge drink – and these figures are climbing. Every time you drink alcohol, it acts as a diuretic and the body excretes vital minerals and vitamins, especially the B-group vitamins, which help keep your nervous system, hormone production, hair and nails in good shape. Moderate consumption (meaning a single unit – one shot of spirits, one glass of wine or half a pint of beer) of alcohol has been shown to be slightly protective against heart disease.

If your cholesterol level is above 4.5, you can justify having an occasional drink – the ideal being a glass of aged red wine. The nutrient-content of alcohol is very low, but many people have a drink believing they are protecting their heart and choose to forget they are elevating their risk of hormonal cancers, particularly breast cancer. Alcohol places an enormous strain on the liver, which reduces its ability to detoxify the body. Over-consumption of alcohol can lead to fatigue and dehydration, as well as disruptive sleep patterns, and can deplete many vital nutrients from the body. Pregnant women risk foetal abnormalities if they consume more than one unit of alcohol a day during pregnancy; alcohol should be avoided if you are trying to become pregnant. During pregnancy, give it up.

Think of your future. When you are young – you think "It will never happen to me" – but believe me it can and does.

Foods to Avoid

- Avoid eating fresh or tinned grapefruit juice if you are drinking, as this will increase the toxicity of the alcohol.
- Saturated fats also place a great strain on the liver. Avoid fatty, heavy, rich meals – especially sausages, cheese (especially melted cheese), rich pâtés, burgers, pre-packaged meat pies, and so on.
- Never ply anyone who is drunk with coffee, as this will further dehydrate the body, which can increase the concentration of alcohol in the system. (See *General Health Hints*.)

Friendly Foods

- Eat plenty of fresh fruits and vegetables especially broccoli, artichokes, cauliflower, beetroot, celeriac, celery, fennel and radicchio to help to detoxify the liver.
- Eat plenty of soluble fibres such as linseeds (flax seeds), oat bran and low-sugar cereals such as muesli or porridge.
- Drink at least 8 glasses of water daily.
- Use unrefined olive, walnut or sunflower oils for salad dressings.
- See also *General Health Hints*.

Useful Remedies

- The herb milk thistle (silymarin) has been proven to help detoxify and regenerate the liver. Take 500mg of the whole-herb supplement twice daily with meals for one month. During this time you need to cut down your intake of alcohol to give the liver time to repair. **SHS**
- If you are an occasional drinker, take 1 high-strength milk thistle capsule before and after drinking. Kudos makes a high-strength capsule at 900mg.
- Take a good quality multi-vitamin and mineral daily; see Kudos 24 in *General Supplements* on p.160. **KVH**
- To avoid hangovers, take 2 grams of evening primrose oil, 1 gram of vitamin C, a B-complex,

plus 500mg of milk thistle with a full glass of water before going out. Repeat this dosage the next morning upon waking.

- To help alleviate hangovers try the formula Intox Rx, containing vitamin C, the amino acid cysteine, the liver-friendly herbs kudzu and silymarin, plus lipoic acid and pyroglutamic acid. Intox Rx has been specifically designed to provide protection from the toxic effects of alcohol. Take one capsule twice daily. **NC**
- The herb Chinese Kudzu extract contains diadzin, which has been known to be beneficial for treating alcoholism. Not only does kudzu extract help reduce the craving for alcohol, but it also acts as a muscle relaxant which helps to overcome some of the withdrawal symptoms. Take 10–20 drops of the tincture or 2 tablets before you take a drink.

Helpful Hints

- For every alcoholic drink, make sure you have a non-alcoholic one in between. Generally drink more water as alcohol severely dehydrates the body. Avoid alcohol when flying because the pressurised cabins cause considerable dehydration.
- Do not give a person coffee to sober them up as coffee is a diuretic, which depletes fluid from the body and makes the alcohol content in the body even more concentrated.
- If you have a hangover you need to raise your blood sugar quite quickly upon waking. Eat a banana or blend various fresh fruits such as figs, dates and raisins and low-fat, live yoghurt (or rice milk) and drink immediately, or drink some fruit juice.
- Drink 3 glasses of water slowly as soon as you wake up, to rehydrate the body.
- Homeopathic Nux Vomica 30c. Take one before bed and another upon waking to help reduce a hangover. This really helps. **OP**
- Bingeing on alcohol is extremely dangerous – it creates too much shock in the liver. Vomiting is an indication that the body has reached a danger level and you must stop drinking.
- If you must drink, have a couple of drinks daily – but do not drink to excess. Better quality red wine seems to confer the most health benefits, owing to antioxidant substances called polyphenols present in the skin of red grapes. The grapes' skins are discarded during the processing of white wine.
- Dandelion root tea tastes bitter, but is excellent for cleansing the liver
- The liver detoxifies most efficiently between 1 and 3am – but for it to do this you need to be lying down so burning the midnight oil and beyond adds even greater strain on your liver.
- Remember it takes 20 minutes for alcohol to have an effect and more than one hour for the body to process each unit (one unit = half a pint of beer, a small glass of wine or a single measure of spirits). If you are concerned about the amount that you (or a member of your family) are drinking, call Drinkline on 0800 917 8282 for advice and information. The line is open 24 hours a day, seven days a week. All calls are treated in the strictest confidence and Drinkline provides a full support service for people with drink problems as well as their families. Otherwise contact Alcohol Concern on 020 72640510. Website: www.alcoholconcern.org.uk

ALLERGIC RHINITIS (see also *Allergies* and *Hayfever*)

Typical symptoms include a runny nose, sneezing, sinus congestion plus itchy and watering eyes. Unlike hayfever allergic rhinitis tends to affect people all year round, although symptoms can worsen at certain times of year when pollen counts are high. In some individuals it is triggered by a food intolerance. This will need to be addressed for the problem to be resolved, otherwise you can take all kinds of herbs and supplements in efforts to relieve the problem, or worse still antihistamines but this will not address the root cause of the condition. For example, when I eat a high-sugar food, my nose starts running within seconds, which is a shame as I have a sweet tooth! But this demonstrates how immediate any effect can be. This condition can also be linked to candida and/or leaky gut syndrome.

Foods to Avoid
- Avoid sugar and high mucus-forming foods, such as full-fat dairy products, cheese and chocolate.
- Reduce white flour and pasta, orange juice, tomatoes and any other foods to which you may have an intolerance.
- Wheat and dairy produce from cows are known to be triggers for this condition, but it could just as easily be bananas.
- Wine can also trigger this problem in some people.

Friendly Foods
- Include plenty of garlic, onions, horseradish, root ginger and freshly squeezed fruit and vegetable juices (but not carton juice) in your diet.
- If you have an intolerance to wheat, try rye, rice or amaranth crackers and oat cakes. Ask at your health shop for wheat-free bread and pasta.
- Dairy alternatives include organic rice, soya, goat's, almond or oat milk. Soya milk does trigger excess mucus in some people.

Useful Remedies
- When the symptoms are acute take up to 5 grams of vitamin C in an ascorbate form daily plus 500mg to 2 grams of pantothenic acid (vitamin B5).
- Take a Bioflavonoid complex: 500mg to 2 grams.
- Take 500mg of bromelain – an enzyme from pineapple, which helps to break down mucus and reduce the allergic response, which reduces the discomfort.
- Nettle tincture or tea three times a day helps to alleviate symptoms.
- Quercetin another flavonoid helps to reduce the allergic response: 400mg 3 times daily whilst symptoms are acute.
- Oralmat is an extract of the rye plant. It contains naturally occurring compounds, such as Beta 1, 3 glucan, matairesinol, genistein, squalene and co-enzyme Q10. This liquid extract supports healthy respiratory function by strengthening the body's natural defences against allergens. Dr Princetta, an allergy specialist in Atlanta, Georgia, reports impressive results with allergy and asthma patients saying: "The South-eastern United States, and Atlanta, Georgia, in particular, is a well-known allergy area of the world. Even some of my worst allergy patients responded very well to the drops and suffered a minimum of 50% less this past spring. It's certainly worth a try and you can take 3 drops under the tongue (hold 30 seconds or longer) 3 times daily. Children should use 1 drop." **NC**

Helpful Hints
- Until you are able to identify any food intolerance or external allergies, take 400mg of the bioflavonoid quercetin 3 times a day, which helps to reduce the allergic response.
- During an acute attack, a homeopathic nasal spray called Euphorbium Spray is extremely effective. It helps to relieve a runny nose, congestion and headaches. **NC** and **SL**
- Dust and other airborne allergens can be reduced in your immediate environment with an ioniser.
- Try New Era tissue salt Nat Mur for alleviating allergic rhinitis.

ALLERGIES

(see also *Leaky Gut* and *Liver Problems*)

Allergy problems, such as asthma, eczema and rhinitis, are now responsible for an estimated 12.5 million GP consultations a year and 20 million people in the UK alone are thought to have either an allergy or sensitivity to various substances. Allergies or sensitivities to various foods or substances are the most common triggers for a multitude of symptoms from coughing, itchy skin, skin rashes, wheezing, runny nose, sneezing, watery eyes, chronic sore throats and so on. The severest form of allergy triggers anaphylactic shock – which is life threatening and needs immediate medical attention. People with severe allergies usually carry an injection of adrenaline, which would need to be injected immediately.

Approximately 1 in 3 people in the West now suffer some form of food intolerance. Allergies from external sources such as pesticides, food additives, paints, pollution, perfumes, animal hairs, grass, plant and tree pollens are also widespread. There are more than 3,500 foods and product additives in use today and an average person ingests 14kg of toxins through their skin alone each year. Allergies and sensitivities are the body's way of saying "I have had enough and cannot cope with any more toxins." Hence why symptoms appear when the system becomes overloaded with toxins and/or stress. Also, many people only partially digest food proteins, which can sometimes break through the gut wall. The body treats these particles as it would an infection and attacks them as an enemy, which if left untreated can cause a myriad of allergic-type symptoms. The secret to controlling allergies and sensitivities is by reducing your exposure to all pollutants.

Foods to Avoid
- Eggs, dairy produce from cows, wheat, oranges, corn and soya are all very common allergens.
- All food additives found in mass-produced foods.
- Caffeine, peanuts, chocolate, beef, yeast and shellfish.
- It is important to have an allergy test to find your worst offenders. One of the best I have found is available from the York Test Laboratories. Tel: 0800 458 2052 or log on to www.yorktest.com; or IWDL (Individual Wellbeing Diagnostic Laboratories) do a FACT test which looks for inflammatory markers indicating that the body is reacting to certain substances. Tel: 020 8336 7750. Website: www.iwdl.net

Friendly Foods
- This is a possible minefield until you know which foods are your problem, but generally eat more brown rice, pears, lamb, cabbage, lentils, celery, papaya, leeks, green peas, mung beans, Golden Delicious apples and sweet potatoes which are usually well-tolerated.
- Include more flaxseeds (linseeds), sunflower seeds and organic sunflower and olive oil in your diet. These foods are a good starting point that very few people react to.
- It's worth noting that the foods you tend to crave and eat the most are usually the ones that are causing most problems. Wheat and cow's milk are the most common.
- Papaya is rich in digestive enzymes. Live, goat's or sheep's yoghurt contain friendly bacteria and are more easily digestible than cow's milk.
- Raw cabbage juice is high in L-glutamine, known to help to heal a leaky gut. Try making fresh juices daily that include a little chopped raw cabbage, a tiny piece of root ginger, celery, carrots, apples and add half a cup of aloe vera juice. Drink immediately after blending while all the enzymes and nutrients are still active.
- Drink liquorice tea, which helps heal the gut. Nettle tea helps reduce the allergic response.

Useful Remedies
- Histazyme, a complex containing calcium, vitamin C, zinc, bromelain, silica, vitamin A and

manganese, acts as a natural antihistamine. **BC**

- HEP 194 contains various herbs, the enzyme lipase, the amino acid methionine, and B-vitamins, which all help to support the liver. **BC**
- Two acidophilus/bifidus capsules daily after food to help replenish healthy bacteria in the gut and aid digestion.
- Betaine hydrochloride – stomach acid – is often lacking in people suffering allergies, HCl is available from most health stores – take one capsule just as you begin eating your main meal. Not to be taken if you have active stomach ulcers, in which case try a digestive enzyme (without HCl) tablet available from all health stores.
- The amino acid L-glutamine can help heal a leaky gut, take 500mg 3 times daily 30 minutes before main meals until symptoms ease.
- A good quality multi-vitamin and mineral daily.
- Once you have identified your intolerance the above can be reduced to the multi-vitamin and mineral and the HCl or digestive enzyme daily.
- A common homeopathic remedy for runny eyes and nose is Allium 6c, or if there is swelling is Apis 6c, taken 3 times daily.
- There is now good evidence showing that taking healthy bacteria (probiotics) regularly will reduce the amount of 'allergens' from food that may pass through the gut wall. For details ask at your health shop or speak to the nutritionist at BioCare. **BC**

Helpful Hints

- Subscribe to a magazine called *A* – which is especially for allergy sufferers. Log on to www.allergymagazine.com for more details.
- It is vital to chew food more thoroughly.
- Avoid large meals, which overload the digestive system and can trigger an allergic response.
- Many toothpastes, shampoos, soaps, detergents and perfumes contain a myriad of chemicals. Buy products in their most natural and unadulterated state. For anyone who suffers dermatitis or skin allergies, The Green People Company makes organic skin, hair and body lotions, sun screens and toothpaste. Advice line tel: 01403 740350. Email: organic@greenpeople.co.uk. Website: www.greenpeople.co.uk
- The Organic Pharmacy also makes some fabulous creams and their team of homeopaths is always very helpful in suggesting herbal or homeopathic remedies. **OP**
- To test if you have a food sensitivity, first take your resting pulse rate. Then for at least 14 days completely avoid the food you want to test, for example wheat. Then try eating the food you have avoided on its own, for example Weetabix in water or plain brown toast. Take your pulse at 15, 30 and 60 minutes after eating the specific food. If your pulse has increased by more than 10 beats a minute, it is likely that you have sensitivity to the test food. Or have a blood test such as The York Test – details above.
- Nutritionist Stephanie Lashford has specialised in allergy medicine for 25 years. Initially she asks all patients for 7 days to eat only foods and drinks they have not ingested for the previous 6 weeks – except for water – and even that has to be bottled. And during the first 7 days no flour, dairy or sugar from any source is allowed. This triggers a real detox, and for the first few days you may feel worse, but the benefits are profound. After the 7 days when any food to which you have an intolerance is re-introduced, symptoms are immediate. They have clinics in Cardiff, Manchester and London. For details of The Lashford Technique log on to www.sandford-clinic.co.uk; or call 029 2074 7507

- Many allergic and chemically sensitive people can benefit enormously by switching from tap water to mineral or filtered water. Tests in the US found that 98% of environmentally ill patients improved by eliminating tap water. Reverse osmosis water is extremely pure and helps cleanse pollutants and chemicals from the body. For details call The Pure H2O Company on 01784 221188. Email: info@purewater.co.uk. Website: www.purewater.co.uk
- *The Allergy Handbook* published by *What Doctors Don't Tell You* magazine is a good investment for anyone suffering allergies. Tel: 0870 4449886. Website: www.wddty.co.uk
- Dr Jean Monro who has worked at the Breakspear Hospital in Hertfordshire in the UK for 25 years says, "Before the industrial revolution conditions such as hayfever did not exist. But since then we have done a great job of polluting our atmosphere and thus our bodies. We now know that an accumulation of a variety of pollutants, such as paint sprays or pesticides (there are hundreds of others), act as the initial trigger – and these chemicals became the sensitizers – and in most cases the membranes within the nose and throat begin to react and become inflamed. Then, the next thing that comes along, such as grass pollens, the body treats as a threatening foreign invader, which increases any inflammation and induces allergic type symptoms. But it's the chemicals that sensitize the body in the first place. Chemicals can have a local affect such as on the skin – and then this effect is communicated to the rest of the body by neural (nerve) pathways and a sensitivity is born.

  The neural pathway is extremely important because it is the body's sense of awareness, which firstly triggers the dendritic cells, which then send a message to the automatic nervous system that controls pulse, breathing and temperature.

  And if someone suffering a severe reaction to say peanuts – reacts, even if that peanut happens to be in someone's pocket across the room – we now know that this instantaneous effect is triggered not only by particles of the peanuts but also by the *frequencies* emitted by the peanut, which have an instant effect. It's important for people to realize that not only do we all emit our own unique signature range of frequencies – but so does everything around us from asbestos to our foods. And if you have a specific substance/food or whatever emitting a frequency, which is incompatible with your own, then symptoms will eventually show up.

  After 20 years' research, we have developed new vaccines based on frequencies that can help to neutralize any reaction to substances found to trigger a response, and these vaccines are proving very effective. This is the medicine of the future.

  Also, the more that people stay away from synthetic chemicals and reduce the body's toxic overload, the less allergies and sensitivities will occur."

  This is fascinating research and for anyone who wants more details about allergy and environmental medicine, log on to www.breakspearmedical.com; or call 01442 261333.

ALOPECIA (see *Hair Loss*)

ALZHEIMER'S DISEASE (see also *Memory*)

Three in every 10 people over the age of 70 say they suffer with poor memory or concentration, or with confusion. The good news is that most of us have similar problems if living a hectic life, but only about 1 in every 15 actually has Alzheimer's. Alzheimer's affects approximately half a million people in Britain with 60,000 new cases every year and these figures are expected to rise as the population ages. Experts estimate that within 30 years more than half the population over 85 will suffer with Alzheimer's Disease (AD).

AD is a progressive, degenerative disease that attacks the brain, triggering symptoms such as memory loss, especially of the short-term memory, and a decrease in intellectual functioning. It is the loss of memory of how to do everyday tasks that tends to make a familiar life almost impossible.

In the early stages AD-sufferers have symptoms of absent-mindedness and an inability to learn new things. Judgement and intellectual and social functioning begin to go awry. Later there is loss of logic and memory and poor co-ordination. Speech deteriorates and symptoms of paranoia may appear. In the final stages the AD-sufferer completely loses touch with their surroundings and becomes unresponsive.

Needless to say this is very traumatic, not only for the sufferer but also their family. The tragedy is that AD is a preventable disease and can even be reversed to a degree, sometimes remarkably so. If we could all eat a healthier diet, reduce our exposure to pollution, take the right supplements and so on, much heartache could be avoided and billions of pounds saved.

The key to prevention is to understand the numerous contributing factors. Many people state that they can do nothing, thinking that AD is mostly inherited. Of course you can inherit a tendency for a particular ailment, but if you change your lifestyle and diet then you can stack the odds in your favour. But if you eat too many of the wrong foods, are stressed, and so on, and there is some genetic influence, then the accumulation of factors may eventually overwhelm your body's ability to cope, resulting in AD.

One of the commonest theories for a cause of AD is aluminium toxicity. A 1980 study of 647 Canadian gold miners who had routinely inhaled aluminium since the 1940s (a common practice thought to prevent silica poisoning), all miners tested in the 'impaired' range for cognitive function, suggesting a clear link between aluminium and memory loss. And while aluminium is certainly harmful to the brain, there are other key factors that can lead to degeneration of the brain.

Researchers have found a significant imbalance of metals in AD patients, especially mercury, mainly deposited in areas of the brain related to memory. Mercury is known to cause the type of damage to nerves that is characteristic of AD, and researchers have found that early-onset AD patients have the highest mercury levels of all (see *Mercury Fillings*).

Another factor is homocysteine, a toxic compound produced during the metabolism of proteins and an increased homocysteine level is a strong, independent risk factor for the development of dementia and AD. The higher the homocysteine level, the greater the damage to the brain. Homocysteine is readily recycled or broken down within the body by vitamins B6, B12 and folic acid. Therefore, by taking a B complex daily, homocysteine levels can be kept in check. There is also a home test kit from York Test that will give you your Homocysteine level. For details call 0800 458 2052 or log on to www.yorktest.com

Cortisol, the stress hormone, can also harm the delicate balance of your brain, as cortisol causes the connections between brain cells to shrivel up which contributes to AD (see also *Stress*).

Free radicals and an excessive intake of refined, processed foods, low in antioxidant vitamins such as A, C and E are also contributing factors. Basically the more pollutants and refined foods we are exposed to, the more vital minerals and vitamins are excreted from the body and brain function deteriorates. Eating the right foods, taking supplements that nourish the brain, and taking more exercise increases circulation to the brain, and memory can often be improved. (See also *Memory*.)

Foods to Avoid

- Avoid refined grains in products like white bread, rice and pasta. These grains have had most of their nutrients, including B-vitamins, removed in the refining process, and remember that elevated homocysteine levels can be controlled by taking more B-vitamins.
- Avoid foods containing traces of aluminium such as commercial chocolate, desserts, baking powder, processed cheeses, chewing gum and pickles.
- Eliminate any food containing the food additives aspartame (an artificial sweetener), Monosodium Glutamate MSG, which are suspected neuro-toxins.
- Avoid ready-made meat pies, cakes, and pre-packaged meals that are not only cooked in aluminium containers but also packed with saturated fat, sugar and salt.
- Reduce your intake of saturated fats found in fatty meats and full-fat dairy produce.
- Reduce your intake of caffeine, sugar and alcohol, which can all deplete vital nutrients and interfere with brain function. Sugar is particularly deadly for brain function and contributes to beta amyloid deposits, which are now thought to be the main problem for AD patients. Ronald Reagan's notorious sweet tooth may have led to his AD.

Friendly Foods

- AD patients are often lacking in the vital brain nutrient acetylcholine, which is manufactured by the body, found in organ meats, oats, soya beans, cabbage and cauliflower.
- Sprinkle a tablespoon of soya lecithin granules over breakfast cereals, into yoghurt or over fresh fruit. Lecithin is rich in acetylcholine but make sure the brand you choose contains at least 30% of this nutrient. Other foods containing this vital brain nutrient are egg yolks and fish, especially sardines.
- Essential fats are vital for proper brain functioning and reducing inflammation within the brain (and body), as brain inflammation is also linked to AD. Use organic flax, or sunflower oil for your salad dressings, and don't heat these oils. I know this is awful, but foxes and many other animals instinctively will often eat only the heads of their prey – that's because the brain is rich in essential fats.
- Include organic wild salmon (if you can find it), herrings, mackerel and tuna in your diet, which are rich in omega-3 essential fats. Include plenty of organic linseeds, sunflower and pumpkin seeds, which are all rich in healthy fats. Sprinkle them into breakfast cereals, and toasted or raw with salads and vegetables, these seeds are delicious (see also *Fats You Need To Eat*).
- Include antioxidant-rich foods such as berries, dark green leafy vegetables, and any other brightly coloured fruits and vegetables. (See *General Health Hints*.)
- Garden sage has been found to prolong and improve memory functioning, owing to its powerful anti-inflammatory and antioxidant effects. Sage also inhibits the enzyme that breaks down acetylcholine. Use plenty of fresh sage over cooked foods or make sage teas. But don't use sage if you are pregnant as it stimulates the uterus.
- Use fresh coriander over salads and sprinkle over cooked dishes, as coriander helps to remove toxic metals from the body.

Useful Remedies

- Take a multi-vitamin/mineral/essential fats/antioxidant formula daily that also contains brain nutrients. I suggest you try Kudos 24 (see *General Supplements* on p.160). **KVH**
- Magnesium 300mg daily and potassium phosphate 75mg daily are important for nerve connections in the brain. **BLK**
- Silica helps to eliminate aluminium from the body. Take 75mg per day. Fiji mineral water is especially pure and rich in silica.
- Natural-source, full-spectrum vitamin E x 600iu and vitamin C x 1g taken 3 times a day with meals have been shown to slow the progress of Alzheimer's and to help prevent onset of

dementia. Placebo-controlled studies have shown that vitamin E is more effective than drugs in reducing the symptoms of Alzheimer's. However if you're on blood-thinning drugs check with your doctor before taking vitamin E, as it thins the blood naturally.

- Ginkgo biloba is a herb from leaves of what the Chinese call the memory tree. Try 120–240mg daily, which helps to increase circulation to the brain. In rare cases ginkgo can cause a rash in which case you would need to stop taking it. A study published in 1997 by the Journal of the American Medical Association said that ginkgo biloba was shown not only to prevent AD degeneration, but also actually to improve many cases of the disease.

- Phosphatidylserine (PS) is another vital brain nutrient. The body can manufacture PS but only if you tend to eat lots of organ meats. If like most people you avoid organ meats, which are often high in antibiotic residues, then take 100mg of PS twice daily.

- B-vitamins are destroyed by stress and alcohol, but are needed for the formation of acetyl-choline and for the manufacture of other neuro-transmitters within the brain and nervous system, so take a high strength B-complex daily, especially if you're stressed.

- Curcumin, a substance found in the spice turmeric (widely used in curries), may be part of the reason AD is uncommon in India compared with Western countries. Studies in India found a less than 1% incidence of AD in the over-65s. Rat studies undertaken in California are reported to show that curcumin reduces brain amyloid (the protein deposit found in AD) and also reduces the degenerative, inflammatory responses to amyloid. Try 1 or 2 curcumin standardised extract capsules daily.

- Chlorella, which helps to remove heavy metals from the body. Try taking 1 tsp of powder daily in juices or take 500mg capsules twice daily for a couple of months.

Helpful Hints

- Avoid stress. Stress stimulates the adrenal glands to produce a hormone called cortisol, which can damage your brain. Learn to relax regularly, and walk regularly which is very relaxing, or try yoga, T'ai Chi, massage or meditation.

- Stop smoking – research indicates that smokers are twice as likely to develop dementia in later life. Avoid drugs such as cannabis and Ecstasy, which are associated with memory loss if used in the long term.

- Regular exercise has helped many sufferers restore some functions especially memory.

- If you have mercury fillings you are advised to have them removed. It is imperative this is done by a dentist who specialises in this procedure, as increased mercury poisoning can result if the proper precautions are not taken to protect you during the filling removal (see *Mercury Fillings*).

- Because of the link between aluminium and AD, avoid aluminium cooking utensils and pans, and food stored in aluminium containers. Use stainless steel or glass cookware. Many antiper-spirants contain aluminium, so use natural deodorants such as PitRok, or tea-tree based products, available from all chemists and health stores.

- Simple antacids are often based on aluminium salts and should also be avoided. Aluminium is also found in toothpastes, some cosmetics, processed cheeses, baking powder, buffered aspirin and table salts often contain aluminium, which is used as a pouring agent. If our mineral levels are low, then the body tends to absorb more aluminium, so this is another reason to include a good multi-mineral in your every day health regimen.

- Chelation therapy helps to remove all deadly metal toxins from the body. I give full details of this treatment in my book *500 of the Most Important Ways to Stay Younger Longer* (Cico Books). There are several clinics in the UK – for details call 01942 886644 or log on to www.chelation.com Dr Robert Trossell also gives this treatment at 4 Duke Street, London W1U 3EL. Tel: 020 7486 1095. Also try Dr Wendy Denning, tel: 020 7224 2423.

- Use it or lose it. Keep the brain working with simple exercises like doing crosswords and force your brain to work by counting down from 500 each day in multiples of various numbers; such as 500 less 7 = 493, less 7 = 486 and so on. Try writing and using regularly the opposite hand to the one you normally use. Extend your arms out at shoulder level, rotate one hand clockwise and the other anticlockwise and then change over – make your brain work. Buy a dictionary and learn to use and spell at least one new word every day.

- Eat organic food as much as possible and drink filtered or bottled water. Many pesticides are now linked to neurological problems and these chemicals along with aluminium are finding their way into our drinking water, so use a good water filter that removes all of these residues. Contact The Pure Water Company on 01784 221188, or log on to www.purewater.co.uk

- Avoid over exposure to mobile phones and computers. Certain studies have shown that exposure to electromagnetic radiation significantly increases the risk of AD, or makes it rapidly worse. So working with or near computers, VDUs and similar equipment, may harm your brain and evidence of how mobile phones affect the brain is continuing to mount (see *Electrical Pollution*).

- Maintaining circulation to the brain is essential, as poor blood supply to the brain will starve it of oxygen and nutrients. This is why regular exercise like yoga is important.

- Certain prescription drugs are known to cause side effects, which appear similar to symptoms of senile dementia. Anyone who feels that they may have the onset of dementia should immediately consult a qualified doctor, who is also a nutritionist. (See *Useful Information*.)

- Read *The Alzheimer's Prevention Plan,* a brilliant book by Patrick Holford (Piatkus).

ANAEMIA

Anaemia tends to come in two forms – pernicious anaemia and iron deficiency. If you have pernicious anaemia, it is owing to a lack of intrinsic factor needed to absorb vitamin B12. In the past it was always thought necessary to have B12 injections, however, research has now found that 1mg (1000mcg) of B12 taken daily can rectify this deficiency. A number of disorders can create B12 malabsorption including gastritis, and Crohn's and coeliac disease.

If you have been diagnosed as suffering from anaemia the normal procedure is to take a large amount of iron, but it is very important to make sure that the co-factors, which are vitamin B12, folic acid and vitamin C, are taken at the same time to optimise absorption.

Iron deficiency can be brought about by a number of factors, such as losing more blood than the body can replace naturally, common among women who suffer very heavy periods and which should always be investigated by a GP or a gynaecologist. Over-consumption of tea and coffee inhibit iron absorption from your food. Many people take an iron supplement when they are feeling tired, but it is always worthwhile having blood levels of iron checked before you begin supplementing iron, which accumulates in the body. Too much iron in older people is linked to heart disease. Therefore anyone over 50 should not take iron supplements unless they have a medical condition that requires iron. Common symptoms of low iron levels are fatigue, headaches, faintness and pale skin. Generally, vegetarians eat less iron than non-vegetarians. However, in Israel they found that blood iron levels were actually higher in vegetarians, which is probably owing to their high consumption of fruit and vegetables. Vegetarians who do not eat sufficient fruit and vegetables can be low in iron.

Foods to Avoid
- Black tea and coffee, which reduce absorption of iron from food.
- Excessive intake of high-fibre foods will have the same effect, but they are needed for good

bowel health, so if you need iron supplements take them a long time before or after eating high-fibre foods.

Friendly Foods

- Liver and most meats are rich in iron – especially lean steak and venison. Chicken, pheasant, partridge, grouse, pigeon, kidneys, hare and cockles are also good sources.
- Wheat bran and wholewheat flour and wheat germ contain good amounts and most breakfast cereals contain added iron.
- Dried fruits such as apricots, raisins and prunes are also a good source. As dried fruits are high in sugar, soak them for a few minutes in warm water to reduce the sugar content. Drain before serving.
- Almonds, cocoa and curry powder and raw parsley contain moderate amounts of iron.
- Leafy green vegetables such as spinach, kale, cabbage and organic tomatoes are also rich in iron.
- Black Strap molasses is rich in iron, as is Brewer's yeast.
- Prune juice is rich in iron.

Useful Remedies

- Take 1g of vitamin C, plus 400mcg of folic acid and 1mg (1000mcg) of B12 daily as these help to increase absorption of the iron.
- As B-vitamins work together within the body, take a B-complex with the above.
- Take iron ascorbate, 15–45mg, as it is an easily absorbed form of iron. Do not take iron sulphate, which may damage mucous membranes in the digestive tract and can cause constipation.
- Vitamin A and iron together are more effective than taking iron on its own. Take 5000iu. But if you are pregnant only 3000iu of vitamin A can be taken daily and only while symptoms last.

Helpful Hints

- When taking an iron supplement it is generally best to take it with a glass of pure fruit juice, which seems to aid absorption owing to the vitamin-C content in fruit juice.
- Iron is so vital for health that we store it in our bodies, but if taken in excessive amounts, it can become toxic and is known to cause constipation in some cases. The exception to this is women who suffer from heavy periods and are feeling exhausted. Pregnant women can benefit from liquid formulas such as Floradix or Spatone – available from health stores.
- Many scientists now state that no-one over 50 should take a separate iron supplement unless they have a medical condition that requires it, as high levels of iron are linked to an increased risk of heart disease for both men and women. If large amounts of iron are recommended because of anaemia, then it is best to see a qualified nutritionist who can re-balance your diet and supplements (see *Useful Information*).
- As we age our stomach-acid levels fall, which means that nutrients are often poorly absorbed from the foods we eat. Taking a digestive enzyme with meals improves absorption.
- There is a genetic disorder called haemochromatosis, which affects 1 in every 200 women, in which iron and large amounts of vitamin C should not be taken. A simple blood test can detect this condition.

ANGINA   (see also *Cholesterol, Circulation, High Blood Pressure* and *Heart Disease*)

Angina is often experienced as a pain in the chest, most frequently after running up a flight of stairs, but in extreme cases after getting out of a chair. It is brought on by an inadequate supply of oxygen via the blood to the heart muscle. Over many years arteries begin laying down sticky deposits, which harden and eventually cause a narrowing within the blood vessels. Typical symptoms include pain in the centre of the chest, which sometimes spreads to the neck/jaw area and down the left arm. The pain can be accompanied by breathlessness, feeling faint, sweating and/or nausea. If you have these symptoms, please seek medical attention as a matter of urgency. See also *Cholesterol*.

Foods to Avoid
- Drinking 5 or more cups of coffee daily can increase the risk. Try to avoid it completely.
- Cut down on alcohol, which in the long term depletes the body of B-vitamins. When you ingest alcohol, levels of homocysteine, a toxic amino acid linked to heart disease, are raised. Beer contains folate and vitamin B6 – so try an occasional beer instead of spirits and wines.
- Reduce your intake of animal fats, including full-fat dairy produce, pre-packaged cakes, and meat pies, sausages and chocolates.
- Avoid sodium-based salt – use magnesium, potassium-based sea salts such as Solo Salt available from health stores. Or buy some powdered kelp – rich in iodine and minerals and use as a salt substitute.
- Reduce your intake of refined sugars found in cakes, biscuits, fizzy drinks and desserts, which convert to hard fats inside the body if not used up during exercise.
- Avoid all foods that contain hydrogenated or trans fats and fried foods. At all costs avoid mass-produced, highly refined cooking oils. You can see rows of them in plastic bottles at every supermarket and they are usually bright yellow. (See *Fats You Need To Eat*.)

Friendly Foods
- Oily fish such as salmon, tuna or mackerel are rich in omega-3 fats, which help to thin the blood naturally, as do onions and garlic.
- Use a little extra virgin olive oil on salad dressings.
- Include plenty of fresh root ginger in your diet, which improves circulation.
- To help lower cholesterol, often a contributing factor of angina, eat plenty of soluble fibre either from fruit, vegetables, oats or flax seeds (also known as linseeds).
- Dried beans such as haricot, kidney, chickpeas, soya beans and whole grains such as brown rice, buckwheat, millet and barley are all rich in fibre and help to control cholesterol.
- Margarines such as Biona, Benecol and Olivio are healthier alternatives for spreading.
- Use non-dairy, organic rice or soya milk, or try low-fat goat's milk.
- If you can follow a vegan diet with the addition of fish (preferably oily), this would be the ideal solution (see *General Health Hints*).
- Sprinkle a dessertspoon of high potency lecithin granules over cereals and salads to help lower LDL cholesterol levels.

Useful Remedies
- The amino acid L-carnitine taken 1–3 grams daily helps improve functioning of the heart and reduces symptoms associated with angina.
- Co-enzyme Q10 – 150mg a day – has helped angina patients manage more exercise with fewer symptoms.
- Natural-source, full-spectrum vitamin E – 400–500iu a day – taken for at least 1 or 2 years thins the blood naturally. If you are taking blood-thinning drugs have your blood checked regularly by a doctor.
- Fish oils supply EPA and DHA, which are essential fats that thin the blood naturally. Take 3g daily to help reduce chest pain.
- Take 2g of vitamin C daily with 1g of the amino acid lysine, which work together to help reverse atherosclerosis. Many companies now make these in a duo formula.

- Magnesium helps regulate the heartbeat. Begin on 200mg daily and increase to 400mg.
- Include a good quality multi-vitamin and mineral in this regimen.
- Begin using grapefruit pectin fibre called Profibe, over your breakfast cereals or in low-fat yoghurts. In numerous clinical trials regular intake has been shown to lower LDL levels (the 'bad' cholesterol) and to gently remove some of the sticky plaque from artery walls. Available from all good health stores worldwide or call The Nutri Centre. **NC**

Helpful Hints
- Smoking tends to constrict arterial flow – so give it up.
- Remember that negative stress in the long term thickens the blood and constricts arterial flow.
- If you are overweight, then it is wise to lose weight. Rather than going on a strict diet, this is best achieved by eating healthily. See *General Health Hints*.
- With your doctor's permission, embark on a programme of gentle exercise. Start by walking or swimming for 15 minutes daily, gradually building to 30 minutes, and then an hour.
- Intravenous antioxidant therapy (chelation) helps to clear blocked arteries and is well worth a try. For details see either www.chelationuk.com who have 16 clinics in the UK, or I go to Dr Robert Trossell in London at 4 Duke Street, London W1U 3EL. Tel: 020 7486 1095.

ANTIBIOTICS
(see also *Candida, MRSA and Thrush*)

Many people resort to the use of antibiotics whether they really need them or not. Antibiotics kill the friendly bacteria, which have an essential role to play in gut and general health. Bacteria are now mutating and many are becoming resistant to increasing numbers of antibiotics. In the long term, antibiotics suppress our immune system, and along with the loss of healthy bacteria in the gut they often allow fungal infections such as candida to flourish. Whenever you have taken an antibiotic you will need a probiotic. Antibiotics mean anti-life and probiotics the opposite – pro-life. Probiotics are supplements containing friendly bacteria called acidophilus or bifidus.

Many doctors report that patients continue to demand antibiotics for colds and flu – which are caused by viruses – but it's only if you contract a secondary infection such as bronchitis, which is bacterial, that antibiotics may be valid.

Taken in the long term antibiotics can have a very negative effect not only on your immune system, but also on your gut. Eventually this can reduce absorption of nutrients from your food (see also *Absorption*).

Foods to Avoid
- If you have taken antibiotics, for one month avoid foods such as alcohol, sugar and too much fruit (especially bananas, apples, melons and kiwi), which ferment easily within the gut. This tends to lead to an overgrowth of unfriendly bacteria, which can trigger conditions such as thrush and candida.
- Avoid mouldy cheeses, which also cause fermentation in the gut.
- Avoid yeast-based breads and foods, such as Marmite and Bovril.

Friendly Foods
- Fruits that don't ferment are OK to eat – these include berries (blueberries, blackberries, raspberries as well as cherries plus tropical fruits such as papaya).
- Pineapple contains the enzyme bromelain, which increases the effectiveness of many antibiotics. It acts as a digestive aid – so eat a couple of fresh pineapple chunks before meals.
- Eat plenty of sugar-free, live, low-fat yoghurt, containing acidophilus and bifidus.

- Artichokes and beetroots contain inulin, a substance that encourages the growth of friendly bacteria.
- Garlic encourages the growth of friendly bacteria and also kills bad bacteria as well as helping to fight infections.

Useful Remedies
- Acidophilus and bifidus are healthy bacteria. Take 2 capsules daily after food for at least 6 weeks after completing the antibiotics. Keep these sensitive, live, healthy bacteria in the fridge. BioCare also make *Replete* powder which can be dissolved in water, which will help the gut to rebalance quickly. **BC**
- Take a B-complex vitamin that includes 0.5–5mg of biotin daily. Biotin is greatly depleted by antibiotics. Lack of biotin affects your skin, hair and nails.
- Goldenseal tincture (1ml) taken twice a day for up to 2 weeks, or grapefruit seed extract, act like natural antibiotics, and can also be taken to avoid infections in the first place.
- Olive leaf extract is an anti-bacterial, anti-viral and anti-parasitic plant extract that helps to dissolve the coating of bacteria and prevent viral replication. Take up to 4 tablets daily.
- Take 500mg of Milk Thistle 1 to 3 times daily with food to help detoxify the liver.
- Bee propolis is a natural antibiotic used by bees to sterilise their hives. Many therapists and doctors find that two propolis capsules taken every day with at least 1g of vitamin C can lead to a general improvement in health and enhanced resistance to infections.
- A herbal formula containing echinacea, wild indigo, myrrh and low-odour garlic called echinacea compound – take 3–6 capsules daily – helps to boost immune system. **SHS**

Helpful Hints
- Some plastic, mass-produced chopping boards – advertised as being anti-bacterial – are helping to make people resistant to antibiotics, therefore use natural wood chopping boards and simply wash thoroughly in warm soapy water.
- A little dirt never hurt anyone, and our obsession with bleaching and using anti-bacterial cleansers is not only damaging the environment – but is also in the long term weakening our immune systems.
- If you feel low when taking antibiotics, rather than waiting until you have finished the course, with your doctor's permission, start taking the acidophilus as soon as you begin to feel below par. Also take a high-strength, B-complex vitamin.
- A naturopath or nutritionist can help you restore your immune system (see *Useful Information*).

APHRODISIACS – Male and Female   (see *Libido Problems*)

ARTHRITIS – OSTEO AND RHEUMATOID
(see also *Gout* and *Acid–Alkaline Balance*)

Osteoarthritis

In the UK alone 54% of people over 65 suffer arthritis or joint pain. In America a third of adults show x-ray evidence of arthritis in their hands, feet, knee or hips. By the age of 65 as many as 75% of the Western population are arthritic. Women seem to suffer with arthritis far more than men.

Over time the cartilage, which cushions and surrounds the joints, breaks down and the bones can become thickened and distorted which restricts joint movement. In most cases it affects the load bearing joints – hips, knees, spine and hands. There is a popular misconception that exercise makes you more prone to developing osteoarthritis. In reality exercise helps to keep your bones healthier and joints more supple.

Primary osteoarthritis develops when our natural cartilage repair process can no longer keep pace with the degenerative wear and tear we can suffer with age. Secondary arthritis is usually triggered by a trauma, such as a broken joint or a fall, or any underlying joint disease. Arthritis has now reached epidemic proportions in the West.

Weight-bearing exercise such as walking, weight-lifting and so on help prevent bone loss (see *Osteoporosis*). Yoga keeps you supple, but if you play contact sports like rugby, football or hockey then the joints are more likely to be damaged.

The majority of people who suffer osteoarthritis eat too many acid-forming foods. Basically proteins such as meat and dairy produce from cows, plus refined carbohydrates like white bread and pizzas are acid-forming; whereas fresh vegetables and most fruits plus millet are alkalising. And if we could all eat less acid-forming foods, many illnesses could be eradicated. I broke my knee back in 1991 and I really have to keep up my exercises or my joints and spine become really stiff.

People who develop osteoarthritis are frequently told that they should avoid the nightshade family, which includes tomatoes, potatoes, peppers and aubergines. Out of these tomatoes seem to be the worst offender, as tomatoes contain an alkaloid, which can trigger inflammation in the joints. It has been shown that 60–70% of people who avoid these foods for at least 6 months or more see benefits. Being overweight places more stress on joints, which will add to the problem in later life.

In cultures where people eat a mainly wholefood, wholegrain, vegetarian diet, arthritis is virtually unknown.

Foods to Avoid

- Reduce your intake of coffee, alcohol, fizzy drinks and shop-bought cakes, pies, pastries, bread, and pastas that are made with refined white flour and white sugar, which are all acid-forming.
- Avoid known triggers such as tomatoes, potatoes, aubergines and peppers.
- Oranges and orange juice can make symptoms worse in some individuals.
- Greatly reduce cow's milk, red meat, high-fat cheeses (especially Stilton), fried foods, sausages, meat pies and chocolate.
- Avoid all white and malt vinegars, which are highly acid-forming.
- For anyone suffering gout-type problems, also eliminate foods containing large amounts of purines, which break down into uric acid in the body, as excess uric acid can trigger severe inflammation in small joints especially the toes. High purine foods are red meats, alcohol, shellfish, anchovies, mackerel, herrings, sardines and organ meats.

Friendly Foods

- Cherries, plums and blackberries are acid forming, but they help to mobilise uric acid out of the joints, to be excreted in our urine. Cherries and cherry juice are best for gout.
- Pineapple contains bromelain, which is highly anti-inflammatory.
- If you **do not** suffer from gout then eat fresh oily fish such as mackerel, tuna, salmon or sardines 3 times a week. Mackerel and sardines, along with herrings, are high in purines.
- Sweet potatoes are rich in vitamin A and fibre, and are a good alternative to ordinary potatoes.
- Grains such as millet, brown rice, amaranth, spelt, barley, quinoa, buckwheat and so on are all preferable to refined wheat products. Choose wholemeal breads and try pastas made from corn, buckwheat, rice and lentil flours. Try 100% organic rye or amaranth crisp breads, sugar-free oatcakes and low-sugar muesli or porridge.

- Eat more fresh green vegetables to re-alkalise your system. One of the quickest ways to do this is to buy a juicer and juice raw cabbage, watercress, celery, parsley and a little root ginger, and drink immediately. You can also make delicious fruit blends (remember we are blending here, not juicing, so you also get the peel which contains all the fibre). My favourite is half a cup of fresh blueberries, a chopped pear, a chopped apple and a sliced banana, a heaped teaspoon of any organic-source, 'green'-based powder from your health store, a tablespoon of linseeds (flax seeds) and aloe vera juice, all blended with a cup of organic rice or almond milk. Fabulous!
- Fresh root ginger can be made into a wonderful pain-relieving tea. Add a small cube of fresh root ginger to a mug of boiling water, add half a teaspoon of honey and apple cider vinegar and sip when warm.
- Blackstrap molasses is rich in calcium, potassium and magnesium, which all help the joints. Try adding a teaspoon of the molasses to a tablespoon of organic apple cider vinegar or a little lemon juice into a cup of warm water, which helps you to absorb more minerals from your diet and helps to re-alkalise your system. For those who prefer honey, buy organic, preferably locally produced, and if at all possible unrefined, which contains more natural minerals. If your symptoms are severe drink this cocktail up to 3 times daily.
- Use organic, unrefined olive, sunflower, walnut or sesame oils for your salad dressings.
- Eat at least one tablespoon of linseeds (flax seeds), or sunflower, pumpkin or sesame seeds daily, as they are rich in essential fats that are vital for healthy joints. Hazelnuts, cashew, almonds and walnuts are all rich in essential fats to nourish the joints. An easy way to eat more of them is to place 2 tbsp of each in a blender, whizz for 1 minute and store in an air-tight jar in the fridge. Sprinkle over breakfast cereal, fruit salads or into low-fat, bio yoghurts daily.
- Try herbal teas such as devil's claw and nettle and use dandelion coffee.
- Add more turmeric and cayenne pepper in your cooking as they help to reduce inflammation.

Useful Remedies

- One of the best nutritional supplements known to help this condition is the amino sugar glucosamine sulphate. A number of studies have found that taking 1500mg daily can substantially reduce pain and improve mobility. Initially take 1500mg of glucosamine a day until symptoms improve and then lower dose to 500mg daily. This may take several months.
- Studies have found that combining glucosamine and MSM (see below) have an even more positive effect. **NB Glucosamine is usually derived from crab shells, so if you have a severe intolerance to shellfish avoid this supplement. But, it is now a/v in a vegetarian formula derived from corn.** For more details contact Health Perception on 01252 861454, or log on to their website: www.health-perception.co.uk
- Niacinamide (no-flush vitamin B3) x 500mg 3 to 4 times a day is a great alternative to glucosamine, which helps to reduce joint pain. Some people reap the benefits in as little as 4 to 5 weeks, but ideally 3 months to a year is a good time scale to take this vitamin. Incidentally it has been noted that people who take niacinamide over a sustained period of time also have an improved sense of humour. **NB Be sure to ask for the 'no-flush' variety, as common niacin can cause a flushing effect that can be quite shocking if you are unprepared.**
- As all the B-group vitamins work together, add a B-complex to your daily regimen.
- MSM (methylsulfonylmethane) is a form of organic sulphur that is involved with many key functions in the body. Extraordinary results are being reported in terms of pain relief from taking around 2–3 grams daily. It is also available in creams. **HN**
- Nutricol Powder has been developed by Brian Welsby, who designed the health programmes for most of the UK Olympic athletes. It contains glucosamine, MSM and hydrolysed collagen. For details call Be-Well Products on 01778 560868. Fax: 01778 560872. Website: www.be-well.co.uk.

- To help reduce the pain, take a couple of teaspoons of cod liver oil daily, which also includes pain-relieving vitamin D. Or take 3 cod liver oil capsules daily. Many fish oils are now high in toxins that have been pumped into the world's oceans, most notably dioxins, deadly chemicals formed during incineration of plastic and PCBs, persistent industrial chemicals used in electrical equipment and many fish oils contain far too many toxins that can adversely affect hormones. Three of the safest after extensive testing are BioCare's DriCelle Cod Liver Oil powder, Higher Nature's Omega-3 Fish Oil and Seven Seas' One a Day pure cod liver oil. The Seven Seas is available at all health stores and for details of the others, see pages 13–15.
- Natural-source, full-spectrum (with 4 tocopherols and 4 tocotrienols) vitamin E 400iu daily helps reduces pain. (But not if you take prescription blood-thinning drugs as vitamin E naturally thins the blood. Check with your doctor first.)
- Take 1–3g of vitamin C daily in an ascorbate form with meals, which does not irritate the gut and has anti-inflammatory properties. Vitamin C is vital for healthy synovial fluid that surrounds the joints.
- Ginger, curcumin and boswelia are herbs with highly anti-inflammatory properties, take 3–4 tablets a day.
- The formula Ligazyme Plus made by BioCare contains vital minerals such as calcium, boron, magnesium, rutin, silica plus vitamins A and D and digestive enzymes, which all support connective tissue and encourage healthier bones. **BC**
- Sodiphos is a mineral (sodium phosphate) that helps to break down uric acid deposits in joints; especially useful for gout. Take 600mg daily. **BLK**

- Include a good-quality antioxidant formula in your regimen, which helps stabilise cartilage membranes.
- Cayenne pepper capsules are really useful for reducing inflammation and increasing circulation. Take 2–3 capsules daily in the middle of meals. **SHS**
- Homeopathic Rhus Tox 6x helps to relieve stiffness when you first move around. Especially good for people whose symptoms are worse when it's cold and wet.
- Homeopathic Ruta Graveoleans 30c often helps if tendons are sore and if spine and joints feel sore and feel worse when it's cold and wet.
- Use liquid hyaluronic acid (HA). HA is a naturally occurring protein found in all bone and cartilage structures in the body. HA provides the cushioning affect in all joints and it's the high content of HA in young people that keeps their joints (especially the knees) so supple. As we age levels fall. By taking 1ml daily in water you can help restore some of the elasticity in connective tissue and joints. It is also useful for rheumatoid arthritis. For more details ask at your health store or call Modern Herbals on 01274 889047. Website: www.modernherbals.com

Rheumatoid Arthritis (RA)

Rheumatoid arthritis is primarily an inflammatory disease of the smaller joints, such as wrists, ankles, fingers and knees. It is an autoimmune disorder whereby the body's own immune system starts attacking joint tissue. It is a chronic disease and tends to progress with time but many people find the pain and stiffness comes and goes for varying periods of time. RA affects 3 times as many women as men and most often occurs between the ages of 25 to 50. Over-acidity in the body and uric acid deposits in the joints is a contributing factor (see *Acid–Alkaline Balance*).

The pain and stiffness are usually worse upon rising, and tends to wear off as the day progresses. The joints can become warm, tender and swollen. Fatigue, low-grade fever, loss of appetite, and vague muscular pains can all accompany RA.

Researchers have found that at least one third of people can completely control their rheumatoid arthritis by eliminating foods to which they have an intolerance. The most common culprits are any foods and drinks from cows, plus the nightshade group (see *Osteoarthritis*).

Other triggers are a leaky gut, which is when food molecules pass through the gut wall thus triggering an allergic response. Many RA sufferers also have parasites and candida, a yeast fungal overgrowth. There can be a genetic susceptibility (see *Leaky Gut*).

Heavy exercise may cause RA to progress faster, but gentle exercise like swimming, T'ai Chi, yoga, stretching and walking are more helpful. Researchers have found that many rheumatoid arthritis sufferers are deficient in the major antioxidant nutrients, vitamins A, C, E plus the mineral selenium, but particularly vitamin E. The majority of RA sufferer's also appear to be low in stomach acid and supplementing with betaine hydrochloride (stomach acid) can help. (See also *Low Stomach Acid*.) Betaine helps to digest the proteins and most people who have allergies have a problem digesting certain proteins. If you have active stomach ulcers do not take the betaine and use a papaya or pineapple based digestive enzyme capsule instead.

RA is virtually unknown in primitive cultures where the diet is mainly alkaline-forming foods, nor do these people have antibiotics or refined foods, which also contribute to RA.

Foods to Avoid

- Animal fats eaten to excess tend to aggravate RA. Avoiding all dairy produce from cows, plus meat, sugar and eggs helps some people.
- Avoid known triggers such as tomatoes, potatoes, aubergines, peppers.
- Oranges and orange juice can be a problem for some people.
- Coffee, chocolate, peanuts, spinach, rhubarb and beetroot are all high in oxalic acid, which seems to further aggravate RA in some people.
- Greatly reduce your intake of refined sugary foods and drinks.
- Avoid wheat, citrus (especially oranges and grapefruit), corn, food additives, colourings and flavourings. Keep a food diary and note when symptoms are more acute. Eliminate these foods for a month and see if this helps.

Friendly Foods

- Eat more pineapple – a rich source of bromelain, which has anti-inflammatory properties.
- Eat oily fish at least 3 times a week such as wild salmon or mackerel or take a couple of teaspoons of fish oil daily. These omega-3 essential fats reduce uric acid levels. (See also *Fats You Need To Eat*.)
- Use linseed (flax seed) oil plus unrefined olive oil in salad dressings.
- A strict vegetarian – that is, vegan – diet has been shown to help some individuals.
- Root ginger plus the spices turmeric and boswellia have anti-inflammatory properties. These will not alleviate the problem but can substantially reduce the pain and give people more mobility.
- Make a tea using fresh ginger and lemon juice.
- Eat plenty of cherries and garlic and use rice, oat or almond organic milks as alternatives to dairy produce from cows.
- Avocado and raw wheat germ is rich in vitamin E and essential fats.
- Eat lots more green vegetables especially raw green cabbage, kale, spring greens, watercress, parsley, celery and endives or add a green food powder based on wheat grass, spirulina, alfalfa, chlorella and green foods, such as Dr Gillian McKeith's Living Food Energy (available from health food stores) to cereals, juices and desserts.
- Under professional guidance, juice fasts can greatly reduce symptoms.

Useful Remedies

For those who don't like fresh pineapple, bromelain is available as a supplement. Take one capsule

– 500mg – of bromelain on an empty stomach to increase its effectiveness.

- Evening primrose oil can help, but you would need very high amounts and the reason people take EPO is for the GLA (Gamma Linolenic Acid) content. GLA is highly anti-inflammatory and is available as a supplement. Take 1–2 grams daily. Or any high-quality EFA blend such as Udo's Choice Oil can be drizzled over cooked foods or used in salad dressings.
- Vitamin C 1–3 grams daily, plus 400–800iu of natural-source, full-spectrum vitamin E.
- A multi-mineral containing 30mg of zinc, 100–150mcg of selenium plus traces of copper are known to help reduce pain.
- EPA-DHA fish oil 1–2 grams daily
- Many sufferers of RA benefit from taking vitamin B5 pantothenic acid, 500mg can be taken 4 times a day. Pure Royal Jelly has a high B5 content.
- As B-vitamins work together include a B-complex.
- The herbs curcumin, turmeric and boswelia are also available in tablet and capsule formulas, 1200–1600mg of any one.
- Take celery seed extract 300mg daily to reduce uric acid levels.
- L-Glutamine 500mg 3 times daily can help heal a leaky gut. Take between meals.
- Sufferers of RA are often lacking in healthy bacteria within their guts, therefore a daily acidophilus/bifidus capsule after meals can help increase assimilation of nutrients from food and supplements.
- A multi-mineral formula in either a food state or colloidal form taken daily helps to re-alkalise the body.

Helpful Hints for All Types of Arthritis

- If you are overweight this places more strain on the load bearing joints, so lose weight.
- Hot and cold compresses applied alternately will help reduce swelling and pain for 20 minutes at a time. Cold compresses are especially good if the affected joints feel hot to the touch. Moist hot packs help reduce pain and stiffness.
- Joint cartilage needs plenty of fluids, so drink 8 glasses of water daily, which also helps eliminate uric acid. Hard water can sometimes exacerbate arthritic-type symptoms, it is packed with minerals, but in an inorganic form that is hard to absorb. However, fruits and vegetables are able to absorb the inorganic minerals and aided by sunlight converts them to an organic form, and when minerals are in an organic or colloidal form, they become more bio-available to us.
- To ingest the 21 minerals that are essential for life, it makes sense to eat far more fresh fruits and vegetables. But unfortunately thanks to pollution, over-farming and acid rain, most soils (especially in the UK) no longer contain sufficient minerals needed for good health. And if the minerals are not in the soil, they are never going to make it into our vegetables (although organic foods generally contain more minerals). This is why we all need to begin taking a daily multi-mineral.
- The purest forms of water are either distilled water or reverse osmosis (RO) waters, which are extremely pure and free of minerals. These types of waters rehydrate your cells more easily. Really pure waters are filtered in such a way that gives you 99.999% pure H_2O, like the rainwater that fell through an unpolluted atmosphere aeons ago. For further details of reverse osmosis water call The Pure H2O Company on 01784 221188, or log on to www.purewater.co.uk. If you decide to use pure water then you would need to take a chelated multi-mineral supplement daily.
- Numerous people have experienced benefits after taking pure aloe vera juice daily for several months.
- Nettle tea taken regularly has helped reduce the pain and swelling for many people.

- To re-alkalise your system, take a good quality green powder such as Alkalife daily. The same company also make Alkabath salts which are more powerful than Epsom salts and help to eliminate toxins from the joints. They also supply water distillers. For your nearest stockists call Best Care Products on 01342 410303. Website: www.bestcare-uk.com.
- Topically applied oil of wintergreen can help ease the pain and inflammation.
- Homeopathic Apis 30c helps in RA when there is swelling and rheumatic pains that are worse for heat.
- If the RA is in the small joints, ask at your homeopathic pharmacy for Actea Spicata-3c, taken 3 times daily between meals helps reduce the pain.
- Wearing magnets has given pain-relief to many people. Magnets placed on the painful area will increase blood-flow, which brings more oxygen to an injury or area of pain, which helps to reduce swelling and inflammation. For details of Super Magnets call Coghill Laboratories on 01495 752122, or log on to www.cogreslab.co.uk. Email: enquiries@cogreslab.co.uk.
- The Chinese exercise regimes of T'ai Chi or Qigong have helped many sufferers, as these exercises are easy to practise, even with severely impaired mobility. RA seems to be affected by stress, so make sure you stay as calm as possible (see Stress).
- Bioinduction Ltd makes a range of pain relieving machines based on electro-therapy. Tel: 0800 028 1400. Website: www.acticare.com
- Call the Arthritic Association on Freephone 0800 652 3188 or 01323 416550 between 10am and 1pm or 2 and 4pm on weekdays, or log on to their website: www.arthriticassociation.org.uk. This charity provides very good dietary advice and has a great website. Annual membership costs £6.

ASTHMA

(see also *Allergies* and *Leaky Gut*)

Over 5 million people in the UK now suffer from asthma, 1 in every 10 children and 1 in every 12 adults is asthmatic and the problem is escalating. The cost to the NHS is £900 million a year. Asthma affects the bronchial tubes leading to our lungs resulting in periods of wheezing and shortness of breath. Pollution from traffic fumes and overuse of pesticides is without doubt a contributing factor, and during school holidays incidences of attacks are reduced as there is less traffic.

Other atmospheric pollutants such as pollen, cigarette smoke and car exhaust fumes can all be triggers as can house dust mites and moulds. Stressful situations and chronic exhaustion can also trigger an attack as can eating foods to which you have a sensitivity (such as sulphur dioxide, used as a preservative in many dried fruits). You can also suffer exercise-induced asthma. There is also a link between parasites and asthma.

People who take paracetamol every day are twice as likely to suffer asthma, and if you take it twice weekly you are 80% more likely to be affected.

Foods to Avoid
- There is a strong association between asthma and dairy products, especially in children.
- Any foods to which you have an intolerance will make you more susceptible to attacks. For details of good tests see *Allergy*.
- Reduce intake of meat, eggs and full-fat dairy produce, which increase mucus production.
- Sodium-based salt in any foods (some people can have an attack after eating too many crisps).
- Some mass-produced, ready-prepared salads, dried fruits, wines and beers contain sulphur dioxide, which is known to trigger problems in sensitive individuals.

- Avoid sodium benzoate, which is frequently found in soft drinks.
- Generally avoid all mass-produced pre-packaged foods. See *General Health Hints*.

Friendly Foods

- Green leafy vegetables, fresh fruits and honey are rich in magnesium – which helps the airways to relax and a lack of magnesium is linked to breathing problems. Brown rice, avocados, spinach, haddock, oatmeal, baked potatoes, navy beans, lima beans, broccoli, yoghurt, bananas, soya beans, and unrefined nuts are all rich in magnesium.
- Include more lentils, garlic and onions in your diet, which help fight infection and clear the lungs.
- As asthma is often linked by nutritional physicians to a 'leaky gut', include plenty of fresh ginger in your diet, which is very soothing. Cabbage also helps heal the gut (see *Leaky Gut*).
- Eat oily fish three times a week, which is rich in vitamin A. This can reduce the severity and frequency of attacks. Sweet potatoes and pumpkin are also high in vitamin A.
- Use extra-virgin, unrefined olive and sunflower oils in salad dressings and include plenty of linseeds (flax seeds), pumpkin, sunflower and sesame seeds in your diet.
- Turnips, cauliflower, apples, pears, cherries, grapes, kale, and green tea are all great foods for the lungs.
- Try rice, almond or oat milks as non-dairy alternatives to cow's milk, but only if you are not sensitive to these milks – some people are intolerant of almonds.
- Buy a juicer and make yourself a carrot, ginger, cabbage, radish, apple and celery mix – drink immediately. Try different mixes daily, which is a great way to get health-giving nutrients into the body.
- Vine-ripened tomatoes are rich in lycopene, which is great for the lungs (and prostate). Cooking in a little olive oil helps release the lycopene.
- Sprinkle turmeric on your meals or add to cooking, as this herb has anti-inflammatory properties and supports the immune system.
- After an attack drink plenty of fluids to help break up mucus so that it can be expelled.
- Children who eat more fresh fruits and vegetables are known to suffer fewer attacks.
- Eat more edible white membranes in lemons – containing limonene – which is great for the lungs.

Useful Remedies

- Take a good-quality multi-vitamin daily; plus a multi-mineral containing 200–400mg of magnesium; plus 200mcg of selenium as low levels leave you more at risk from an attack.
- Vitamin C in ascorbate form. Take 1 gram 3 times a day with meals to help open the airways.
- Take vitamin B6, 150mg a day; B12, 1,000–2,000mcg a day; plus a B-complex. Asthma medication depletes B vitamins, especially in people who are sensitive to sulphates.
- The enzyme bromelain taken 1,000–4,000mcu a day helps to reduce mucus production and ease breathing.
- Take 60mg a day of natural-source beta-carotene if you suffer exercise-induced asthma.
- The herb ginkgo biloba – 120–240mg standardised extract, or 3–4ml of tincture, taken daily – has been shown to improve circulation and decrease asthma symptoms.
- Oralmat is an extract of rye grass in a liquid formula that has been shown to support healthy respiratory function by strengthening defenses against toxins in the lungs. An Australian study in mild to moderate asthmatics showed considerable lessening of symptoms, for some after only a few days of use. Three drops should be placed under the tongue 3 times daily (hold 30 seconds or longer). Children should use one drop instead. **NC**
- Bronchial-dilating herbs such as euphorbia and grindelia help open the airways. Take 15 drops of each herb 3 times daily in juice. **NC**
- Try Respiratory Drops made from ginger, myrrh, garlic, echinacea and lobelia – 15 drops a day. This helps expand the airways and keep the respiratory tract clearer. **OP**

Helpful Hints

- Avoid chlorinated pools as exposure to chlorine can constrict the airways.
- Use an ioniser in any room in which you are going to spend any length of time, as it can reduce the amount of pollen and dust in the air.
- Use Ultra Breathe, a very handy, inexpensive device that does a great job of exercising the lungs. It costs £16.95 plus £2.95 for p&p. For details call 0870 608 9019, or visit www.ultrabreathe.com
- Try to avoid antibiotics during the infant years, which have been linked to an increased risk of developing asthma in later life.
- Acupuncture has proved useful for many sufferers.
- To check for food and environmental allergens, consult a kinesiologist who can determine what foods and environmental agents you should avoid. Kinesiology is not 100% accurate but thousands have found it a good indicator of which foods and other factors are causing the most problems (see *Useful Information*).
- It's incredible how many people suffer breathing problems simply because they are not using their lungs properly. Most asthmatics benefit from tuition in proper breathing techniques. Every 20 minutes or so remember to take a deep breath down into your lower-abdomen area.
- Shallow breathing is associated with being stressed. Learn relaxation techniques or consult a hypnotherapist who can teach you how to relax (see *Useful Information*).
- Take gentle exercise such as yoga, T'ai Chi, swimming or walking. Exercise reduces stress and helps you to breathe which should help to reduce the incidence of asthma attacks.
- Consult a nutritionist (see *Useful Information*).
- Homeopathy has proved especially helpful for children, but be sure to consult a qualified homeopath. Call the Organic Pharmacy in London on 020 7351 2232 during office hours and have a word with the on-duty pharmacist; or call any homeopathic local pharmacy that you trust.
- Homeopathic Pothos Foetidus 200c can be used if an attack is triggered by animals. Blatta Orientalis 30c can be taken during an attack when catarrh is present. Deeper asthmatic treatment using homeopathy helps reduce the susceptibility for attacks (see *Useful Information*).
- Have a regular massage using essential oils of camomile and lavender.
- A company specialising in indoor, air-quality equipment is the JS Air and Water Centre. Tel: 01903 858657. Website: www.airandwatercentre.com
- Stress is a major factor in asthma – stay calm! (See *Stress*.)
- It may be worth consulting a chiropractor as blocked airways may link back to nerve compression in the spine.
- Scientists in Germany have developed a machine called Air Energy, which makes the oxygen we breathe easier to utilize. The air we breathe contains 21% oxygen – but our body can utilize only around one quarter of the available energy within this amount. Air Energy converts the oxygen into a form that the body can easily utilize. With regular use, this machine is obtaining amazing results for all lung conditions, and clinical trials are ongoing in the UK and Europe. The machine is expensive, starting at £2100, but the results and research to date is very exciting. For more details call 01938 556800. Website: www.biolifesolutions.co.uk These machines are also becoming available at many health clinics and doctors' surgeries – call the above number for your nearest clinic – and treatments start at around £35 an hour.
- Consult the Asthma Helpline. Tel: 08457 010203, 9am–5pm, Monday–Friday.
- For a further range of asthma information contact the National Asthma Campaign, Tel: 020 7786 4900.Website: www.asthma.org.uk

ATHLETE'S FOOT

(see also *Candida*)

Athlete's foot is caused by a fungal infection of the skin and is characterised by itchy, flaking and cracked skin, especially between the toes and on the soles of the feet. This problem can be transmitted in public places such as swimming baths where people walk barefoot, and in moist atmospheres. Wear socks made from natural fibres, such as cotton and silk, which allow the skin to breathe; and change footwear regularly. It is important that feet are dried properly after bathing or exercise. Persistent athlete's foot is often associated with an overgrowth of candida in the gut (see also *Candida*).

Foods to Avoid
■ Avoid sugar when symptoms are acute. Sugars ferment and feed yeasts in the body.
■ Avoid foods containing yeast such as cheese, wine, yeasty breads, beer, mushrooms, vinegar, soy sauce and yeast-based drinks such as Bovril and Marmite.
■ Grapes are high in sugar and may have moulds on the skin.
■ Peanuts should also be avoided.

Friendly Foods
■ Eat plenty of garlic and onions, which are anti-bacterial and anti-fungal.
■ Live, low-fat yoghurt contains acidophlius and bifidus – eat at least 250 grams a day.
■ The herb pau d'arco is anti-fungal – take 6 capsules daily or drink several cups as tea.

Useful Remedies

■ Apply tea tree oil externally, or tea tree oil and grapefruit seed extract (known as citricidal).
■ Black walnut and calendula tincture, applied topically and taken internally twice a day is effective.
■ Try tea tree, manuka and neem cream. Apply twice daily. OP
■ Pierce a low-odour garlic capsule in powder form and sprinkle on the affected area.

Helpful Hints
■ Pau d'arco is the bark from a South American tree and boosts immune function and helps fight fungal infections. It makes a very pleasant tasting tea and is easily available in capsules. It can also be added to a foot wash made with tea tree oil.
■ Add 5–10 drops of citricidal liquid to a footbath and soak feet twice daily.
■ You may not want to try this! Dip an old cloth in fresh urine and wrap around the affected area – urine is a natural anti-fungal. Change the 'bandage cloth' daily.

AUTISM

(see also *Allergies*)

An estimated 535,000 people, mainly children in the UK have autism, with 40% of those waiting at least 3 years for a clear diagnosis. Four times as many boys are affected as girls with symptoms generally beginning in early childhood. Its numerous symptoms include an inability to communicate and concentrate, impaired language and learning, disturbed sleep patterns, hyperactivity, abnormal social relationships, rituals and compulsive behaviour.

Some doctors say that autism is genetic and this is undoubtedly a factor in some cases, but reports are now accumulating which link the huge increase in autism to toxic overload either from vaccines (especially MMR – measles, mumps and rubella), pesticides, PCBs and heavy metals such as mercury, lead and aluminium, plus chemicals in foods such as phenolic compounds and salicylates (see below).

Research shows that incompletely digested particles of wheat and dairy were found in higher amounts in children with behavioural problems and a link is widely acknowledged between neurotoxins in the brain and autism. Problems with digestion, absorption and elimination are often seen. Reduced breakdown of proteins in milk and gluten (wheat, rye, oats and barley) leads to 'neurotoxins' entering the brain and disrupting brain chemistry. Many autistic children have also been given large doses of antibiotics, which in the long term can trigger more gut problems – these in turn can initiate intolerances and sensitivities to many foods (see also *Allergies*, *Candida* and *Leaky Gut*).

Poor immune function and sluggish liver function (see under *Liver Problems*) can contribute to this condition, as can fungal overgrowth (see *Candida*). I have heard of several cases where autistic children have been referred to psychiatrists and when given mind-altering drugs the children's symptoms worsened considerably.

Foods to Avoid
- Remove all gluten from the child's diet. This is in most mass-produced breads, biscuits and cereals. Remember that rye, barley and oats also contain gluten. Many doctors are now happy to prescribe gluten-free products on the NHS. Some children suffered withdrawal-type symptoms and became worse before their parents notice improvements.
- Dairy produce from cows should also be avoided.
- Soya, fish, eggs, citrus fruits, chocolate, peanuts, or any nuts to which there is an intolerance. Shellfish have been found to cause many problems associated with food intolerance/allergy and leaky gut.
- Avoid all pre-packaged, junk-type foods and drinks that are packed with salt, sugar and animal fats. Keep a food diary and note when symptoms become worse.
- Avoiding additives found in packaged and processed foods is a must as they may contain compounds that can be toxic to the brain when the body fails to break them down properly.
- For some children avoiding excitotoxins – chemicals which stimulate the brain – is helpful. Foods rich in salicylates (a form of excitotoxins) are oranges, almonds, apples, apricots, tomatoes, cherries, cranberries, cucumbers, grapes, nectarines, tangerines, peaches, plums, peppers, prunes and raisins. For the full list check out www.feingold.org
- To make sure that your child does not suffer nutritional deficiencies when avoiding foods work with a qualified nutritionist or a nutritional physician (see *Useful Information*).

Friendly Foods
- As far as possible, give your child only organic, whole foods that are free from pesticides and rich in magnesium, vitamin B6 and folic acid; especially green leafy vegetables, beans and liver.
- Gluten-free cereals plus carrots, broccoli, baked beans, parsley, spinach, watercress and sesame seeds are all high in calcium, which will hopefully reduce the incidence of self-injury and have a calming effect.
- Essential fats are vital for healthy brain-functioning. Recent research shows that autistic children have lower levels of the omega-3 fats in the brain – these are found in oily fish, nuts and seeds. Give your child oily fish (salmon, unsmoked mackerel, fresh tuna, herring, sardines and anchovies) at least twice a week, and unrefined, organic pumpkin, sunflower, sesame, flaxseeds (linseeds) and walnuts daily if these are not any of their problem foods. Add cold-pressed organic seed oils to cooked foods and use in salad dressings. See also *Fat You Need to Eat*.

Useful Remedies
- Take magnesium, 15mg per kilo of body weight; and vitamin B6 25–100mg for a child of 2–6 years. Many children with autism have also been found to be low in folic acid – part of the B-group of vitamins, so try to include a B-complex daily. As children do not tend to like tablets, try adding liquid B-vitamins to their food. BioCare make a liquid formula called Vitasorb B. **BC**

(Nature's Plus also make great vitamin and mineral ranges for Children. **NP**)

- Many parents have found that including an essential fatty acid formula has helped their children enormously. Try Efamol's Efalex capsules or Higher Natures tasty Smart Fish, which comes in individual, child-friendly sachets. **NC**
- Dissolve an additive-free vitamin C tablet into water daily to boost immune function. One gram daily for a child aged 2–6 years.
- A good probiotic taken daily will build up the good bacteria in the gut, help to support digestion and begin to squeeze out yeast. BioCare do a powdered one easily sprinkled onto foods. They contain only the probiotic and either freeze-dried strawberry or banana. **BC**
- www.positivehealthshop.com stock Nutri's low-allergy, cherry-and-banana flavoured multi: 'Ultracare for Kids'. It has added digestive support and good fats for brain health. Add a scoop to juice and shake, or add to a fruit smoothie.

Helpful Hints

- For a healthy mayonnaise full of healthier fats add 4 tbsp of live, sugar-free soya yoghurt to 2 tbsp of cold-pressed sunflower oil. Stir in a teaspoon of Lecithin granules available in health food stores. Leave to stand for half an hour and stir again before serving.
- Try to remove all chemicals from the child's environment such as perfumes, chemical cleaning products and toiletries – look out for unnatural flavourings in toothpastes.
- Aspirin has salicylate-like qualities so is best avoided in those that are sensitive to salicylates.
- Beware of colourings and flavourings in cheaper vitamin supplements as even these may cause a reaction.
- Many parents have had some success in using homeopathy to minimise vaccine damage. Call The Organic Pharmacy – on 020 7351 2232 – and ask for a remedy to suit your child's specific symptoms.
- Dr Ben Feingold researched the link between diet and behavioural problems. He is the creator of the very successful Feingold diet, which includes avoiding salicylates. Check out his website full of helpful information and tips at www.feingold.org
- A great book called *Optimum Nutrition for the Mind*, by Patrick Holford, the founder of the Brain Bio Centre, is full of lots of useful information and tips on dealing with autism.
- For further help the National Autistic Society can be contacted on www.nas.org.uk. They also have an autism helpline on 0845 070 4004
- Because each case of autism is so unique, I strongly suggest that before embarking on this programme you consult a nutritional therapist. Search for one at www.autismfile.com or try the Brain Bio Centre, which can be reached on 020 8871 9261, or check out their website at www.mentalhealthproject.com

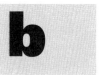

BACK PAIN

Twenty million working days in Britain alone are lost every year thanks to back pain, which affects 80% of people at some point in their lives. This is partly owing to poor posture but more frequently to poor lifting habits. Most companies now train their staff how to lift properly;

without doubt prevention is better than cure. Until recently most people thought that bed rest was the most sensible option, but 'right and light' exercise under the supervision of a professional is definitely preferable.

The centre of the back can be thought of as a column made up of 33 pieces of bone called vertebrae. The spinal column is strengthened by ligaments, which run the length of the spine, and is supported by muscles, which attach to the vertebrae though tendons. It is important to have back pain diagnosed and, in an ideal world, you should see a chiropractor or an osteopath on a regular basis.

I have seen people with ME and chronic fatigue that have received huge benefits by having their back and necks manipulated back into place. I have also seen people who have ended up on crutches or even in a wheelchair when all they needed was a good chiropractor. One lady was given such strong painkillers after continually complaining of back pain that she ended up wandering the streets suffering memory loss. Doctors need to refer more patients with back pain to an osteopath or chiropractor. And if they won't, I suggest you find your nearest practitioner and pay privately. Chronic low-level back or loin pain can also be linked to a kidney infection.

Foods to Avoid
- If you are in pain, it is worth avoiding foods and drinks containing caffeine, which reduces our ability to make endorphins that are the body's natural pain-killing chemicals.
- Reduce your intake of meat, which will exacerbate any inflammation.

Friendly Foods
- Eat oily fish at least twice a week for its anti-inflammatory properties.
- Add fresh rosemary to meals to improve circulation and aid healing.
- Ginger, turmeric and cayenne pepper can all improve circulation and have anti-inflammatory effects.
- Cauliflower, berries, sweet potatoes, fresh fruits (especially cherries) and green leafy vegetables are all rich in vitamin C, which helps to produce collagen which makes up 90% of the bone matrix and also acts as a mild anti-inflammatory.

Useful Remedies
- While symptoms are acute take 1500mg of glucosamine daily. This amino sugar helps to restore the thick gelatinous nature of the fluids and tissues around the joints and in between the vertebrae. This takes time! Once the pain is eased, lower the dose to a maintenance intake of 500mg daily. If you suffer a severe sensitivity to shellfish do not take this supplement, which is usually made from crushed crab shells. Instead look for vegetarian glucosamine, derived from corn. For more details call Health Perception on 01252 861454. Website: www.health-perception.co.uk. Many companies now blend the glucosamine with MSM, an organic form of sulphur, which has been found to be more effective against pain.
- Taking 3–4 tablets a day of a combination formula containing ginger, curcumin and boswelia can also help to reduce the pain and inflammation. **FSC**
- Calcium 500–1000mg, with 500mg of magnesium daily – many companies make them in one tablet. These minerals are known as nature's tranquillizers and help to reduce muscle spasm.
- Take 3 grams of vitamin C over the course of the day, in an ascorbate form – this vitamin helps to produce collagen.
- Try Ligazyme Plus, a supplement devised by a chiropractor containing calcium, vitamin C, bromelain, magnesium and rutin, which all help support the skeletal system. **BC**
- Cayenne pepper capsules can help to reduce the inflammation and increase circulation to the affected area. 3–4 capsules daily with food. **SHS**

Helpful Hints

- As soon as possible after any injury, consult a chiropractor or osteopath. To help reduce the immediate pain and muscle spasm, wrap some ice cubes or a bag of frozen peas in a towel and place on the painful area for 10 minutes every hour.
- Most towns now have alternative health centres that include chiropractic, acupuncture and/or physiotherapy. Go along and see if they can help. They also sell gels that help reduce the pain, gel based packs for the freezer, plus various pain relief ideas. Well worth a try.
- Back pain often has its root in poor posture. This is compounded by the fact that we now tend to lead very sedentary lives, which weakens the supporting structures of the spine and makes them much more prone to injury. Much severe back pain is caused by muscle spasm.
- Before agreeing to any surgery, always consult a chiropractor or osteopath for a second opinion (see *Useful Information*). However, always report severe and persistent back pain to your doctor.
- If you are extremely tired and under stress, not only does your immune system begin to fail but also your body in general. In other words when you stop supporting your body, it stops supporting you. If this is the case, then you need to take a long, hard look at your lifestyle and get more rest. Acupuncture is known to help in many cases and is great for reducing the inflammation and pain.
- Try the Young Living Oils Raindrop Technique. These therapeutic essential oils (especially wintergreen, which is highly anti-inflammatory) have tremendous healing properties. For more details contact Susie Anthony on 01749 679900; or have a look at the Resources Page on her website on www.psalifemastery.com

- For general back maintenance, yoga can be very beneficial as it improves flexibility, strengthens the spine and improves posture, protecting it from injury in the long term.
- Alexander Technique and Pilates teach individuals how to maintain their back and general health through better posture and exercises. After suffering a chronic back problem, Pilates has really helped me. (See *Useful Information*.)
- Walk more – this helps to tighten the abdominal muscles – which in turn supports the back. Treat yourself to a pair of MBT (Masai Barefoot Technology) shoes, which are made using state-of-the-art technology to support the feet. They are used by orthopaedic therapists and physiotherapists the world over. For more details log on to www.mbt-info.com
- Swimming is a great exercise because although the back muscles are worked, they are protected from jarring by the support given by the water. But obviously do not swim if your symptoms are acute.
- Wearing magnets has given relief from the pain to many people. Magnets placed on the painful area will increase blood-flow, which brings more oxygen to an injury or area of pain, which helps to reduce swelling and inflammation.
- Use good bath salts such as Epsom salts or Alkabath to help reduce muscle spasm. Alkabath salts are more powerful than Epsom salts and help eliminate toxins from the joints and re-alkalise the body. For your nearest stockists call Best Care Products. Tel: 01342 410 303. Website: www.bestcare-uk.com
- Have a weekly aromatherapy massage – the essential oils penetrate into the bloodstream and really help calm the muscle spasms, which can leave you doubled up in pain. Roman camomile, lavender, and eucalyptus oils all help reduce pain.
- Use a 'wheat or lavender bag' – these bags are available in most health shops. You heat them in the microwave and apply to painful muscles. Alternate with the ice packs for more relief.
- For further help contact BackCare, 16 Elmtree Road, Teddington, Middlesex TW11 8ST; or call their helpline on 0845 130 2704. Website: www.backcare.org.uk

BAD BREATH (see *Halitosis*)

BEREAVEMENT (see also *Immune Function* and *Stress*)

Losing a loved one at any age can be a devastating blow to your life and wellbeing at every level. Therefore, after a loved one's passing, it is vital for you to express your feelings and let your emotions out. Grief, anger and guilt have a tremendous impact on the physical body. Tears shed in trauma contain high levels of stress chemicals – let them out and don't be afraid to break down. When my mother died in my arms in 1991 I was inconsolable and, like millions of others, I turned to good mediums who were able to give me specific messages that only the two of us knew.

During the past 15 years, I have written regularly about life after death and have received hundreds of letters from people of all ages who have lost a loved one. Their sense of loss and grief is often overwhelming. But how different we might all feel if we knew that our loved ones live on. In April 1998 I went through a near-death experience with a medical doctor present and my story is well documented in my book *Divine Intervention* (Cico Books).

These days I write from a totally different perspective as I have an absolute personal 'knowing' that we all go on. I and many scientists now believe that our unique energy field, which contains all the information about us, simply moves to another frequency or dimension. When you turn on your radio or TV you can tune in to hundreds of different channels or stations and receive or see huge amounts of information. And just because you cannot see these signals it does not mean they are not there! The spirit realms are also on various frequencies, but more sensitive people can hear and see them.

I have interviewed and met dozens of people who by learning to meditate, and stilling their minds into a more receptive alpha state, have after time heard messages from departed loved ones for themselves. Obviously, some people are better at this than others, but we all have the capability to hear other realms. When some people suddenly begin hearing voices they are labelled as being mentally ill – some are – but others have simply begun hearing the spirit world and it is vital that the medical world begins to recognise this possibility. See also *Spiritual Emergency*. I have listed much of the science in my book *The Evidence for the Sixth Sense* (Cico Books).

b

Foods to Avoid
- As much as possible avoid junk, sugary, pre-packaged meals, which place a strain on your immune system, which is already under great stress. But then again, at times of extreme stress, the brain burns more sugar. Therefore, if you don't mind putting on a few pounds, enjoy your treats – but don't go overboard.
- Caffeine, alcohol and sugar place a great strain on your adrenal glands, which further increase the feelings of total exhaustion.

Friendly Foods
- At times of extreme emotional stress it is easy to forget our own health. It is important to eat as healthily as possible, which will not only help your nervous system to cope but also boost your immune system. You help no one by allowing yourself to become ill. Try to eat one meal daily containing quality protein such as fish or chicken with fresh vegetables and fruit.
- Make a fruit smoothie. Add one dessertspoon of Solgar's Whey To Go Protein, one small box of blueberries, one banana, a spoon of linseeds (flax seeds) and sunflowers seeds, a few raisins,

and a chopped apple. Blend all with some rice milk, and drink. This mixture will give you some energy and good nutrients.

■ See also *General Health Hints*.

Useful Remedies

■ Take homeopathic Ignatia 30c and the Bach Flower Remedy Star of Bethlehem, which help to reduce the feelings of shock and grief.
■ Take a B-complex daily to support the nerves.
■ Take a good-quality multi-vitamin and mineral, such as Kudos 24 (see *General Supplements* on p.160). KVH
■ Kali Phos New Era Tissue Salts are excellent for reducing stress. Take 4 tablets under the tongue in-between meals twice daily.

Helpful Hints

■ If you have a friend, colleague or relative who is dealing with the death of a loved one, take time out to shop and prepare the odd meal for them. Not only will this help to support their physical needs but also by having someone to talk to, it also supports their emotional needs.
■ Cruse Bereavement Care, a charity founded in 1959, has 180 branches in the UK. For their helpline call 0844 477 9400 (9.30am–5pm weekdays). Website: www.crusebereavementcare.org.uk
■ The Compassionate Friends is a nationwide organisation of bereaved parents offering under-standing, support and encouragement after the death of a child or children. Members of TCF receive regular issues of *TCF News* and a quarterly newsletter. For further information, contact The Compassionate Friends' helpline on 08451 232304 (10–4pm and 6–10pm). Email: info@tcf.org.uk Website: www.tcf.org.uk
■ To find a medium in your area contact the Spiritualist National Union, Redwoods, Stansted Hall, Stansted, Essex CM24 8UD. Tel: 0845 458 0768. Website: www.snu.org.uk If they are unable to locate a medium, they are happy to give details of your nearest spiritualist church.

BLADDER PROBLEMS
(see *Cystitis*, *Incontinence* and *Prostate Problems*)

BLEEDING GUMS
(see also *Fluoride*)

Bleeding gums can be triggered by over-enthusiastic brushing or by gum disease, but they can also indicate a lack of vitamin C or bioflavonoids, either in the diet or through supplementation. To make sure you are not suffering with anything more serious, go along and see your dentist. Make sure you see an oral hygienist at least twice a year for a proper scale and polish. When plaque builds up gum disease, such as gingivitis, can take hold. If left unchecked you can lose your teeth. Believe me, after all the problems I have suffered with my teeth during the last decade, I know your own teeth are very precious and should be taken care of at all costs.

Foods to Avoid

■ The plaque-forming bacteria that cause chronic gum disease thrive on sugar. Young children especially should be allowed only small amounts of fizzy drinks, sweets and puddings that are high in sugar.
■ Keep refined carbohydrates including biscuits, cakes and sweets to a minimum.
■ Avoid all foods and water containing fluoride, which is a by-product of the plant fertiliser industry. Fluoride may have reduced the number of cavities, but it is a poison and in my opinion should not be allowed into our drinking water. This is mass medication without consent.

Friendly Foods

- Foods containing plenty of fibre such as leafy green vegetables, brown rice, fresh fruits like apples, figs and cherries are all rich in vitamin C, which supports healthy teeth and gums.
- Garden sage makes a great mouthwash for inflamed or bleeding gums, an inflamed tongue, mouth ulcers or a sore throat. Simply add 1–2 tsp of chopped leaves to a cup of boiling water. Allow to cool. Place in a screw top jar and use twice daily as a mouthwash. You can also gargle with this mixture whilst still warm. **NB As sage stimulates the muscles of the uterus, DO NOT use sage during pregnancy.**
- Chew liquorice sticks regularly to keep teeth and gums clean and reduce bacteria in the mouth.
- Drink at least 6 glasses of filtered water daily.
- Dilute concentrated fruit juices at a ratio of 1 part juice to 4 parts water.
- Thai foods such as lemon grass, coriander and garlic help keep teeth healthy and the coriander helps eliminate heavy metals from the body.

Useful Remedies

- Co-enzyme Q10 is well known to improve gum health. Take 60mg a day.
- Vitamin C with bioflavonoids, 1 gram a day with food.
- A good-quality multi-vitamin and mineral powder, such as Kudos 24 (see *General Supplements* on p.160). KVH

Helpful Hints

- Mercury from amalgam fillings is also known to cause swollen, bleeding gums (see *Mercury*).
- Eat a piece of fruit after main meals. This increases saliva production, which is alkaline and neutralises the acid produced by the bacteria, which is responsible for dental decay. Apples are excellent, but if you eat sweet or highly acid fruits after a meal, such as oranges, then simply swill your mouth with water immediately afterwards. If you clean your teeth directly after fruit, you can brush away weakened enamel and cause erosion.
- Also if you eat very sugary desserts, swill the mouth with water. Don't brush for at least an hour.
- Toothpaste containing sodium lauryl sulfate can thin the lining of the cheeks and may weaken gum tissue.
- Gengigel, a gel and mouthwash containing hyaluronic acid – a natural substance that forms an important part of gum formation. This gel helps to reduce inflammation. For details call Revital on 0800 252 875, or log on to www.revital.com
- Vitamin C supplements containing sugar when chewed will attack tooth enamel and weaken the lining of the mouth.
- Use a good electric toothbrush.
- Practise good daily dental hygiene by using floss and a natural tea tree mouthwash. Clean your teeth and gums daily using a water pick appliance, adding a few drops of tea tree oil and 1 drop of clove oil, which is an excellent antiseptic, to the warm water. Water Tooth Cleaners are available from large chemists including John, Bell and Croydon in London. Tel: 020 7935 5555.
- There are now numerous herbal toothpastes containing everything from co-enzyme Q10 and vitamin K to support your gums, to red clover and herbs known to help ladies through the menopause! Find one that suits your needs.

BLOATING

(see *Candida, Constipation* and *Flatulence*)

BODY HAIR, EXCESSIVE (Hirsutism)

Many women suffer this problem after going through the menopause; some can be affected when they are much younger. This problem usually begins with extra hairs on the face and sometimes hair begins growing in-between the breast area. It is normally owing to an excess of male hormones called androgens, which are produced by the ovaries or the adrenal glands. It is important to consult your doctor if you have unexplained excess body hair. But this condition can often be helped if you can balance your hormones naturally (see *Menopause*). The condition is often related to polycystic ovarian syndrome (see *PCOS*).

Foods to Avoid
- Cut down on alcohol and excess caffeine, which can affect hormone levels
- Reduce animal fats from dairy and red meat.
- If you cook food in plastic containers, buy food wrapped in cling film or use cling film at home, then chemicals within the cling film can leach into your food, especially if it is heated in a microwave. The chemicals that are released from the cling film can have an oestrogen building effect within the body, which in turn can trigger a whole host of hormone-related problems.
- If PCOS is a factor, reduce sugar to a minimum as this leads to surges of insulin, which is needed to balance sugar levels in the body. As far back as 1980 researchers found that an excess of insulin is linked to higher testosterone levels.

Friendly Foods

- Include more hormone-regulating foods, such as tempeh, chickpeas and fennel.
- Eat more beans, lentils, and leafy greens including broccoli, cauliflower, cabbage, artichoke and beetroot, all of which help cleanse the liver of toxins and help to balance hormones.
- Eat more linseeds (flax seeds), sunflower and pumpkin seeds, plus Brazil nuts rich in essential fats, which also help regulate hormones.
- Fill up on fibre, which binds to excess hormones so that they can be easily removed from the body. Oat or rice bran, fruit (especially apples), whole grains, such as brown rice would be ideal. Fresh root ginger is also rich in zinc.
- Make sure you drink plenty of water.

Useful Remedies
- The herbs that have proved most useful for reducing excess body hair are dong quai and agnus castus, which help to normalize hormonal levels. Take 500mg of either or both daily. Try the Agnus castus in the first instance. Femarone contains blessed thistle, squaw vine, and black cohosh; take 2 capsules 3 times daily with food for 3 months. (Femarone also comes in drops.) SHS
- Black cohosh taken 500mg twice a day has been used successfully to inhibit and reverse facial hair growth in women. Many companies now sell all these herbs in one formula – try 500mg twice daily or take 1ml of a tincture.
- Herbs used for the related condition PCOS are liquorice, saw palmetto, paeonia and agnus castus. Take 5mls of each daily.
- Zinc helps to balance blood-sugar levels and is also necessary for good hormone function. Take 15mg daily.

Helpful Hints
- A study of women with excess body hair found that acupuncture reduced both hair density and length and significantly reduced their levels of androgens – male sex hormones. See *Useful Information*.
- If you are overweight, this can add to the problem. See *Weight Problems*.

■ Women with excessive body hair may be short of the hormone progesterone, which helps balance the male hormones that women also produce in small quantities. Many women don't ovulate regularly (but still have periods), often triggered by stress, excess pollution in the environment or foods containing herbicides, which have an oestrogen-like building effect. As progesterone is produced only after ovulation or during pregnancy, progesterone deficiency is becoming more common; hairier legs and chins are one sign. Natural progesterone, made from yams in a cream can reduce hairiness when used for some time. It is available on prescription in the UK (but freely available in the US). The natural progesterone information service has more details about the use of progesterone and contacts for doctors who will prescribe it in the UK. Check out www.npis.info. Or call them on 07000 784849. You can order natural progesterone creams for your own use by calling Pharm West. **PW**

BODY ODOUR

We are all covered in bacteria and in certain parts of the body such as under the arms and between our legs bacteria can accumulate. Unpleasant body odour is usually associated with poor hygiene habits but it can also indicate internal toxicity. The skin is a route of elimination that is used by the body when other routes – such as the liver, bowels and kidneys – are struggling to cope and become overloaded. Also if you eat too much garlic, the smell begins to ooze through your pores. It's very healthy for the person who has eaten it, but not so pleasant for those around you!

b

Foods to Avoid
■ Reduce the amount of low-fibre foods you eat such as jelly, ice cream, white breads and pastas, cakes, biscuits and so on.
■ Avoid full-fat dairy produce which triggers mucus production and can exacerbate constipation.
■ Any foods that ferment in the gut, such as mouldy cheeses or high-sugar fruits, can eventually trigger body odour. Therefore eat fruit in-between meals.
■ Cut down on sugar and alcohol.
■ Red meat and heavy fatty meals are hard to digest and slow your digestion and elimination.
■ Avoid any foods you are intolerant to – especially wheat and cow's milk, which trigger constipation in many people. See *Constipation*.

Friendly Foods
■ Drink at least 6 glasses of filtered water daily to help flush toxins from the body and reduce constipation.
■ Add a tablespoon of soluble fibre to your breakfast cereals such as linseeds (flax seeds), hemp seeds, psyllium husks, or oat or rice bran – all available from health stores.
■ Treat yourself to a blender and a juicer. To help cleanse your system blend any selection of fruits you like with a tablespoon of added linseeds (flax seeds), a dessertspoon of oat or rice bran, plus a teaspoon of a good-quality green food powder. My favourite smoothie is organic blueberries, a banana, a chopped pear and a kiwi or apple, to which I add some flax seeds, sunflower seeds, oat bran, a couple of organic dried apricots, some of Dr Gillian McKeith's Living Food Energy Powder and a cup of organic rice milk. If you drink this cocktail instead of having an evening meal or for breakfast, it really helps to clear you out! If you add half a teaspoon of powdered essential fats it helps even more. Omega Plex EFA formula is available from BioCare. **BC**

- On alternate days, juice any green foods, plus artichoke, celery, apple, raw beetroot, a little fresh root ginger and aloe vera juice, which will all help to detoxify your system.
- Generally eat more artichokes, chicory, beetroot, watercress, alfalfa sprouts, broccoli, cabbage, kale, fennel, leeks and onions – which all aid detoxification.
- Adding fresh coriander to these juices and meals helps keep the bacteria that can cause unpleasant body odour under control.
- Eat more pineapple and papaya, which are rich in digestive enzymes.
- Kelp, almonds, buckwheat, millet, brown rice, and figs are all rich in magnesium – often lacking in constipated people.

Useful Remedies
- Healthy bacteria acidophilus/bifidus help improve gut functioning – take 2 capsules daily after meals.
- A deficiency of the mineral zinc is related to excess perspiration – take a multi-vitamin and mineral daily, which usually contains 15mg of zinc, and then take a further 15mg before bed.
- Any organic green food supplement powder containing chlorella and/or wheat grass is a great way to increase elimination.
- The mineral silica really helps to reduce body odour. Take 75mg daily. **BLK**

Helpful Hints
- When the bowels are moving frequently the body doesn't have to try to eliminate toxins through the skin.
- Fresh, live yoghurt with acidophilus and bifidus eaten on a regular basis keeps gut flora in good shape.
- Take a shower every day and change underwear regularly.
- Dry-skin brushing will help to break up and remove toxins stored under the skin, so that the body can eliminate them. Combine this with an Epsom salt bath to really help flush out toxins that may cause odour. Use 1 cup per 60lbs of body weight and add to a warm bath. Soak for 15–20 minutes and rub your skin all over with a wash cloth. Don't rinse off before getting out of the bath tub. Just dry off and retire for the evening. Keep some water handy by the tub as a warm bath can make you thirsty.
- Colloidal silver has anti-bacterial actions so it can be helpful to spray under the arms. Higher Nature make an excellent spray – which can also be used for sore throats! **HN**
- Wear cotton or silk next to the skin, which enables the skin to breathe.
- If persistent, body odour may indicate liver dysfunction, digestive problems and/or yeast infections, which are probably best investigated by a qualified nutritionist or a doctor who is also a nutritionist (see *Useful Information*).
- Try PitRok – the natural, odourless mineral salt deodorant, which prevents bacterial growth without the use of harsh chemicals or aluminium. Just wet the crystal and glide it over the skin. It is also available in a spray. For your nearest stockist call PitRok Ltd. Tel: 0208 563 1120. Website: www.pitrok.co.uk

BOILS
(see also *Immune Function* and *Liver Problems*)

Boils are normally triggered by an acute bacterial infection of a hair follicle caused by the bacteria staphylococcus aureus. If you suffer from boils on a regular basis, it's the body's way of telling you that your immune system is run down, you're consuming a very poor diet and you are full of toxins. Boils are more common in diabetics and AIDS patients and may be accompanied by a slight fever. The secret to controlling boils is to keep your liver clean, as once the liver is overloaded, or you become constipated, then toxins are dumped into the skin. See also *Constipation*.

Foods to Avoid
- Any foods and drinks high in sugar, which will lower immune function.
- Reduce your intake of red meats and full-fat dairy produce especially cheese, chocolates, double cream and so on.
- Avoid all pre-packaged meals, and mass-produced cakes, biscuits and snacks containing hydrogenated or trans fats.
- Eliminate mass-produced burgers, fried foods and oily take-away meals.

Friendly Foods
- Eat more soluble fibres such as linseeds (flax seeds), or oat or rice bran to encourage faster elimination of toxins from the bowel.
- Include more garlic and onions, which have antiseptic properties that help cleanse the gut.
- Eat more fresh beetroot, fennel, celeriac and artichokes, which help to cleanse the liver.
- Eat plenty of fibre in the form of lightly steamed vegetables, jacket potatoes, brown rice and fruits with the peel left on where practical. Apples are great for the skin – but make them organic.
- Eat low-fat, live yoghurt, which contains healthy bacteria acidophilus and bifidus.
- Drink at least 6 glasses of water daily.
- See *General Health Hints*.

Useful Remedies
- Zinc is a vital mineral for healing the skin and stimulating the immune system. Take 30mg a day.
- Vitamin C: take 1 gram in an ascorbate form 3 times a day with meals for one month and then reduce to 500mg daily.
- Vitamin A is also great for healing the skin. If you are not pregnant or planning a pregnancy, take up to 30,000iu daily for 7 days. Then reduce to 3000iu daily, which is also an acceptable dose if you are pregnant.
- Place some Goldenseal tincture on a cotton swab and apply it directly to the boil. Goldenseal helps to kill off the bacteria staphylococcus aureus.
- Apply a little tea tree oil on a cotton swab to the boil once it has burst.

Helpful Hints
- Goldenseal can also be used as a poultice. The boils don't normally rupture if you use this herb.
- If you do want the boils to come to a head and possibly rupture, 2 dessertspoons of Epsom salts in half a pint of hot water can be applied directly to the boil to enhance draining.
- Try a mixture of silica, arnica and belladonna 30, which will help to reduce pain and help the boil pop. Once it has popped clean it with tea tree oil and Goldenseal. **OP**
- After the boil has come to a head and suppuration has finished, take a mixture of hypericum and calendula 30 twice a day to help it heal.
- Recurrent boils would benefit from a detox.
- Get plenty of exercise, which helps detoxify the skin, and wash as soon as possible after exercise.
- Saunas help to clear blocked pores and drain toxins from the body.
- A wonderful book for people suffering from skin problems is *Super Skin* by Kathryn Marsden (Thorsons).

BREAST CANCER

(see also Cancer)

Today there is a lot we can do to help prevent and heal breast cancer. Nevertheless figures for women contracting breast cancer are still climbing. By 2015, 1 in 8 women will have had a diagnosis of breast cancer at some point in their lives and it remains the most common cause of death in women aged between 35 and 54.

A few women are so frightened of contracting breast cancer, as their mother, sometimes their grandmother and other relatives died of this disease, that they have their breasts removed as a precaution. My mother died from breast cancer, but I would not undergo such radical surgery unless I actually had cancer. Our inherited genes control the structure and function of our body but if our genes stay healthy then our body can stay healthy. If you live a healthy lifestyle you can mostly change which genes are expressed. In other words if your parents and grandparents died of heart attacks, or cancers, you may well have a pre-disposition for heart problems and cancer. But if you live a different lifestyle and eat healthier foods, you can help change the chemistry within the body and stack the odds more in your favour.

Meanwhile, risk factors for breast cancer include orthodox HRT, the contraceptive pill, excessive intake of saturated animal fats, dairy products, alcohol, pesticides, herbicides, and a low intake of protective fruit and vegetables, which are rich in antioxidants.

Also, many young women overproduce oestrogen and this is one of the reasons they suffer with symptoms of pre-menstrual syndrome. If you eat a healthy diet the body excretes these hormones via the liver. However, if the diet is high in saturated and animal fats or alcohol, not only is it harder for the body to excrete these oestrogens, it tends to recycle them into an aggressive form, which begins attacking tissue.

Residues of pesticides and herbicides known to trigger various cancers are now in our food chain and drinking water and these toxins live in fatty tissue within the body, so the more you avoid contact with such substances, the more you reduce your chance of contracting cancer.

Foods to Avoid

- Reduce your intake of alcohol to no more than one unit a day. See *Alcohol*.
- Animal fats should be kept to a minimum, eat lean organic meats.
- Reduce your intake of dairy, especially from cows, sheep and goats and if you do eat diary make sure it's low fat.
- Pesticides and plastics in the body act like strong oestrogens within the body, which are known to trigger certain cancers; hence why you need to eat organic food as much as possible. Never re-heat a pre-packaged meal in its plastic container as the chemicals leach into your food. Transfer them to glass or stainless steel cookware before heating.
- There has been much misinformation in the media about soya, saying that it causes hormone activity that is non-beneficial to health. Whilst this argument is ongoing it is generally accepted that fermented soya in the form of miso or tempeh is beneficial. Cooked tofu is fine, but if in doubt avoid unfermented soya products such as soya yoghurt or milk. Soya isoflavones act like a weak oestrogen, which helps block stronger negative oestrogens in our environment and therefore soya isoflavones in capsule or tablet form are fine.
- Avoid all fried foods.

Friendly Foods

- As a preventative measure soya beans, chickpeas, lentils, beans (dried beans are best), and fermented soya products, such as tempeh are fine. Japanese and Thai women have a much lower incidence of breast cancer and this appears to be due to their regular consumption of fermented soya-based foods, which are rich in phyto-oestrogens and isoflavones, which contain genistein. And genistein helps inhibit the growth of cancer cells. Eat organic and/or GM-free soya in its traditional form – tofu, miso, soy sauce and tempeh. If you have breast cancer (or any hormonal cancer) then avoid all soya products, or discuss with your health professional.

- Broccoli, cabbage, Brussels sprouts and alfalfa sprouts all contain substances that are protective against breast cancer.
- Raw linseeds (flax seeds) sprinkled regularly onto meals contain a fibre called lignan, which helps to protect breast tissue.
- Eat more essential fats – see under *Fats You Need to Eat*.
- My favourite way to ingest a lot of nutrients quickly is by juicing. Juice some organic raw carrots, cabbage, apple, fresh root ginger, raw beetroot, radish and celery, add to this a teaspoon of any organic green food supplement and some organic source aloe vera juice.
- In cancer the only problem with juicing is that some of the live enzymes and nutrients and almost all of the fibre is left in the juicer, so scrape them out and add them to your juice, it makes the mix thicker but you then receive far more nutrients. For this reason I use my blender quite a lot as then you get the whole fruit including the peel. A great meal replacement is to chop a banana, an apple (remove the pips), a small box of blueberries, a teaspoon of soya lecithin granules, some green food powder with a couple of fresh or dried figs. I throw in some sunflower seeds and linseeds (flax seeds) and a cup of low-fat organic rice milk and whiz this for a minute; it makes the most deliciously healthy and filling shake.
- Replace margarines containing hydrogenated and trans fats with healthier spreads such as Biona or Vitaquell.
- Many patients with cancer have low levels of the carotenes. Apricots, sweet potatoes, asparagus, French beans, broccoli, carrots, mustard and cress, red peppers, spinach, watercress, mangoes, parsley, tomatoes are all rich in carotenes. Fresh, organic carrot juice is a great source, but don't overdo the carrot juice as your skin may turn orange!
- Take extra fibre daily, which keeps toxic wastes and old hormones from being absorbed from the colon into the bloodstream. The colon must be kept clean and bowels emptied regularly for healing to occur in the body. Starting with a low dose and gradually increasing – mix 1 tsp increasing to 1 dessertspoon of psyllium husks in a full mug of cold water – twice daily. Take the mix at different times from other supplements; it can cause bloating, which is why you start with a small dose. If the husks don't suit your system, then add a tablespoon of oat or rice bran (or flax/linseeds) to the fruit blends and drink daily – and remember to include more water in your regimen.
- Drink plenty of water to aid elimination.
- Add more curcumin (extracted from the spice turmeric) to your foods. It is highly anti-cancerous. **NB: If you are undergoing chemotherapy – then check with your GP before taking large amounts of this spice.**
- Drink more organic green tea, which has been shown to have anti-cancer properties.

Useful Remedies to Prevent and Heal Breast Cancer

- See details of WFK1 under Cancer section. This Quinone treatment is a real breakthrough.
- If you don't like soya-based foods, many companies now make isoflavone supplements. **HN**
- If you have cancer, you can take 5–10 grams of vitamin C daily in an ascorbate form for a few weeks. In such doses you may experience loose bowels in which case cut the dose by 500mg. For maintenance take 1 gram daily.
- Take a high-strength antioxidant formula that contains vitamins A, C and E plus zinc and selenium.
- If you have breast cancer take Co-enzyme Q10 x 200mg twice a day. This important co-enzyme

has been shown to inhibit cancer-cell growth and protect breast tissue. To aid prevention take 100mg daily.

- Reishi, shiitake and maitake mushrooms are available either as tincture or as tablets and should be taken 3 times a day. They have been shown to have great immune-enhancing properties and to inhibit the growth and spread of cancer cells. **NC**
- A good quality multi-vitamin/mineral.
- Indole 3 Carbinol (I3C) is a phytochemical supplement isolated from cruciferous vegetables (broccoli, cauliflower, Brussels sprouts, turnips, kale, green cabbage, mustard, pak choy, and so on), which has been shown to inhibit the growth of oestrogen-receptor-positive cells. This supplement has huge anti-cancer potential. To ingest therapeutic quantities of indole would require eating enormous amounts of raw vegetables as cooking tends to destroy these phytochemicals. Take one tablet 2–3 times a day. **NC NB: Pregnant women should not take this supplement as oestrogen is needed for healthy foetus growth.**
- With your doctor's permission start taking the hormone melatonin. A high percentage of women with oestrogen-receptor positive breast cancer have low plasma levels of melatonin. Begin by taking 3mg nightly and gradually increase. This can trigger vivid dreaming, so increase dosages slowly. Your GP can give you a prescription for melatonin, or it can be bought freely in the US. **PW**

Helpful Hints

- Examine your breasts once a month. If you find even the hint of anything unusual or any type of lump see your doctor immediately. Remember the earlier any problems are detected, the greater your chance of a complete cure. Many lumps are simply benign cysts, so the sooner you see your doctor, the better.
- Some scientists believe that antiperspirants may be linked to breast cancer. Many sprays contain chemicals that are absorbed into the body and they also stop you from sweating, but this is nature's way of getting rid of many unwanted toxins. The majority of breast cancers occur in the part of the breast nearest the armpit. Use natural tea-tree based antiperspirants or ones that are free from aluminium such as Pit Rok Crystal.
- Avoid wearing a bra for too much of the day. Women who wore a tight fitting bra for 14 hours or longer a day were 50% more likely to develop breast cancer. At the very least find yourself a comfortable loose fitting bra that doesn't block lymph drainage.
- Some women who have had their breasts removed find that any remaining lymph glands, especially under the arms can be really painful. Manual lymph drainage can often relieve the discomfort (see *Useful Information*).
- Keep your stress levels to a minimum (see *Stress*).
- As much as possible take regular exercise, but not to excess.
- Breast cancer is more common in people who are overweight and obese. Take steps to control your weight (see *Weight Problems*).
- Oxygen therapies are well worth looking into (see Helpful Hints in *Cancer*).
- Read Patrick Holford's book *Say No to Cancer* (Piatkus). If you have specific queries that you need help with log on to www.patrickholford.com.
- Read Dr John Lee's book *What Your Doctor May Not Tell You About Breast Cancer* (Warner Books).
- Another wonderful book is *Your Life in Your Hands; Understanding Preventing and Overcoming Breast Cancer* by Jane Plant (Virgin Books).
- Read *The Breast Cancer Prevention and Recovery Diet* by Suzannah Olivier (Penguin).
- Contact Penny Brohn Cancer Care (formerly the Bristol Cancer Help Centre), Chapel Pill Lane, Pill, Bristol BS20 0HH. Helpline: 0845 123 2310 (9.30am–5pm weekdays).

Email: helpline@pennybrohn.org; website: www.pennybrohncancercare.org
■ The Naturopathic Cancer Therapy Trust (NCTT) have a network of practitioners all over the UK and elsewhere who can support you through their protocol for dealing with cancer without drugs. Website: www.defeatingcancer.co.uk

BREAST PAIN and TENDERNESS

(see also *Breast Cancer* and *Pre-menstrual Tension*)

Tender breasts are a common symptom of pre-menstrual tension (PMT; also known as pre-menstrual syndrome or PMS) when they can become increasingly swollen and tender prior to menstruation. Breast pain is often associated with other symptoms such as fluid retention, abdominal bloating and an excess of the hormone oestrogen. Tender breasts during the first few months of pregnancy are quite common. But if breasts are tender the whole month or if the discomfort becomes severe, it is important to see a doctor. If you find any lumps of any size or shape in your breasts seek medical attention immediately. Exercise is one way of reducing the symptoms of PMT as this encourages lymphatic drainage. On the other hand, wearing a bra for more than 12 hours a day can reduce the body's ability to drain the lymph nodes.

Foods to Avoid
■ Caffeine – complete avoidance can reduce the symptoms of breast pain. Moderate reduction doesn't always work; it does need to be complete elimination. Remember that caffeine is not just in tea and coffee but also in cola, chocolate and some over-the-counter cold remedies.
■ Alcohol should be kept to a minimum as it can increase breast pain.
■ Sodium-based salt tends to aggravate fluid retention, which can exacerbate breast tenderness. Ask at your health shop for a magnesium-based sea salt and use sparingly.

Friendly Foods
■ Eat plenty of sunflower and sesame seeds and linseeds (flax seeds), which all contain essential fatty acids, which should help reduce breast tenderness. See *Fats You Need To Eat*.
■ Eating organic, fermented soya-based foods such as tempeh on a regular basis can also reduce the tendency to painful breasts and help to balance hormones.
■ Drink herbal teas, such as red clover, plus dandelion coffee.
■ Add kombu seaweed to bean dishes. It contains iodine, which helps reduce mastitis-type pains.
■ Eat more broccoli, cauliflower, kale and cabbage, which help to balance hormones naturally.

Useful Remedies
■ Take 400mg of magnesium for its muscle relaxing qualities.
■ Full-spectrum vitamin E, 200–600iu a day for 3–4 months.
■ A good-quality B-complex contains 50mg of B6 – take another 50mg of B6 separately. The dose should total 100mg daily.
■ Evening primrose oil is useful for this problem, but you would need around 2–3 grams daily. Therefore it would be easier to take 250mg of Mega GLA. **BC**
■ The herb agnus castus; 500–2000mg a day or 2ml of tincture should help regulate hormone levels more naturally.
■ Take a good-quality multi-vitamin and mineral for women.

Helpful Hints
■ In Chinese medicine breast pain is often caused by liver congestion; see *Liver Problems*.
■ Regular exercise (running or walking 1–3 miles a day) can relieve tenderness. Many women find it uncomfortable to run when their breasts are tender, but if you exercise on a regular basis

b

tenderness should not be so much of an issue for the 7–10 days prior to a period. Wear a sports bra.

- Exercise improves circulation and aids drainage of the lymph system. Mini-trampolines are wonderful, as is any vigorous exercise such as fast walking, swimming or dancing.
- Lymphatic drainage massage is known to improve drainage, thereby reducing swelling and pain (see *MLD* [manual lymphatic drainage] in *Useful Information*).
- Sometimes breast pain is due to an imbalance of oestrogen and progesterone, which causes tender breasts and breast cysts, known as fibrocystic breast disease. It is becoming increasingly common because of the high levels of oestrogen pollutants we are exposed to from excess pesticides and herbicides. Using a natural progesterone formula found in creams and capsules may reduce the cysts and tenderness in a few months. You need a prescription for natural progesterone in the UK. For details of natural progesterone call Pharm West. **PW**
- If, after three months, there is no improvement on the above regimen, see a qualified nutritionist who is also a doctor (see *Useful Information*).

BRITTLE NAILS

(see *Nail Problems*)

BRONCHITIS

(see also *Immune Function*)

This common problem is triggered when the bronchial tubes – your airways – become infected. Older people with compromised immune systems are more likely to be affected.

Bronchitis can have a viral or bacterial origin and symptoms normally occur when you have an upper respiratory tract infection. Bronchitis is more common during winter months. If you contract a cold or flu, immune function can become very low indeed – thus allowing any infection to take hold and spread down towards the lungs. For some sensitive individuals, tobacco smoke is enough to set them off, but with other people exposure to pollens and other toxins they inhale can lead to an attack of bronchitis. The effects of stress greatly deplete immune function, and fatigue, nutrient deficiencies and lack of exercise can also make you more prone to bronchitis. This is because at such times you rarely take deep breaths. Some cases can be managed without the use of antibiotics, but if you find it painful to take a deep breath, have a temperature for more than 48 hours or can hear a rattle in your chest when you breathe or cough, you must see your doctor. If the infection reaches your lungs it can become pneumonia.

Having suffered bronchitis a couple of times in the past which resulted from colds caught on long plane journeys I can assure you this condition is no laughing matter. Once you have the weakness you really need to look after yourself. If my immune system had been in better shape I would have been more able to fight off these infections. See also *Immune Function*.

Foods to Avoid
- Greatly reduce your intake of any foods containing sugar – this includes concentrated fruit juices – as sugar reduces your immune system's ability to fight infections.
- Whilst symptoms are acute, avoid all dairy products from any source including chocolate, plus refined carbohydrates such as cakes, pastries, biscuits, and for some people soya products – all of which create more mucus.
- Avoid any foods and oils containing hydrogenated or trans fats – as they trigger inflammation in the body and are linked to asthma.

Friendly Foods

- Eat plenty of fresh fruits and vegetables. When you feel this poorly, your digestive system can labour under the strain. Therefore eat fresh vegetable soups, which are an easy way to ingest nutrient dense foods. Thickening them with sweet potatoes, pumpkin, carrots or squash – all rich in vitamin A – also helps boost your immune system.
- Papaya, mango and apricots are also great lung foods.
- Apples are great for lung health but can be sprayed with many different pesticides – go organic and eat 2 apples daily for breakfast to support your lungs.
- Garlic and onions are really cleansing and have antiseptic properties.
- Vine ripened tomatoes are rich in lycopene, which is great for your lungs. The lycopene is released when the tomatoes are cooked in a little oil.
- Eating fish regularly helps to reduce the frequency and severity of bronchial attacks and if you are undergoing one, the oils in fish can provide a strong anti-inflammatory effect. Guavas and pink grapefruits are also rich in lycopene.
- Quercetin – a protective flavonoid – helps defend you from the harmful effects of pollution and smoke. Found in apples, pears, cherries, grapes, onions, kale, brocolli, garlic, green tea, and red wine.
- Limonene found in the rind and edible white membrane of citrus fruits – oranges, lemons, limes, tangerines, and grapefruit may help to protect the lungs.
- Increasing vitamin B1 (thiamine) found in peas, wholegrain rice, sunflower seeds and pine nuts is essential for maintaining the health of the lungs.
- Brown rice, avocados, spinach, haddock, oatmeal, baked potatoes, navy beans, lima beans, broccoli, yoghurt, bananas and unsalted nuts are all rich in the mineral magnesium, which is also vital for healthy lungs.
- As zinc has anti-viral properties that fight colds and flu – eat more oysters, pumpkin seeds, fresh root ginger and unrefined nuts.
- As you are likely to be running a temperature, drink at least 6 glasses of water daily.
- Make teas with fresh lemon juice, a small piece of root ginger and a little honey. Drink lots of herbal teas such as liquorice, fenugreek and elderberry.

Useful Remedies

- Include a high strength multi-vitamin and mineral in your daily regimen – see details of Kudos 24 in *General Supplements* on p.160. **KVH**
- Whichever multi you take, make sure it contains 400mg of magnesium, as studies have found that people who take more vitamin C and magnesium tend to have healthier lungs.
- Bromelain, extracted from pineapples, is extremely effective for bronchial conditions as it improves lung functions and helps loosen any mucus. While symptoms are acute take 1,000–4,000mcu of bromelain, plus 1–4 grams of vitamin C in an ascorbate form with meals.
- N-acetyl cysteine (NAC) helps to break up mucus and reduces the bacterial count for people suffering with bronchitis. Take 500mg twice a day. Studies have shown that people who take NAC on a regular basis suffer less incidence of bronchitis. NAC also helps to support the liver.
- For 7 days, you can also take 25,000iu of vitamin A (if you are pregnant only take 3000iu).
- Useful herbs for boosting immune function and reducing bacteria are echinacea, goldenseal and elderberry.
- Liquorice is anti-inflammatory, anti-viral and can be very useful with bronchial conditions.
- Zinc Gluconate lozenges really help to reduce the coughing and sore throat.
- Olive Leaf Extract has powerful anti-bacterial qualities, which have been shown to help with respiratory conditions – take 3 capsules daily to help boost your immune system.
- Expectorant herbs that help to clear any 'gunk' in your lungs are garlic, white horehound and euphorbia. They can be taken either in capsules or as a tincture. **OP**

Helpful Hints

- Inhaling steam is really helpful for opening up the lungs. Add a few drops of Olbas oil or any pure eucalyptus oil into a bowl of boiling water. Place a towel over your head and really inhale the steam through your nose. If you do this 4–5 times daily it helps to loosen your chest.
- If you have a tendency to suffer bronchitis, take a 3-month programme in the autumn to boost the lungs and clear any mucus out of the lungs. The herbs in the programme include elecampane, golden rod, thyme and pau d'arco. **SHS**
- Echinacea taken regularly helps prevent viral bronchitis from progressing into a more dangerous bacterial infection. A good formula is Ultimate Echinacea Complex which includes astragalus and wild indigo, which boost the immune system. To order log on to www.holoshealth.com
- The herbs mullein, wild cherry bark, liquorice and lomatium are useful expectorants and have anti-viral properties. These herbs are available as tinctures and taken on a regular basis can help loosen mucus, reduce the coughing and help fight the infection. **FSC**
- If the infection becomes serious and you are prescribed antibiotics, as soon as you finish the course begin taking the healthy bacteria acidophilus and bifidus for at least 6 weeks to replenish healthy bacteria in the gut, which in turn helps immune function. **BC**
- Don't exercise near main roads – and learn to exercise your lungs. Professional singers rarely catch a cold – they use their lungs more. Sing along to your radio and give your lungs a workout!
- In general terms, whenever you are suffering from a bronchial infection, you should stay in bed and rest for at least 2 days. The more you try to struggle on, the slower your recovery.
- Use an Ultra Breathe, a very handy, inexpensive device that does a great job of exercising the lungs. £16.95 plus £2.95 p&p. For details call 0870 608 9019 or visit www.ultrabreathe.com

BRUISING

The discolouration of the skin is caused by blood leaking from damaged blood vessels into the tissues of the skin. It is a normal process but some people bruise excessively, especially older people. Excessive bruising is often due to a deficiency of vitamin C and/or bioflavonoids, the water-soluble pigment in fruits. But if you suffer regular bruising not associated with a hard knock or injury – it can indicate rarer underlying problems such as leukaemia, so if in any doubt check with your GP.

Foods to Avoid

- Avoid all highly processed foods such as mass-produced cakes, biscuits and pre-packaged meals, which are generally lacking in any nutrients.
- Don't cook foods for too long as cooking greatly reduces nutrient levels.
- See *General Health Hints*.

Friendly Foods

- Eat plenty of foods high in vitamin C such as kiwi, cherries, peppers, blueberries, pineapple and papaya.
- Include more leafy green vegetables in your diet, especially kale, cabbage, spinach and pak choy.
- See also *General Health Hints*.

Useful Remedies

- Take 1–3 grams of vitamin C in an ascorbate form daily plus 500–2,000mg of bioflavonoids, to help strengthen capillaries.

- Rutin Complex includes bromelain, a flavanoid extracted from pineapple. It has an anti-inflammatory effect. Take 500mg of bromelain daily until bruising disappears.
- The herb horse chestnut is excellent for bruises. Take 500mg daily until symptoms disappear.

Helpful Hints
- For bruising after a trauma such as surgery, homeopathic arnica is a wonderful remedy. If you have had surgery of any kind, you can take Arnica 30c every 4 hours until the bruising fades. Arnica cream or witch hazel gels used topically are really helpful for reducing the swelling.
- For deeper tissue damage use Ledum 30c 3 times daily for 4–5 days.
- Comfrey ointment speeds up soft-tissue healing.
- For sprains and injury-type swellings use an ice pack to help reduce the immediate swelling. In an emergency, I use a bag of frozen peas, wrapped in a towel and placed directly over the swelling for 10 minutes every hour.

BURNS, MINOR

First-degree burns affect the very top layer of the skin. Second-degree burns leave blisters but usually heal without scarring or infection. Third-degree burns are far more serious and affect the full thickness of the skin, leaving it charred or white. These burns need urgent medical attention to reduce the risk of infection and scarring. Also, if you come into contact with acid, solvents or chemicals that burn the skin, as quickly as possible dowse the area with running cool water to lessen the damage. If a child drinks any chemical such as bleach that burns the oesophagus, do not encourage vomiting as it will also burn on its way back up. If possible allow the patient to drink milk and seek **immediate** medical help.

b

Foods to Avoid
- Avoid too many foods and drinks containing sugar or alcohol, as they will slow the healing process.
- Generally, avoid highly processed, refined foods, which contain almost no nutrients.

Friendly Foods
- High-quality protein is vital in the initial stages for tissue healing. Include plenty of organic free-range chicken, fresh fish, beans and lentils or even a good-quality whey protein powder (such as Solgar's Whey To Go) in your diet, which is a very digestible form of protein that will help to speed skin-healing. Or ask for a whey powder that includes extra L-glutamine an amino acid that will also help with tissue healing.
- Unprocessed, preferably organic nuts and seeds, such as sunflower and pumpkin seeds, are rich in essential fats and zinc, which are vital for healing the skin.
- Wheat germ and wheat germ oil are rich in vitamin E, which aids skin-healing and reduces scarring.
- Eat plenty of fresh fruits and veg high in natural carotenes to help heal the skin such as apricots, sweet potatoes, spinach. Cantaloupe melons, carrots and green leafy vegetables are good too.

Useful Remedies
- The herb gotu kola has been used to aid healing of burns for centuries. You can either take 500mg daily or take 1–2ml of tincture.
- Take natural-source vitamin E; 500iu twice a day until the wound heals.
- Vitamin C is vital for the production of collagen, take up to 3 grams daily with food – buy a formula that also contains bioflavonoids.
- Also take a good-quality vitamin and mineral supplement that contains 30–60mg of zinc, which

aids skin-healing and boosts immune function. See details of Kudos 24 in *General Supplements*.

■ MSM (organic sulphur) encourages wound healing and is anti-inflammatory – take up to 400mg three times daily.

Helpful Hints

■ You can bathe the burn in cold water for up to 30 minutes, if necessary. Dry with a clean sterile dressing and smother with sterile aloe vera gel.

■ Try Dr Christopher's Burn Paste. This consists of a mixture of runny honey, preferably Manuka, and wheat germ oil (which you buy and mix for yourself), to which you add comfrey root powder. When spread on the skin this really aids to speed the healing process. **SHS** (for the comfrey powder).

■ Take Bach Homeopathic Rescue Remedy every few hours to reduce the feelings of shock.

■ Cover the area with a thin layer of Manuka honey and cover with a sterile gauze. Honey is a very effective antiseptic, is anti-bacterial and can also speed the healing process. You can now buy Manuka dressings from large pharmacies – made by Comvita.

■ In India, fresh potato peelings are placed on burns. The wounds heal more quickly and infection is reduced.

■ Papaya pulp has been shown to be effective in sloughing off dead tissue, preventing wound infection. Papaya is rich in enzymes that aid healing.

■ Calendula cream helps to soothe the pain and promote tissue repair.

■ Lavender oil helps to aid burn healing.

■ Homeopathic Cantharis 6x, taken two or three times daily, will help to reduce the blisters.

■ Aloe vera gel or calendula cream can be applied topically.

■ MSM cream (organic sulphur cream) containing vitamin A and E, B5, aloe vera and comfrey extract, can be applied topically to aid healing of minor burns. **HN**

BURSITIS

This is also commonly known as tennis elbow or housemaid's knee and is an inflammation of the bursa, the sac-like membrane containing the fluids responsible for lubricating the joints. It is most common in the shoulder, elbow, hip and knees and can cause severe pain or tenderness, particularly when the person places any weight on that joint. Orthodox medicine offers anti-inflammatory drugs and sometimes cortisone injections. My husband has suffered tennis elbow, which was triggered by too much weight lifting, and after the injections he found great relief – but within 3–4 months, the pain and tenderness returned and was even worse than before. He has found some relief by resting his elbow completely and when he is under less stress or on holiday the pain recedes.

Foods to Avoid

■ Reduce your intake of caffeine and alcohol, which can increase inflammation within the body.

■ Cut down on animal-based foods and junk-type meals, which are very acid-forming.

■ Avoid plums, rhubarb, prunes, and orange juice, which are acid-forming.

Friendly Foods

■ Eat more foods that re-alkalise the body such as fresh vegetables – the greener the better. See *Acid–Alkaline Balance*.

■ Include plenty of fresh fruits in the diet.

■ Millet and buckwheat are alkaline foods – sprinkle the fine grains over a low-sugar breakfast cereal or use for baking.

- Eat more fresh ginger and oily fish, which have anti-inflammatory properties.
- Use turmeric and cayenne pepper in meals as they have anti-inflammatory properties.
- See also *General Health Hints*.

Useful Remedies

- Take 1–3 grams of vitamin C with bioflavonoids daily until symptoms ease.
- Fish oils have anti-inflammatory properties: take 1–3 grams a day of fish oils that contain EPA and DHA, which are key essential omega-3 fatty acids.
- Take 1,000–4,000mcu of the enzyme bromelain, extracted from pineapple, for its anti-inflammatory properties.
- Boswelia Complex contains the herbs ginger, boswelia, curcumin, which all have anti-inflammatory properties. Take up to 4 tablets daily. **FSC**
- Glucosamine sulphate, an amino sugar with MSM (an organic form of sulphur), helps to restore the gelatinous fluids around the joints. Take 1500–2000mg daily and once symptoms are alleviated reduce to 500mg daily. If you are allergic to shellfish, ask for the vegetarian version by Health Perception, available from all health stores.
- Manganese; 10mg daily helps to speed up tendon repair and ease pain.

Helpful Hints

- N Acetyl glucosamine gel with cayenne pepper applied locally can help ease the inflammation. From Health Perception or **FSC**.
- Apply a bag of frozen peas wrapped in a tea towel to ice the painful area for 10 minutes every few hours. This really does help to reduce inflammation and pain. You can alternate the cold compress with a warm ginger compress – simply add a piece of root ginger to boiling water. Let it steep for 10 minutes, soak a cloth in this mixture and press on the painful area for 10 minutes. Make the compress as warm as possible without burning yourself! Otherwise use a warmed wheat or lavender bag.
- Use an elasticated bandage during the day to limit swelling. Elevate the affected area above the level of the heart to encourage drainage of fluids out of the injured area.
- Avoid weight-training when pain is acute, as this will further aggravate the problem.
- Acupuncture works really well for this condition.
- Gentle aromatherapy massage using oils such as Roman camomile, ginger, marjoram and geranium can also help to relieve the pain.
- Ask at a local sports shop or good chemist for a magnet pad to wear around the affected area. Magnets help increase circulation, which brings more oxygen to the area and thus speeds healing.
- Check out www.repetiveusetherapy.com – this site gives some great tips and exercises that really help these types of problems.

b

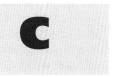

CANCER

(see also *Breast Cancer*)

Although cancer can strike at any age, the great majority of cancer patients are 70 and over. Current figures show that almost 1 in every 2 men and 1 in 3 women will contract a type of cancer at some point in their lives. Cancer remains the biggest killer in the Western world, ending the lives of over 6.5 million people annually – that's one in every four people. But there are plenty of things you can do to reduce your risk, and if you contract cancer, to help yourself. Without doubt, prevention is preferable to cure.

Newer screening methods and earlier diagnoses have meant that surviving cancer (which technically means surviving for 5 years after diagnosis) is becoming far more commonplace. Thousands of people recover every year and there is always hope.

There are more than 200 types of cancer, but the biggest 4 killers are lung, breast, bowel and prostate. It is now known that many cancers are triggered by environmental factors including excess free radicals, radiation, viral infections and chemicals.

Free radicals are unstable molecules that are formed within the body during normal metabolic processes, though more are produced by stress, excessive exercise, pollution, fried food, radiation and so on. Known risk factors for cancer are diets that are high in saturated fats, sunbathing to excess, exposure to toxic chemicals found in burnt food, petrol fumes, pesticides, preservatives, excessive hormones, multiple nutrient deficiencies, and over-exposure to certain electromagnetic fields (see *Electrical Pollution*).

And just because a family member died of cancer and you can indeed inherit a tendency towards certain cancers, you still can change which genes are expressed by stacking the odds more in your favour – by eating a better diet and living a different lifestyle. Eating healthily, staying physically active and maintaining a healthy weight, can cut your cancer risk by 40–90%, depending on whom you listen to. Various cancers have been linked to over-consumption of specific foods; for example, people who regularly consume overly processed foods such as hot dogs and mass-produced burgers are more likely to develop bowel cancer. And excessive intake of dietary animal based fats results in higher levels of oestrogens, a known risk factor for cancers especially of the breast and ovaries.

Emotions affect our health too and tragic stories of people who suffer a major shock in life like the loss of a partner through death or divorce, and develop cancer within a few years, are common. My mother was angry and bitter after my father died aged only 50 from a heart attack. In later life she developed a cancer that killed her, and I firmly believe it was her overall attitude to life that eventually caused her death. Hence I believe that healing emotional scars as well as physical ones is crucial to our long-term health.

There are always exceptions. Some people eat healthily, exercise and really take care of themselves, but still develop cancer. Others smoke until they are almost 100 and are fine. We all carry within us our own genetic strengths and weaknesses, and if our genetic ability to adapt is exceeded by our diet, lifestyle, pollution overload and so on, then naturally occurring genetic errors can accumulate and overwhelm our body's ability to correct the damage.

The orthodox approaches to cancer treatment mainly rely on surgery (cut it out), chemotherapy (drug it out) and radiotherapy (burn it out). Unfortunately these approaches place a considerable additional burden on our bodies and often have negative side effects.

However, the picture has begun to improve. Dr Keith Scott-Mumby, a nutritional physician based in California says "At last there have been attempts to try and understand the mechanics of the life process, and tumour growth in particular, and how nature's wisdom can be harnessed to our advantage. One such idea has been to bond the damaging chemo-substance onto some inactive carrier that makes it harmless to the ordinary cells. But by using cancer cell antibodies (your natural immune response to cancer cells), the chemo-substance is delivered and released ONLY in the tumour, which is where it is needed. It's like addressing a parcel bomb to the exact house you want to demolish, leaving the rest of the street intact. An even simpler idea is to set the 'bomb' to go off when oxygen levels drop, because cancer cells don't like oxygen and live only where there is less of it. Another idea has been to use the antibody weapon to trick the tumour into taking up a substance, which sensitises the cancer cells to light and then shining lasers on the tumour. As before, the ordinary cells are left unharmed. And these treatments are now coming on line."

"Meanwhile, don't leave everything to medical 'experts'. There are many steps that you can take, if you are to have the best chance of surviving the crisis and going on to enjoy a happy, productive life. Make no mistake, all cancers are a challenge, and surviving and thriving after cancer can mean that healing yourself becomes a full-time occupation. So a holistic strategy should include elements such as detoxification, an optimum diet, nutritional supplements, specific anti-cancer remedies, and mental, emotional and spiritual healing."

Dr Scott-Mumby adds, "The single most important thing you can do that offers you the best chance of avoiding or beating cancer is to eat a healthier diet – starting NOW. According to The World Cancer Research Fund (WCRF), eating at least 5 portions of vegetables and fruits each day could, in itself, reduce cancer rates by 20%. The WCRF asserts that half of all breast cancer cases, 3 out of 4 cases of stomach cancer and 3 out of 4 cases of colon cancer could be prevented by dietary measures alone. It must be your choice whether you go the natural route, the conventional route, or to try a combination of both. There are no guaranteed results; but the more right actions you take, the more positive re-actions you are likely to see."

Foods to Avoid
- All non-organic meat. If you want to eat red meat then have no more than 3–4oz (75–100g) twice weekly.
- Reduce or eliminate all dairy produce, especially from cows. If you do eat dairy, make it organic and low-fat.
- Eliminate white flour, rice and pasta.
- Limit your alcohol intake, to say, one glass of organic red wine a day.
- Sugar, coffee, sodium-based salt, and any pre-packaged, tinned and mass-produced foods, such as burgers or take-aways. Especially reduce sugar, as cancer cells feed on sugar.
- Don't re-heat pre-prepared foods in plastic containers, as the plastics they release into your food can have a negative effect on your hormones.
- Avoid fried, burnt or smoked foods. This is a good way to cut down on your exposure to free radicals.
- Reduce your use of sodium-based table salts, use an organic sea salt and add a little to the food on your plate (see *Anti-cancer Diet* below).

Friendly Foods – Anti-cancer Diet
- Eat more organic foods and if you have cancer *only* eat organic. This is because many non-organic foods contain up to 11 pesticides that are either carcinogens or hormone-disrupters. They are allowed on food only because the levels are very low – and no negative effect is

expected. This might seem reasonable accept that we do not know of their accumulative cocktail effect.

- Eat more pineapple and papaya, they contain the enzymes bromelain and papain. These enzymes help dissolve away the protective protein coating that surrounds most cancer cells.

- Most anti-cancer diets recommend juicing, but the pulp contains healthy phospholipids, which are essential for healthy tissues. Therefore chop all the ingredients and blend, or if you have a juicer, then scrape out the pulp and add this to your juice mix; it will be thicker, but healthier.

- For cancer prevention eat soya in its traditional, fermented form – such as tofu or miso – and the soya is best cooked. Soya contains anti-cancer compounds. A healthy amount is around 2–4oz (50–100g) of fermented soya in total a day. Soya is without doubt beneficial to adults but it should not be given to small infants and children. Infant soya milk formulas give the infant a daily dose of phytoestogens, which helps to protect adults against cancer, but for infants the levels are too high. The obvious first choice is to breast-feed infants for the first year. Soya lecithin granules are also a great food for adults, as lecithin lowers LDL (the bad cholesterol), improves memory and helps protect against many cancers.

- Eat more organic Brussels sprouts, cauliflower, cabbage, spring greens, kale and garlic, which all help to fight cancer. A great quick anti-cancer soup includes: 2 carrots, 2 heads of broccoli, half a pack of tempeh, a tablespoon of vegetable stock and some water in the blender for a delicious immune boosting soup. Add almond milk if you want it creamy, and spices such as curcumin if you like it hot. Heat and serve.

- Drink plenty of filtered water, which helps to wash out toxins from the kidneys. Use reverse osmosis or distilled water, as the last thing you need is any fluoride. Look at www.purewater.co.uk

- Boil, steam or bake, eating most of your food raw or lightly cooked. Try 'steam-frying' food using a watered down soya sauce, plus herbs or spices for taste. Barbecued and char-grilled foods, especially if fatty, are also best avoided because they contain relatively high concentrations of cancer-causing substances called carcinogens.

- Non-organic carrots, lettuce and many other healthy foods are overloaded with pesticides and herbicides that are associated with an increased risk of cancer. Throw away the outer leaves when preparing non-organic vegetables like cabbage or lettuce and always wash these vegetables thoroughly.

- Just one serving of crisp or raw cabbage each week can help reduce the risk of colon cancer by as much as 50%. Make more coleslaw: grate raw cabbage, carrot, apple, and add a few raisins, pumpkin seeds and a small amount of low-fat mayonnaise.

- Eat at least 5 pieces of fresh whole fruit a day. Vitamin C and natural beta-carotene and lycopene are potent anti-cancer nutrients. Lycopene is a carotenoid found in tomatoes which has been shown to reduce the risk of many cancers, especially prostate cancer but also reduced the risk of cancers in the colon, rectum, pancreas, throat, mouth, breast and cervix. If you are not allergic to tomatoes eat 6–10 servings weekly. When the tomatoes are heated in a little olive oil more lycopene is released. Otherwise guava or pink grapefruit contain plenty of lycopene.

- All foods that are rich in carotenes help reduce the risk of cancer. These include carrots, apricots, cantaloupe melons, asparagus, sweet potatoes, parsley, mustard and cress, red peppers, spinach, spring greens, watercress, raw mangoes, French beans and tomatoes.

- To ingest highly absorbable nutrients quickly, place a selection of your favourite fruits into a blender with a tablespoon of organic green food powder (see *General Supplements*) a dessertspoon each of mixed seeds: sunflower, sesame, linseed (flax seed) and pumpkin, adjust the amount for your personal choice – and whiz with a cup of organic rice or almond milk. If you are undergoing chemotherapy or radio therapy add at least a tablespoon of pure whey powder to this mix. Whey is a highly absorbable form of protein containing the amino acid L-Glutamine, which helps to soothe an irritated gut. As weight loss is often a problem with cancer, whey is a very useful food. I use Slogar's Whey to Go. I drink this blend every day either for breakfast or as a meal replacement at supper. My favourite blend is blueberries, apple, a slice of pineapple and a banana. To ring the changes I add a pear or strawberries to the blend. It's delicious.

■ Strict vegetarians seem to develop fewer cancers than non-vegetarians as proteins feed cancer cells. People who live in Thailand and Japan have much lower incidence of most cancers so adopting a Far Eastern diet may well be a good way of staying healthy – fewer refined foods, less meat and more fish.

■ Drink more organic green tea, it contains powerful antioxidant polyphenols that have been investigated for their cancer-protective effects and found to be even more powerful than vitamins C and E. It is believed green tea consumption, on average 3 cups a day, may be another reason behind the relatively low rate of cancer in Japan. Otherwise try white tea, a variant of green tea from the plant, *Camellia sinensis*. Clipper Teas make several varieties.

■ Eat whole foods, unprocessed nuts, beans and seeds. Anything in its whole form, such as oats, brown rice, lentils, almonds or sunflower seeds are high in the anti-cancer minerals zinc and selenium. Buy a pack each of sunflower seeds, pumpkin seeds, sesame seeds, hazelnuts, Brazil nuts, almonds, walnuts and linseeds (flax seeds), whiz a tablespoon of each at a time in a blender and keep in a jar in the fridge. Sprinkle daily over fruits, cereals, soups and desserts.

■ Whole grains, such as brown rice, contain substances called phytates, which offer some protection against cancer. They are now available as an isolated substance called Inositol Hexaphosphate or IP6, which is extracted from brown rice. **NC**

■ If you eat bran to keep your bowels regular, avoid wheat bran, which can irritate the gut. Try oat or rice bran instead.

■ Minimise alcohol. Alcohol is associated with an increased risk of cancer. Red wine does however contain antioxidant nutrients called polyphenols, which are associated with a reduced risk of heart disease. One glass a day is the recommended maximum. Red grape juice contains the same antioxidants without the alcohol.

■ Animal fats are a major contributing factor in cancers; greatly reduce your intake of saturated fats from meat, full-fat dairy produce, chocolates, cheeses, sausages, meat pies, cakes and so on. Avoid any foods containing hydrogenated or trans fats. Once you start reading labels you will be appalled at how much saturated fat you are ingesting. Never fry with mass-produced, highly refined oils. Use only organic sunflower, sesame, walnut or olive oils for salad dressings. Eat more oily fish, which are rich in omega-3 fats, especially sardines, salmon, mackerel, herring and fresh tuna (see *Fats You Need To Eat*).

■ Cut down on stimulants like sugar and caffeine. Sugar has been shown to lower your immune function for up to 5 hours after consuming it.

■ The World Cancer Research Fund offers an online library of healthy recipes. Have a look at www.wcrf-uk.org

Useful Remedies

■ WFK1 – is a high dilution Quinone, (which is similar to, but more powerful than, the vitamin-like substance Co-enzyme Q10 that the body makes naturally). This liquid form is made in the laboratory and it helps to normalise the metabolism of aberrant cells bringing them back to their normal oxygen-breathing pathway. Quinone helps repair cancer cells rather than killing them. This is an exciting breakthrough in the way cancer may be treated in the future. For details log onto www.cogreslab.co.uk; or Tel: 01495 752122. In 2003 the *British Journal of Cancer* published a study of 66 patients with colorectal cancer treated with this Quinone – and the treated patients started to recover with virtually no (metastasis) secondaries. Quinone can be taken alongside orthodox treatments and in Hungary this has been granted Government approval as an adjuvant alongside chemotherapy.

- Some cancer specialists state that vitamins and minerals can prevent the orthodox treatments from working, but numerous studies show that the right nutrients support your immune system and help fight the cancer.
- IP6 a substance extracted from brown rice has been shown to inhibit the growth of certain cancers. There is 20 years medical research behind IP6 and trials to date have proven very exciting indeed. 6000mg (6 grams) daily, needs to be taken on an empty stomach 30 minutes before food. **NC**
- Vitamin C, 3 or more grams a day in an ascorbate (non-acidic) form.
- MGN-3 is a blend of the outer shell of rice bran with extracts of shiitake, kawaratake, and sue-hirotake mushrooms. These 3 mushroom extracts are the leading prescription treatments for cancer in Japan. They increase Natural Killer (NK) cell activity. It is the activity of NK cells that determine whether you get cancer or a virus infection, rather than their number. In one study of 27 cancer patients, the NK activity increased from 100% to 537%, depending upon the kind of cancer, in only 2 weeks. If you have cancer, take 4 capsules 3 times daily with meals for 2 weeks, then 2 capsules twice daily for maintenance. Two capsules twice daily may be taken for prevention. **NC**
- Maitake mushrooms available in capsule form have been shown to stimulate the immune system and seem to reduce the effects of chemotherapy.
- Selenium x 200mcg daily.
- A high-potency multi-vitamin/mineral without iron, as iron has been linked to cancer cell growth – see details of Kudos 24 in *General Supplements* on p.160.
- Take 1200mcg of folic acid plus a daily B-complex, which helps to stabilise genes.
- Indole 3 Carbinol (I3C) is a phytochemical supplement isolated from cruciferous vegetables (broccoli, cauliflower, Brussels sprouts, turnips, kale, green cabbage, mustard, pak choy, and so on), which has been shown to inhibit the growth of oestrogen-receptor-positive cells, which are linked to hormonal type cancers. This supplement has huge anti-cancer potential. To ingest therapeutic quantities of indole would require eating enormous amounts of raw vegetables as cooking tends to destroy these phytochemicals. Take 250mg twice daily. Available from all good health stores. **NB: Pregnant women should not take this supplement as oestrogen is needed for healthy foetus growth.**
- The Organic Pharmacy make a liquid formula containing the herb astragalus (proven to help boost white blood cell count and help the body cope with chemo), cat's claw (anti-inflammatory and boosts natural killer cells), turmeric and shiitake (immune-boosting and antioxidant); 15 drops twice daily. **OP**

To Help Prevent Cancer

- Take IP6 – an extract of brown rice that has proven positive affects on cancers, most especially leukaemia – 2 grams can be taken daily on an empty stomach (if you think you're at high risk). **NC**
- Take a good-quality, high-strength multi-vitamin/mineral every day.
- Additionally, take a good, high-strength, antioxidant complex daily.
- 1 gram of vitamin C daily, more if you're stressed or ill.
- Take 200mcg selenium daily.
- Take 400iu of natural-source, full-spectrum vitamin E.
- Take alpha lipoic acid; 200mg daily.
- Also see details of MGN3 and I3C above.

Helpful Hints

- First, with professional help, detox your body. To find a qualified nutritionist see under *Useful Information* at the back of the book.
- If at all possible begin taking regular saunas as heat helps to eliminate toxins from the body. Don't use them if they are packed with too many other people, as you may pick up other people's toxins. Ask if you can have the sauna on a lower heat (120–140°C) and then you can stay in for a few minutes longer.
- Minimise your exposure to pollution. Remember, anything that is combusted produces free radicals, so reduce your exposure to car exhaust fumes. Electrical pollutants can also cause problems, only use mobile phones for 10–15 minutes at a time at most. Reduce your exposure to other electrical pollutants: microwaves, TVs etc, and don't sleep with an electric clock by your bed (see *Electrical Pollution*).
- Never use chemical pesticides and herbicides in your garden and home. Ask for environmentally friendly natural products. Greatly reduce or eliminate your exposure to non-organic foods, cleaning fluids, garden sprays, insect sprays.
- If you smoke give it up and stay away from smoke-filled rooms, as passive smoking has now been shown to trigger cancer.
- Type A blood-types and ABs need to be more careful with their diets as their blood has a tendency to become sticky and therefore it is very important to ensure that their livers are kept clean (see *Liver Problems*).
- If you consult a naturopath who uses a dark field microscope, they can tell a lot about your blood regarding cancer. Contact The Association of Naturopathic Practitioners via www.naturopathy-anp.com. I see a brilliant naturopath Bob Jacobs at The Society for Complementary Medicine in London who uses a dark field microscope – which can see details that are not normally found in blood tests. Bob's office is on 020 7487 4334.
- Curcumin, found in turmeric, used in most curries and Eastern dishes is a great anti-cancer spice. It enhances immune function and helps inhibit new blood vessel growth that occurs as tumours grow. It is especially useful for skin cancers, liver and colon cancers. It also helps remove toxic metals from the body and helps block pesticide type pollutants from entering cells. Add to your diet. It can be found in capsule form in most health shops. If you are undergoing chemotherapy, make sure that you check with your GP before taking high dosages of this spice.
- If you are already undergoing any type of cancer therapy, Dr Rosy Daniel (the former Medical Director of the Bristol Cancer Help Centre) says that nutrition is vital to help bring back up the white blood cell count. She advises patients to eat plenty of organic fresh fruit and vegetables along with whole foods like brown rice and brown bread. All animal fats should be avoided. She also recommends that cancer patients take a good antioxidant formula, which contains vitamins A, C and E, plus natural beta-carotene complex, and zinc and selenium. Dr Daniel stresses that fear drains energy levels and advocates any therapy that can reduce anxiety, such as spiritual healing, Reiki, relaxation exercises, visualisation, acupuncture or homeopathy. Dr Daniel has written a wonderful book called *Living With Cancer*, available from the Centre 0117 980 9500 for £7.99 (Constable Robinson).
- Contact the charity Killing Cancer run by David Longman, which focuses on informing cancer patients about the alternatives to chemo- and radiotherapy – using Photo Dynamic Therapy (PDT), which eliminates the need in some cases for any radical intervention and drugs. Well worth looking at their site at www.killingcancer.co.uk
- Laugh a lot. Watch films and programmes that make you laugh; laughter boosts your immune system. Stay as positive as possible, without doubt the patients with the more positive outlook

heal and recover more quickly. This does not mean that you cannot shed tears, as tears release stress chemicals, and you are not meant to be a positive saint all the time! An inspiring book that uses this theme is *Love, Medicine and Healing* by Bernie Siegal (Rider).

■ Oxygen Therapies are well worth looking into. Dr Otto Warburg in the US won a Nobel Prize for Medical Research for discovering that if the body has sufficient oxygen then cancer cells cannot proliferate. You can use an ozone cabinet and some doctors are working with hydrogen peroxide injections (for details see under MRSA). Many therapists who offer these treatments have been harassed by various government bodies. I can only surmise that some people would prefer people not to know that there is an inexpensive non-drug based treatment that really does help. Mark Lester in London uses an ozone cabinet and therapies to treat patients. He also uses oxygen supplements to great effect. Tel: 020 8349 4730 or log on to www.thefinchley-clinic.com

■ For further information I suggest you read *Oxygen Healing Therapies* by Nathanial Altman (Healing Arts Press), or *Flood Your Body with Oxygen* by Ed McCabe (Energy Publications). Both are available from Mark Lester as above.

■ At the Hospital Santa Monica in Mexico, Dr Kurt Donsbach has used intravenous hydrogen peroxide for years. For details log on to www.cancure.org/donsbach_clinic.htm.

■ In the UK some of these therapies (as well as high dose intravenous nutrients such as vitamin C) are used by Dr Patrick Kingsley in Leicestershire on 01530 223 622; Dr Fritz Schellander in Tunbridge Wells on 01892 543 535; Dr Wendy Denning in London on 020 7224 2423; or Dr Robert Trossell at 4 Duke Street, London W1U 3EL on 020 7486 1095.

■ Many associations offer help, counselling and advice. One of the best is The Penny Brohn Cancer Care (formerly the Bristol Cancer Help Centre), Chapel Pill Lane, Pill, Bristol BS20 0HH. Helpline: 0845 123 2310, Email: helpline@pennybrohn.org, Website: www.pennybrohncancercare.org

■ Read Patrick Holford's *Say No to Cancer* (Piatkus). If you've realised you need to fully educate yourself about cancer and how to avoid it, this book is a great place to start. Or log on to www.patrickholford.com. There are hundreds of excellent books on cancer – for more details call the Nutri Centre Bookshop on 020 7323 2382.

CANDIDA

(see also *Allergies, Antibiotics* and *Thrush*)

Candida albicans is a yeast that is responsible for the condition known as thrush. Common symptoms include itching in the vaginal area, odour and discharge. Doctors estimate that at least 75% of women will experience it at some time in their lives. Although commonly found in the vagina, candida can also occur in the throat, mouth and gut. Normally, relatively low levels of candida are present in the gut as they are balanced by large amounts of healthy bacteria, which helps to keep the yeast in check. Problems arise when the yeast begins to overgrow in the gut. This ultimately triggers a variety of symptoms including bloating, wind, constipation/and or diarrhoea, food cravings (especially for sugar and wheat-based foods), headaches, mental confusion, mood swings, skin rashes, persistent coughing, regular bouts of thrush, arthritis-type aching joints and chronic fatigue. Candida can change its form and burrow through and irritate the gut lining, which increases the risk of food sensitivities and an exacerbation of the symptoms above (see *Leaky Gut*).

It is crucial to kill the candida or keep it under control by using herbs, supplements and, most importantly, dietary changes. One of the primary triggers for candida is overuse of antibiotics, others are long-term use of the Pill, and steroids, chemotherapy, diabetes, HIV and pregnancy.

Many women believe that you cannot have candida if you don't have thrush, but the majority of women with candida do not have thrush. Men are also sufferers. Dr Gwynne Davies, a clinical ecologist based in the UK, an expert on candida says, "Candida now affects up to 75% of the population. It can become a serious condition if left untreated and is little understood by many doctors." He is right. During my teens I was given dozens of antibiotics for my acne, thrush and ear infections. Every time the thrush returned, I would be given more antibiotics, which in the long run made the vicious cycle worse. I strongly advise that anyone testing positive for high levels of candida should consult a doctor who is also a nutritionist (See *Useful Information*).

Foods to Avoid

- Initially remove all yeast and fermented food from the diet – this includes breads, all aged or mouldy cheeses including Stilton, Brie, Camembert and so on. Alcoholic drinks – especially beer and wine, ginger beer, vinegar and foods containing vinegar (ketchups, pickles, salad cream, baked beans), soya sauce, gravy mixes (many contain brewer's yeast), miso, tempeh and mushrooms.
- I know it's hard, but try and avoid all white-flour products for at least one month, including crackers, pizza and pasta.
- Sugar feeds the yeast – so for a month avoid sugar in any form including honey, maltose, dextrose or sucrose and really sweet fruits such as grapes, peaches, kiwi and melon. I know it will be hard as sugar is highly addictive but you also need to avoid dried fruits, fruit juices and canned drinks for this period as they are high in sugar. Artificial sugars such as aspartame should also be eliminated.
- Avoid malted products – found in some breakfast cereals, brown Ryvita and malted drinks like Ovaltine and Horlicks.
- Avoid peanuts and peanut butter which tend to harbour moulds.
- Avoid cow's milk for 1 month.
- If you have really severe candida, for the first two weeks also avoid courgettes, carrots, corn, and any of the squash family as they quickly convert to sugars in the gut.
- Avoid any foods you know you are intolerant to.

Friendly Foods

- Garlic has potent anti-fungal action; raw is best. If you're worried about your breath, chew on some parsley.
- Eat fresh fish and shellfish, chicken, turkey and lean meats, eggs, cooked tofu and pulses.
- Research shows that a candida infection leads to inflammation – to help combat this eat more oily fish: salmon, mackerel, herring, anchovies and fresh tuna, along with nuts (unsalted and not peanuts) and lots of organic, unrefined seeds, which are also rich in essential fats.
- Include more artichokes, asparagus, aubergine, avocado, broccoli, cabbage, cauliflower, Brussels sprouts, celery, green beans, leeks, lettuce, garlic, onion, parsnips, spinach, tomatoes and watercress. Fruits that I found OK during my detox were apples, pears (not over-ripe), raspberries, blueberries, bilberries and cherries. Papaya is good too, if not too over-ripe.
- Use a **low-sugar**, organic rice or soya milk instead of cow's milk.
- Eat live, plain unsweetened yoghurt, which contains the healthy bacteria acidophilus and bifidus.
- Brown rice, lentils, corn, millet, buckwheat or rice pasta, oat cakes, soda bread, scones made with a little butter are all OK. As a wheat substitute, try yeast-free rye bread. It can take some getting used to but for a month it's acceptable.
- Coriander is a great herb for helping control this infection, so use liberally in soups and stews.

Useful Remedies

- Bio-acidophilus forte (healthy bacteria) will help replenish gut flora; begin by taking 1 daily and after 2 weeks increase to 2 daily for a further 6 weeks. **BC**
- Take 1 yeast-free B complex.
- Take a good multi-vitamin and mineral (see Kudos 24 in *General Supplements*; p.160). **KVH**
- Take AD 206, containing ginseng and pantothenic acid, to support adrenal function, which is often exhausted in candida patients. **BC**
- To help cleanse the liver, take 1 HEP 194 and 1 gram of vitamin C. **BC**
- Take a good digestive enzyme. Such as Polyzyme Forte with main meals. **BC**
- Floraguard is a duo-pill that combines anti-fungals such as oil of oregano (which is 100 times more potent than the commonly used caprlyic acid) on the outside with good bacteria on the inside. Research has shown it to be effective against a huge range of yeasts and parasites. Do not use this if you suffer from ulcers. **BC**
- Take 1 pau d'arco plus a formula made specially to help eliminate the fungus. **BC**
- Take black walnut, pau d'arco and calendula tincture, 2–4ml twice a day. **FSC**
- Glutamine is great for healing and calming an irritated and inflamed gut. Take up to 5 grams twice a day half an hour before food. **HN**
- I realise I have suggested numerous supplements here – there is certainly no need to take them all, I am simply giving you plenty of choices!

Helpful Hints

- Follow the yeast-free diet for 2–4 weeks before you add in any anti-fungal supplements or you may kill off the candida quicker than your body can dispose of it – this could lead to a general feeling of malaise. Should this happen at any time drink more fluids, up your vitamin C and reduce your anti-fungals for a day or two.
- If indigestion and bloating are a problem and digestive enzymes do not help, you may still be low in stomach acid – see *Indigestion* and *Low Stomach Acid*.
- As candida is usually linked to multiple food intolerances, consider a food intolerance test. Contact Individual Wellbeing Laboratories. Tel. 020 8336 7750; or check out www.iwdl.net
- A comprehensive stool test and parasitology can also check for evidence of candida (plus other yeasts) in your body in addition to parasites and your levels of good bacteria. Check out www.smartnutrition.co.uk. Tel: 01273 737000 for details about the test.
- Many women who suffer candida are very stressed and exhausted – the best thing you can do to help boost immune function is to go away for at least a week.
- Avoid compost heaps, cut grass and staying too long in moist, humid atmospheres where moulds can thrive.
- Women who wear nylon underwear are twice as likely to suffer with thrush as those who wear cotton underwear.
- Bubblebath can aggravate any thrush so is best avoided. A better choice is to add a few drops of tea tree essential oil to your bathwater. It has powerful anti-fungal and antiseptic properties. **NB: do not use neat.**
- For further help contact the National Candida Society, PO Box 151, Orpington, Kent BR5 1UJ. Tel: 01689 813039. Website: www.candida-society.org.uk – full of heaps of information. Email: info@candida-society.org.uk. Membership is £15 annually, and includes a helpline on Thursdays along with lots of extra support.
- Recent research indicates that people who have persistent and chronic candida may have intestinal parasites. Herbal combinations containing wormwood, tincture of black walnut hull and cloves, plus the amino acids ornithine and arginine help eliminate parasites. For details of this candida cleansing formula call G&G Food Supplies on 01342 312811. Email:

sales@gandgvitamins.com. Website: www.gandgvitamins.com
■ Read Erica White's *Beat Candida Cookbook* which has more than 250 recipes, many of these are quick and easy to prepare.

CARPAL TUNNEL SYNDROME (CTS)

Carpal tunnel is caused by the compression of the median nerve that runs under tissues in the wrist. People who use keyboards and other machinery on an everyday basis are the most frequent sufferers; symptoms range from pain to numbness or tingling in the fingers. CTS is relatively common in pregnancy and more women suffer than men, it is also linked to an underactive thyroid, weight gain and arthritis. The single most successful supplement for this condition is vitamin B6.

Foods to Avoid
■ Because this problem is often associated with fluid retention, avoid adding too much sodium-based salt to food. Use a little magnesium-based sea salt for cooking.
■ Reduce your intake of salty foods, such as crisps, pre-packaged meals, pies, soy sauce and so on.
■ Foods containing monosodium glutamate (MSG), often found in high amounts in Chinese take-aways and used in many Japanese restaurants, dehydrate the body. MSG depletes vitamin B6 from the body, as does the contraceptive pill.
■ In some people, foods such as oranges, tomatoes and wheat further exacerbate the problem.

Friendly Foods
■ Foods rich in vitamin B6: liver, cereals, lean meat, green vegetables, unrefined organic nuts – especially walnuts and Brazil nuts, fresh and dried fruits.
■ Eat more brown rice, beans, lentils, pulses, wholemeal pasta and breads.
■ Eat oily fish such as salmon, tuna, mackerel, herrings and sardines, which are rich in omega-3 fats that have anti-inflammatory properties.
■ Use unrefined linseed oil, rich in omega 6 fats, with organic extra virgin olive oil for salad dressings.
■ Eat pineapple before meals, which contains bromelain that helps to reduce inflammation.
■ Bilberries, cherries and blueberries are rich in bioflavonoids, which have anti-inflammatory properties.
■ Cook with more ginger, turmeric and cayenne.
■ Drink at least 8 glasses of water a day.
■ Drink more organic green tea.

Useful Remedies
■ Take B6, 100–400mg, plus a B-complex daily whilst symptoms are acute.
■ Take magnesium, 200–600mg, which nourishes nerve endings and relaxes muscles.
■ Take a good multi-vitamin and mineral (see Kudos 24 in *General Supplements*; p.160). **KVH**
■ Take 1–2 grams of evening primrose oil or 500mg of Mega GLA. **BC**
■ The herbs white willow bark and devil's claw are highly anti-inflammatory; 1–2 grams daily whilst symptoms are acute. **NB: if you are allergic to aspirin do not take this supplement.**

Helpful Hints
■ Glucosamine gel applied topically can help reduce the inflammation.
■ If you are a regular computer user, try to find an ergonomic keyboard, which will be easier to use.

C

- If symptoms are severe, buy a wrist splint containing magnets, which are available from good pharmacies and health stores.
- Sleeping heavily on your side, with your wrists under you, can also cause this. If you wake up with numb hands, immediately shake them and give them a massage to restore circulation.
- Acupuncture and daily massage with homeopathic Rhus tox ointment are also helpful.
- Log onto www.repetitiveusetherapy.com, a really useful site with some great information, and good exercises to help alleviate this condition.

CATARACTS
(see also *Eye Problems*)

As we age, the normally clear and transparent lens of the eye oxidises to become cloudy, which can severely impair vision. Many people who live in the Tropics develop cataracts and they are a major cause of blindness in developing countries. Cataracts are becoming more common in the West in people who tend to take too much sun. A poor diet lacking in antioxidant nutrients, smoking, diabetes and overuse of steroids and other prescription drugs can all cause cataracts. As with so many other conditions, cataracts are much easier to prevent than to cure. Once you have cataracts, the normal approach is laser treatment, however, some individuals claim to have reversed their cataracts with a combination of herbs and nutrients.

Foods to Avoid

- Smoking, fried foods and sugar speed up the oxidation process and make cataracts more likely to develop.

Friendly Foods

- Bilberries, cherries and blueberries are very rich in bioflavonoids, which help protect the eyes.
- Leafy green vegetables, in particular spinach, contain lutein, the powerful antioxidant found in most green vegetables that has specific properties for protecting the eye.
- Sweet potatoes and butternut squash have high levels of carotenes, which convert to vitamin A within the body. Other good sources of carotenoids are carrots, green vegetables, tomatoes, apricots, cantaloupe melons and pumpkin.
- Include plenty of oily fish in your diet, which is rich in vitamin A.
- All foods high in vitamin C, E and selenium help to support the eyes. These include wheat germ, avocado, sprouting seeds such as alflafa, sunflower, pumpkin and linseeds, eggs, nuts, lean meats, wholegrain cereals and fresh fruits, especially cherries, kiwi fruit and green peppers.

Useful Remedies

- People who take vitamin C on a regular basis over a number of years are at a much lower risk of developing cataracts. Take 1 gram daily in an ascorbate form with food.
- People with low levels of vitamin E are nearly four times more likely to form cataracts, so take 400iu of natural source vitamin E a day included in a good-quality multi vitamin mineral, such as Kudos 24 (see *General Supplements*; p.160). **KVH**
- Take Bilberry Eye Formula 1–2 capsules a day. People who consume bilberry on a regular basis have a much lower risk of forming cataracts. **FSC**

Helpful Hints

- Anyone concerned about developing cataracts should protect their eyes from bright sunlight with sunglasses that have been verified for UV filtering ability. If you work outside, wear a hat to protect your eyes. UV filtering contact lenses are also available, ask your optician for details.

CATARRH

(see also *Allergic Rhinitis* and *Allergies*)

Catarrh, or chronic congestion, can be caused by an inflammatory response to airborne pollutants (from pesticides, paints, insect sprays, chemical based air fresheners etc) – and the inflammation can then be further aggravated by other substances such as grass pollens, house dust mite or cat fur, but in most cases it is triggered by foods that you eat on an everyday basis, such as cow's milk, wheat, cheese or chocolate. Many people assume that dairy products cause catarrh, but in reality this is only the case if you have an intolerance to these foods. Catarrh can just as easily be caused by wheat, eggs, citrus or any foods to which you have an intolerance. It is important to get to the root cause of the problem, so if you are suffering with a lot of catarrh look at the foods you eat daily. Cut out one food at a time and keep a diary of the results. After a few weeks it is usually easy to find the culprit (see also *Leaky Gut*).

Foods to Avoid
- Avoid any foods to which you have an allergy or intolerance. Typically this might include cow's milk and produce, especially full-fat cheeses, yoghurts and chocolate, plus caffeine, citrus fruits and juices, peanuts, wheat, and foods from the nightshade family which includes tomatoes, potatoes, aubergines and peppers.
- I personally also find that goat's cheese and too much soya milk or yoghurts tend to leave me feeling very 'bunged up'. Also avoid rich, creamy sauces.
- Avoid foods containing too much sugar, which weaken the immune system making you more susceptible to food intolerances. And most foods high in sugar are high in saturated fats.

Friendly Foods
- Garlic, ginger, horseradish, onion, cayenne pepper, pineapple and pears can help the body fight an infection if there is one and loosen up mucus so the body can expel it more easily.
- The herbs thyme, rosemary and fenugreek make great expectorants, which help relieve congestion. Either make a strong tea and drink, or add these herbs to foods.
- Eat plenty of whole grains such as brown rice, lentils, fruits, and fresh vegetables.
- When people go on a cleansing diet, the catarrh usually disappears.

Useful Remedies
- Take Garlic, Ginger and Horseradish Winter Formula, use 1ml of tincture 3–4 times a day. **FSC**
- New Era make tissue salts specifically for catarrh.
- Take Muccolyte, a complex containing bromelain, potassium plus vitamins A, C and D to help support the mucus membrane and loosening up existing mucus. **BC**
- Take 1 gram of vitamin C with added bioflavonoids daily with meals.
- Sinus and cattarh pills containing a homeopathic mixture of Kali Bich, Pulsatilla, Merc Sol, Thuja, Chamomilla, Hydrastis Canadensis 30 that help address infected green or yellow mucus are suitable and safe for babies and adults. Cough and Mucous tincture contains elecampane, coltsfoot, pulmonaria, liquorice, mullein and helps clear coughs and mucus (even stubborn ones). **OP**
- An excellent nasal spray is Weleda's Aloe Nasal Spray.

Helpful Hints
- Ask at your health store for a nasal spray such as Salcura – which really helps to clear the sinuses.
- Make a soup from 6 onions, a whole bulb of garlic, a small spoon of honey, 1in (2.5cm) of fresh root ginger and if you're brave a bit of cayenne pepper, in a vegetable or chicken stock. This will fight most infections and help clear catarrh.
- Invest in a humidifier/air filter or ioniser to help keep the air free of potential allergens.

- Many people have found that limeflower tea is useful for reducing catarrh.
- If your ears are blocked due to excess mucus, use warm 'hopi' ear candles, which gently remove excess wax and congestion. For details, call Revital Tel: 0800 252 875. Website: www.revital.com

CELLULITE

(see also *Circulation*)

Cellulite is suffered by nearly nine times as many women as men. This is partly due to the different structure of the skin, and the fact that women have more underlying fat. Cellulite is mainly due to water retention plus an accumulation of toxins in the body, which have weakened the connective tissue just below the surface of the skin. It is much less common in female athletes who have very low body fat.

Foods to Avoid
- High-fat foods, refined carbohydrates such as mass-produced cakes and biscuits plus meat pies and pastries.
- Foods with a high salt content such as tinned foods, pre-packaged foods and take-aways, which also tend to contain a lot of saturated fats.
- Also avoid too much coffee and alcohol, which place a strain on the liver, which is already struggling to deal with the toxins from your diet. The more you take care of your liver, the more your skin will improve. (See *Liver Problems*.)

Friendly Foods
- Eat plenty of complex carbohydrates like beans, lentils, fruits, vegetables, and brown rice. These foods help increase the rate of metabolism, making fat deposits less likely and increase elimination of toxins from the body.
- Make sure you drink plenty of water and add organic seeds like sunflower, pumpkin and linseed to fruits salads and cereals.
- Pectin in apples helps to absorb and eliminate toxins – eat an organic apple daily.

Useful Remedies
- The herb gotu kola is by far the best-researched and most successful remedy for cellulite when taken orally. Try 500mg 3 times a day for 2–3 months.
- A multi-vitamin and mineral daily.
- Horse chestnut cream, gel or lotion applied twice a day reduces some of the swelling and discomfort and helps to strengthen the connective tissues, which tend to be damaged when you have cellulite. Available from all good health stores.
- Cellulite tincture contains bladderwrack, alfalfa, horse chestnut, dandelion and gotu kola to improve micro circulation, elimination and oxygenation, as well as speeding up the metabolism. OP
- A formula which helps to clean the lymph is Essential De-Tox combination containing clivers, blue flag, burdock and yellow dock. For details log onto www.holoshealth.com

Helpful Hints
- Massage in any form is beneficial as it increases circulation and lymph drainage. If you are not able to treat yourself to a massage on a weekly basis, invest in a skin brush, which increases circulation and helps eliminate toxins from the body. Skin brushes are available from all health shops and the Body Shop.
- Detox body oil (juniper, rosemary, grapefruit and fennel) helps detoxify and firm the body by improving microcirculation, oxygenation and elimination. Juniper and fennel are natural

diuretics. Use with a skin brush every morning. **OP**
- Begin taking more exercise to encourage circulation and elimination of toxins. Rebounding on a mini-trampoline and yoga are great for reducing cellulite.
- If you need to lose weight do it gradually, as losing weight too quickly can make the appearance of cellulite much worse.
- Try the Lashford 7-day Detox (see *Allergies*).

CHILBLAINS
(see also *Circulation* and *Raynaud's Disease*)

Chilblains are caused by poor circulation and are characterised by red inflamed areas that affect the extremities. Chilblains can cause intense itching, swollen toes and sensitivity to heat and cold. Some unfortunate individuals suffer in both hands and feet. It is more common in cold weather, because the small blood vessels in the skin naturally constrict when it is cold. If you tend to suffer with chilblains every winter then you should improve your circulation. To prevent chilblains in the long term you should make sure your circulation is as efficient as possible.

Foods to Avoid
- Anything that worsens circulation – this inevitably means foods which tend to encourage hardening of the arteries such as animal fats, full-fat dairy produce, low-fibre foods such as ice cream, jelly, fatty puddings, chocolates and cakes. See diet in *Circulation*.

Friendly Foods

- Oily fish, cayenne pepper, garlic, onion, ginger, soluble fibre such as linseeds (flax seeds) plus oat and rice bran. All of these foods can help either to improve circulation or help reduce levels of LDL (the 'bad' cholesterol), which in the long-term will help your circulation. (See *Fats You Need to Eat* and *General Health Hints*.)

Useful Remedies
- Ginkgo biloba, 120mg of standardized extract twice a day or 1ml of tincture twice a day, increases circulation to all extremities.
- Vitamin E, 400iu a day, helps to thin the blood naturally.
- Take niacin (vitamin B3), 30mg–100mg daily, which pumps blood into the minor capillaries. But beware if you are taking niacin for the first time, only take 30mg and slowly increase to 100mg daily. Niacin causes a flushing sensation in the skin. This is simply blood moving into the small capillaries, but it can make you look like a freshly cooked lobster for a few moments. As all the B-vitamins work together, also take a B-complex.
- Udo's Choice Oil is a blend of omega-3 and -6 fats, which help to keep one's blood healthy. Use 1 dessertspoon a day over cooked food. To find your nearest stockist. Tel: 0845 0606070.
- Include a multi-vitamin and mineral in this regimen plus 1 gram of vitamin C with bioflavonoids, which helps to strengthen small capillaries.

Helpful Hints
- Smoking restricts circulation – so give it up.
- Have a regular massage or reflexology. Essential oils such as black pepper or rosemary (do not use black pepper undiluted) can be rubbed into your feet every morning to improve circulation.
- Regular exercise such as walking, rebounding and skipping all increase microcirculation.
- I used to suffer chilblains every winter, after having varicose veins removed years ago. The surgeon told me that I would still have plenty of veins left, but the legacy has been poor circulation. Obviously the key would have been for me to have avoided varicose veins in my

youth! Keep this in mind and wear bed socks during winter months.

- Never wear tight-fitting shoes as this really aggravates chilblains by restricting circulation to the toes. Invest in fur-lined boots during cold weather.
- Try massaging homeopathic *Tamus* cream into the chilblains. This cream is made from wild black bryony root, and has helped many people.
- Homeopathic Agaricus 3x or 6x can be taken 2 or 3 times daily. This is a classic homeopathic remedy for chilblains.
- Sixtuwohl Thermo Activ Anti Cold Foot Balm is based on Alpine herbs known to increase circulation. Available to order from JICA Beauty Products Ltd. Tel: 020 8979 7261. Website: www.jica.com
- Magnets increase circulation, which brings more oxygen to the affected areas. If like me you suffer cold feet, wear magnet insoles in your shoes and in the depths of winter wear bed socks with the inserts inside them. For details ask at your local health store or pharmacy or call John Bell & Croydon, a large pharmacist in London on 020 7935 5555.

CHOLESTEROL, HIGH AND LOW

(see also *Heart Disease* and *Strokes*)

Every year in Britain alone, more than 200,000 people die from a heart attack or stroke, and a high cholesterol count increases your chances of becoming one of these statistics by more than 60%. Cholesterol is a fatty substance manufactured by the liver and is a vital component of every cell.

There are two types of cholesterol HDL (high density lipoproteins) and LDL (low density lipoproteins). The HDLs are good for us – the easy way to remember this is H is for healthy. The LDLs are generally bad for us – L stands for lethal.

A high-LDL cholesterol level is one of the major risk factors for developing heart disease and stroke – whilst low cholesterol is associated with depression.

Ideally, 20%–40% of your total cholesterol should be HDL. There is also a type of cholesterol, VLDL (very low density lipoprotein), which is extremely bad for you. Ideally, your cholesterol reading should be between 3.0mmol/l and 5mmol/l. As soon as your cholesterol reading goes above 5.2 you are at a higher risk of contracting heart disease. If, on the other hand, your cholesterol reading is below 3.0, it tends to indicate that your liver is not functioning properly and there may be an underlying problem such as undiagnosed food intolerances. When cholesterol is high your liver is not breaking down the LDL cholesterol properly, so it is important to keep your liver as healthy as possible. Low cholesterol can also denote an imbalance in the liver.

Some families seem genetically predisposed to manufacture more cholesterol, which means that they need dietary cholesterol even less. Then there are people who seem to live on fatty foods and still maintain a normal cholesterol level. There are always exceptions. From a dietary point of view it is very important to reduce saturated fats and increase soluble fibres. The former tend to increase the levels of LDL cholesterol and the latter reduce them.

If you do have a high cholesterol level, two of the most important supplements you can take are vitamin E, which helps to prevent the cholesterol oxidising, and B-group vitamins including B12, B6, B3 and folic acid, all of which prevent the elevation of homocysteine levels (see below), which again tends to oxidise cholesterol and leads to plaque formation in the arteries. Thanks to eating too much animal fat many children in the West now have raised cholesterol and arterial plaque by the age of 10. But, while cholesterol levels have been used for many years as a possible way to predict our risk of heart attacks and strokes – it's only part of the story. Medical science is now beginning to re-think the role that cholesterol plays in heart disease and strokes.

Homocysteine levels are now also being recognized as an important indicator for heart disease and stroke. Homocysteine is a toxic amino acid produced during the metabolism of proteins and high levels are associated with an 80% increased risk for heart disease and strokes, even if you have a healthy cholesterol level. The good news is that there is now an easy way to test your own homocysteine levels (see *Helpful Hints*), and you can lower levels naturally, by simply taking more B vitamins (see under *Useful Remedies*). If your level of homocysteine is high and you are taking B-vitamins to lower it, retest your levels periodically to see if you are taking sufficient dosages.

High plasma levels of homocysteine cause damage to artery walls, then LDL cholesterol (the bad cholesterol) can easily stick to them – which triggers the cascade of events that leads to heart disease and strokes. It is also linked to numerous other age related conditions from Alzheimer's and diabetes, to obesity and mental health problems such as schizophrenia.

Another important indicator of heart-disease risk is the level of LDL cholesterol. An ideal level would be less than 2.6mmol/L. If your level is between 2.6 and 3.4mmol/L it is OK but a little high. If your level is 3.5 to 4.2 mmol/L, it is borderline high and between 4.21 and 4.89 is high. Levels of LDL cholesterol above 4.90 are too high and would need attention.

Cholesterol is not all bad! You need cholesterol for healthy cell membrane production and the manufacture of hormones. It is also needed to help in the synthesis of bile acids for the digestion of fats and for production of vitamin D. Low cholesterol levels are linked to depression and in rare cases suicide, hence why fat free diets are definitely not a good idea. For years we have been told to avoid certain foods, especially eggs, because they contain cholesterol. In fact, blood levels of LDL cholesterol, are more affected by eating too much fat and sugar, rather than foods like eggs which contain cholesterol (see Friendly Foods).

Eating too many barbecued or burnt foods, especially meat, hard margarines, fried foods and so on, causes cholesterol to oxidise which makes it more dangerous, and once oxidised it begins attaching itself to artery walls. And as we age cholesterol tends to oxidise at a faster rate, therefore the more antioxidants we eat, the less cholesterol oxidises, triggering health problems.

Around 20% of the body's total cholesterol is obtained from the diet, and the body manufactures the rest. Studies have shown that overweight people produce 20% more cholesterol than people of normal weight for their age, usually triggered by eating too much fat and sugar, stress and smoking. However, if you have a persistently raised cholesterol level but eat a healthy diet, you may have an under active thyroid. Also, people with blood type A are more susceptible to high total cholesterol.

Optimum liver function helps you to make more good cholesterol, therefore the more you look after your liver, the more likely you are to have a healthy level (see *Liver Problems*). About 1 person in 500 has a genetic predisposition to high blood cholesterol levels and even this can be helped through diet and taking the right supplements.

Foods to Avoid
- Cut down on your intake of animal fats and full fat dairy produce and eat more essential fats (for a full list see *Fats You Need To Eat*).
- Read labels – and as much as possible avoid mass-produced foods and oils that contain hydrogenated or trans-fats.
- Refined carbohydrates, white rice and pastas, processed white breads, cakes etc, can reduce the production of HDLs and white bread eaters usually have higher cholesterol levels than those

who eat mainly wholemeal varieties.

- Sugar, if not burnt for energy during exercise, converts to fat in the body and resides on your hips – and in the long run raises LDL cholesterol.
- Eggs contain cholesterol, but this is balanced by a high choline content (great for memory), which breaks down the cholesterol. However, some scientists say that if an egg is fried – this causes oxidative damage – and it's the frying that causes the problems not the eggs themselves. It makes sense then to boil or poach eggs. Buy organic or eggs containing omega-3 fats, which are now available in all major supermarkets.
- Alcohol and coffee (especially if microwaved), taken to excess has been shown to raise cholesterol levels.
- Greatly reduce the amount of sodium-based salt you use.

Friendly Foods

- Generally you need to increase your fibre intake. Eat more oat or rice bran, rolled oats, wheat germ, and any beans and peas such as soya beans, red kidney beans, lima beans, broad beans, chickpeas and lentils, whole grains such as brown rice, whole wheat, barley, rye, millet and quinoa are great for controlling cholesterol.
- For even more fibre add 1 tsp of psyllium husks to a glass of warm water and drink daily in-between meals. This tastes awful, but the husks help to remove bile salts that in turn will lower LDL cholesterol levels. Some people are not keen on these husks – and if they cause bloating, simply use various brans over cereals, in soups and smoothies until you find one that suits your system.

- Increase your intake of fresh fruit and vegetables (raw, steamed, roasted or stir fried, not deep fried or boiled). Green vegetables are especially rich in magnesium and potassium, as are cereals (also rich in B-vitamins) honey, kelp and dried fruits like dates.
- A couple of raw organic carrots or apples per day can lower cholesterol levels.
- Eat porridge for breakfast. Make with half low-fat milk (or even better rice milk) and half water. Add a chopped apple and a few raisons to sweeten, rather than sugar.
- Buckwheat, which is high in glycine, has been shown to lower cholesterol levels. Buckwheat flour makes great pancakes.
- Fermented soya products, such as natto, miso and tempeh, can help raise HDLs and lower LDLs. Soya lecithin granules are a great way to help lower LDL and help to control the growth of kidney and gall stones. Sprinkle a tablespoon daily over cereals, into yoghurts and onto fruit salads.
- Increase your intake of healthier fats found in olive oil, avocados, sunflower, pumpkin, sesame and linseeds, plus walnuts and Brazil nuts and their unrefined oils (see *Fats You Need To Eat*).
- Oily fish such as salmon, trout, mackerel, herring and sardines contain a fatty acid known as eicosapentaenoic acid (EPA). This helps to make the blood less sticky thus lowers the risk of coronary heart disease. Garlic and onions do the same.
- Look for spreads that are free from hydrogenated and trans-fats such as Biona or Vitaquell. Benecol spread has also been shown to lower cholesterol as it contains plant sterols.
- Vegetarians tend to have lower cholesterol levels.
- Use an organic mineral-based sea salt available from all health stores.
- Look for Columbus eggs, which are high in healthy omega-3 essential fats. Columbus chickens are fed on seeds that are rich in essential fats and therefore they lay healthier eggs!
- Use dandelion root tea, which helps liver function; and green tea, which lowers cholesterol levels.
- Globe artichoke and fennel stimulate liver function and cell regeneration and can help lower blood cholesterol.

- Eating more live, low-fat, plain yoghurt containing lactobacillus/acidophilus, which lowers blood cholesterol levels by binding fat and cholesterol in the intestines.
- A glass of red wine per day is also helpful.
- Drink plenty of water – at least 6 glasses daily.

Useful Remedies

- If you are taking statin drugs, which are now available over the counter from pharmacies, these drugs block the enzyme that makes cholesterol. The same enzyme also makes CoQ10 (Co-enzyme Q10), a vitamin-like substance, which is needed to protect against heart disease. Therefore, if you are taking statins **it is really important** that you also take 150mg of CoQ10 per day. Research shows people on statins (lipitor, lescol, mevacor, zocor) have low levels of CoQ10.
- As a base take a good-quality multi-vitamin and mineral such as Kudos 24 (see *General Supplements*, see p.160). **KVH**
- HMB – Hydroxy-beta-methylbutyrate – is generally used by body builders, but studies show that this amino acid metabolite helps to lower overall cholesterol – especially LDL. Take 3 grams daily.
- One of the best and easiest ways I have found for lowering cholesterol is to take grapefruit pectin fibre. The best one I have found is Profibe, which has been shown to reduce LDL if taken daily, even in people who refuse to change their high-fat diets. For details contact any health shop, or The Nutri Centre. **NC**
- Plant sterols are available in a tablet called Lestrin. Taken daily, Lestrin can help to maintain normal cholesterol levels – without adding more dairy fats to your diet. Initially take 2 tablets twice a day with meals but after a few weeks intake may be reduced to 2 tablets daily. **NC**
- Take 1–2 grams of fish oil daily.
- Evidence has shown that taking garlic each day could help lower overall cholesterol blood levels and increase the levels of HDL over LDL cholesterol. This is especially true if you are an A or an AB blood type. Kudos make a high-strength one-a-day. **KVH**
- Include a high-strength antioxidant formula that helps prevent the cholesterol oxidizing. **HN**
- Co-enzyme Q10, 60–100mg daily – combined with 100iu of natural source full spectrum vitamin E, has been shown to be more effective in protecting LDL against oxidation, than vitamin E alone.
- Folic acid, B12 and B6 all lower levels of homocysteine in the blood, thus reducing our risk of heart disease. A good B-complex should contain 400mcg folic acid, 10–20mg B6 and 50–100mcg B12.
- The mineral chromium 200mcg per day, can help elevate HDL levels whilst reducing cravings for sugary foods.
- The minerals calcium and magnesium are useful for reducing cholesterol. Take 1000mg of calcium and 600mg of magnesium.

Helpful Hints

- There is now an easy test to discover your plasma homocysteine levels. Made by York Laboratories and backed by The British Cardiac Patients Association – it's a simple pinprick method that can be done by post. For details call York Labs on 0800 074 6185, or log on to www.yorktest.com.
- Exercise is vital for controlling cholesterol, it can raise HDL levels and lower LDL. Try and walk for at least 30 minutes daily and do some kind of aerobic exercise 3 times a week.
- Smoking increases oxidation of LDL.
- Eating smaller meals every 3–4 hours, rather than 3 big meals per day, can help lower cholesterol.

CHRONIC FATIGUE

(see *Exhaustion* and *ME*)

CIRCULATION

(see also *Chilblains, Cholesterol* and *Raynaud's Disease*)

It is amazing how many conditions are linked to poor circulation. Common symptoms range from cold hands and feet to leg ulcers and varicose veins. Hair loss can be triggered by poor circulation to the head – hence Uri Geller practices a yoga headstand daily to keep his thick hair in tip-top condition.

If you laid out your blood vessels end to end, it is estimated that they would encircle the globe twice over – that's a lot of miles. No wonder we end up with so many circulatory problems.

Our circulation becomes less efficient as we age and therefore fewer nutrients and oxygen are delivered to the cells, which in turn reduces our cells' ability to eliminate toxins.

Numerous conditions associated with ageing – leg ulcers, memory loss, atherosclerosis, cold hands and feet – are all linked to poor circulation. This is why keeping your circulation in tiptop condition is vital to your health.

Our arteries make up a major part of our blood circulatory system and contain about 15% of our blood supply at any given moment. Healthy arteries have thick, muscular walls, which are necessary for the pressure of the blood moving through them. Your heart weighs just 280–310 grams (10–11ozs) and it is about the size of a clenched fist. The left side of the heart forces blood into the arteries, which carry the bright red, nutrient rich, oxygenated blood through the body.

The oxygen (from the lungs) and nutrients (absorbed into the arteries via the gut) are taken up by the cells, before the blood (now a darker, bluish colour) is returned to the heart via the veins, and the right chamber of the heart then pumps it through the lungs. Veins are more numerous and hold more of the body's blood (about 70%) and they transport blood laden with waste products, and partly depleted of oxygen, back to the heart.

From the lungs the re-oxygenated blood returns, purified, to the left chamber, ready for redistribution and the whole cycle begins again. Veins are forced to move against gravity much of the time. In order to maintain normal blood pressure, an adequate supply of blood must be returned to the heart from the peripheral vessels. Two main factors are responsible for this 'uphill' flow from the legs and abdomen to the heart. Firstly, muscular contractions compress veins, thus squeezing the blood along. When a person stands still for a long time such as soldiers on sentry duty, the blood pools in the lower limbs due to the force of gravity and in the long-term as the leg valves become weaker, can trigger varicose veins. This pooling of blood means that there is insufficient blood returning to the heart to maintain blood pressure, and less blood makes it to the brain. In extreme cases fainting can result, which forces the person into a horizontal position, which alleviates the problem.

Secondly, as we get older, especially if we have a sedentary lifestyle, we tend to breathe more shallowly which has a direct effect on our circulation. Coronary heart disease is almost always due to a condition called atherosclerosis in which fatty deposits attach themselves to the insides of the arteries. Arteries that were once smooth and elastic become rough, inflexible and narrow (see *High Blood Pressure*). With this narrowing, the volume of blood arteries can transport is reduced. Factors that contribute to atherosclerosis are high blood pressure, cigarette smoking, high cholesterol, a high-fat diet, excessive salt, and so on.

Once an area has been damaged, fats from the blood, including cholesterol, accumulate and build up a thick fatty layer called plaque. This plaque narrows the artery and a clot may detach itself and if it causes an obstruction inside the coronary artery, a heart attack can occur. If it blocks an artery leading to the brain, it can cause a stroke.

This slow build-up of plaque and consequent narrowing of the artery can also lead to a condition called angina, which is very common after 50. The pain of angina (which can vary considerably) is generally felt when the person is under stress or more demands are put on the heart muscle during exercise. The pain of a heart attack is a more 'crushing' pain in the chest, which can radiate to the jaw or down the left arm (see *Heart Disease*).

Blood pressure tends to increase with age. Normal blood pressure depends on a number of factors including the elasticity of the arterial walls, amount and consistency of the blood, digestion, smoking, weight and stress. High blood pressure can cause heart attacks and strokes. An aneurysm can occur when there is a weak spot in an arterial wall which balloons out and releases blood into surrounding tissues; hence why looking after the integrity of your veins and arteries can help keep you healthier at any age.

Foods to Avoid

- Salt hardens your arteries (which need to be elastic) and although essential to life, most people consume too much inorganic salt in the form of sodium chloride. Too much salt can result in high blood pressure because where salt goes water follows! It is found in most tinned, pre-packaged mass produced foods, burgers, crisps, laxatives, antacids and carbonated drinks, especially canned fizzy drinks.
- Reduce animal fats such as red meat, full-fat milk and dairy produce, cheese and chocolates.
- Pies, pastries, cakes and foods made with saturated/hydrogenated trans fats, such as lard and margarines, should be avoided or reduced (see *Fats You Need To Eat*).
- Avoid or greatly reduce your intake of fried foods. Never fry with mass-produced vegetable oils.
- Avoid coffee, caffeine and other stimulants, which can ultimately lead to a constriction of blood vessels.
- Avoid excessive alcohol. A glass of red wine with meals however, can be beneficial.

Friendly Foods

- Try chopping up seaweeds such as kelp over your food instead of salt.
- Use organic mineral rich sea salt, but only over the food that is in front of you! I use Himalayan Crystal Salt, which is rich in natural minerals.
- Vitamin C is vital for healthy circulation. Foods naturally high in vitamin C include kiwis, blue-berries, cherries and capsicum – all fruits and vegetables.
- Garlic and onions help to thin the blood naturally.
- Wheat germ, avocados, nuts and seeds are all rich in vitamin E, which also helps to thin the blood naturally.
- Foods rich in rutin help to strengthen the small blood vessels. So eat more buckwheat, the peel of citrus fruits, rose hips and apple peel.
- Silica rich foods such as lettuce, celery, millet, oats and parsnips help to strengthen arterial and vein walls. Fiji mineral water is rich in silica.
- Linseeds (flax seeds) and sunflower and sesame seeds, and fish oils contain essential polyunsatu-rated fatty acids, known as omega-3 and omega-6 fatty acids, that have been shown to lower the bad fats and thin the blood. Try eating at least 3 portions of fish a week such as wild salmon, mackerel or fresh tuna.
- Unrefined Brazils, walnuts, hazelnuts, almonds, seeds and their unrefined cold oils, are excellent sources of essential fats, and enjoy one avocado a week, a rich source of mono-unsaturated fats.
- Sprinkle GM-free lecithin granules, which emulsify bad fats, over your breakfast cereals, into yoghurts or over fruit to help lower LDL cholesterol.

- People on high-fibre diets are four times less likely to suffer from circulation problems and heart disease. Soluble fibre (that is, beans and lentils) consists of compounds which bind to bile salts and this helps lower cholesterol levels.
- Psyllium husks are a good source of soluble fibre and a level tablespoon mixed into a large glass of water and taken each morning is a great preventative for high cholesterol. Make sure that you drink plenty of water throughout the day to help the psyllium work properly. If previously you have been on a low-fibre diet, begin with a teaspoon and gradually increase the dose. Otherwise use more oat or rice brans in your diet.

Useful Remedies

- The herb gotu kola helps increase circulation to the extremities such as feet and hands through its vasodilatory action on peripheral blood vessels. Take 500mg twice daily.
- The herb butcher's broom is high in rutin, a bioflavonoid, which helps to tone the vein walls. It is therefore very beneficial in treating varicose veins. As butcher's broom is a vasoconstrictor (the opposite to gotu kola), caution should be taken if you suffer from high blood pressure. Take 500mg twice daily.
- The herb horse chestnut has a similar action on varicose veins as its components help strengthen the small capillaries. Take 500mg daily.
- V-Nal contains butcher's broom, horse chestnut, B-vitamins and rutin. Made by Bional and available from all health stores. All the above herbs are usually used for varicose veins, as they strengthen veins, have anti-inflammatory properties, reduce swelling, thus making venous return to the heart more efficient.
- The herb ginkgo biloba is beneficial for helping to increase blood-flow to the head as it promotes microcirculation to the brain. Poor circulation to the head can trigger hair loss, memory loss and eventually dementia.
- Studies have shown that patients suffering with visual and hearing problems linked to poor circulation have demonstrated improvements after taking ginkgo biloba for 3 months. To save taking several capsules daily, Kudos make a high-strength, 900mg one-a-day. **KVH**
- Vitamin C with bioflavonoids helps to strengthen capillaries. Take 1 gram daily with food.
- Vitamin E helps reduce stickiness in the blood, take 200iu daily of full spectrum natural source vitamin E. This is especially true for type A and AB blood types, which tend to be 'stickier' than other blood types.
- Niacin (vitamin B3) increases circulation but can induce a short-term 'flushing' or reddening of the skin, so begin with 30mg and work up to 100mg daily.
- Ginger helps to warm the body so make a ginger tea infusion daily and add grated fresh root ginger to stir-fries and fruit salads.

Helpful Hints

- Exercise is a wonderful way to help increase circulation. Just taking a brisk walk every day can be very helpful. Skipping, dancing, rebounding and power walking all help by gently pounding the feet.
- Massage and reflexology are important, especially for people, who for health reasons, cannot exercise much or lead a more sedentary lifestyle. Aromatherapy massage using essential oils such as rosemary, black pepper or ginger can be very effective in aiding circulation.
- Skin brushing also aids circulation. Work upward from the feet and hands towards the heart, rubbing briskly and try to do this 5 times a week in the bath or shower.
- Long-term stress constricts blood vessels, which will impede circulation.
- Magnets increase circulation by drawing blood to them. Magnetic insoles (placed in your shoes) can aid in circulation to the feet. As our peripheral circulation tends to lessen as we age, this can be very effective in winter.

- If you smoke give it up as it impairs breathing and hence circulation.
- Acupuncture has a long history in the treatment of poor circulation and high blood pressure. The action of the needles promotes better circulation through unblocking stagnation of both *qi* and blood (see *Useful Information*).

COELIAC DISEASE (see also *Absorption* and *Leaky Gut*)

Coeliac sufferers cannot break down a protein called gluten, which is present in wheat, rye, barley and oats. However, most coeliacs appear to be able to tolerate a small amount of oats and spelt. This condition often goes undiagnosed for several years. Symptoms include frequent indigestion, abdominal pain, loss of weight and depression. Because fat is poorly absorbed, the stools can be pale, frothy and foul smelling. It is very important that if you suffer with any or some of these symptoms over a period of several months that you see a doctor. The longer you suffer with coeliac disease, particularly if it goes undiagnosed, the more likely you are to do more damage to the gut lining. This greatly reduces the body's ability to absorb adequate levels of nutrient, which can even lead to malnutrition. Coleliacs are also at a higher risk for osteoporosis, due to mineral malabsorption.

Foods to Avoid
- Any foods containing wheat, rye and barley are absolutely crucial to avoid. Quite a few people with coeliac disease also have a problem with cow's milk and dairy products or soya foods.
- You will also need to avoid cakes and desserts.
- Until the condition is under control also avoid fatty meats, sausages, pies and processed meat products as they often contain wheat.

Friendly Foods
- Fortunately, these days, there are plenty of gluten-free foods available, most of them fairly palatable. Some will be high in sugar so be sure to read labels carefully – sugar converts to fat in the body if not burned up during exercise and in coeliac sufferers, fat is poorly absorbed. Look out for the gluten-free Orgran or Barkat ranges of products.
- Look for breads, instant foods, and flours made from grain alternatives like quinoa, spelt, amaranth, millet, corn, rice, buckwheat and lentils.
- Dairy alternatives to cow's milk include rice, oat, pea and almond.
- Eat plenty of leafy greens, which are rich sources of magnesium and calcium. Cabbage is rich in the amino acid L-glutamine, which helps to heal the gut – try making fresh vegetable juices that include raw cabbage, a little root ginger, which is very soothing, plus any vegetables you have to hand. If you cook cabbage in water, save the water and make gravy with it. Or add cabbage to stews and soups.
- Try to eat more fish to provide vitamin D, which is often deficient in coeliac sufferers.
- Eat plenty of unrefined organic nuts, seeds and fish; and free-range, low-fat meats such as venison, pork and turkey to keep up zinc intake often deficient in coeliacs. Try to use only organic meat.
- Essential fats are needed to heal the gut, so use a little organic sunflower, sesame, olive or walnut oil for salad dressings.
- Eat an avocado once a week, as they are rich in vitamin E.

Useful Remedies
- None of the supplements suggested will cure coeliac disease, it's just that the vast majority of these nutrients are often deficient in coeliac sufferers. It is very important to increase your intake

of these nutrients to prevent deficiency.

- Calcium 500mg and magnesium 250mg are vital minerals, as many coeliac sufferers have a low bone density.
- Folic acid – 400–800mcg; and vitamin B6 – 50–100mg.
- Vitamin A – 20,000iu daily (if you are pregnant no more than 3000iu daily); vitamin D – 400–1200iu a day.
- A high-strength multi-vitamin and mineral to make up for any other nutritional deficiencies such as Cantamega 2000. **FSC**
- Essential fatty acids, 1–3 grams a day of Efalex or 10–20ml of Udo's Choice Oil (before taking any fats and oils, see *Fats You Need To Eat*).

Helpful Hints

- Breast-fed children are much less likely to develop coeliac disease than those fed on cow's or soya milk formulas. Formula milks are harder to digest and potentially can cause health problems later on.
- The Village Bakery in Cumbria make great wheat-, rye- and barley-free breads and cakes. Sold at most health stores. Tel: 01768 881811. Website: www.village-bakery.com
- Research from Finland shows that small amounts (50–70 grams) of oat-based products can be tolerated by coeliacs without damaging intestinal absorption.
- Slippery Elm tablets help to reduce the irritation. Take one tablet with each meal.

COLDS and FLU

Colds and flu are caused by viruses and the secret to avoiding them is to keep your immune system in great shape. See also *Immune Function*.

Flu symptoms are usually far more severe and symptoms include a fever, aching joints and dreadful headaches. With colds there is plenty of congestion, often accompanied by a headache. With heavier bouts of flu your joints ache, and all you want is bed rest, which is one of the fastest routes to recovery. If you have a temperature, take paracetamol every four to six hours to help bring it down. Only if you contract a secondary bacterial infection – meaning if it hurts to breathe and you are wheezing – may antibiotics be warranted; see also *Bronchitis*.

We become more susceptible to colds and flu if we overwork, over-train or consistently eat a poor diet high in saturated fats and sugars. For example, if you eat a sugar rich pudding and a bar of chocolate, and are then immediately in contact with someone suffering with a cold or flu, you have doubled your chances of picking it up.

Foods to Avoid

- All sugars plus refined carbohydrates such as white bread, cakes pies and biscuits plus high-fat foods, alcohol and caffeine. All of these can weaken the immune system and make us more susceptible to infection.
- Generally while you have a cold reduce your intake of mucus-forming foods such as cheese, chocolate and full-fat dairy produce. Mucus will also form as a reaction to any foods to which you have an intolerance; see *Allergies* and *Catarrh*.

Friendly Foods

- Garlic and onions are great foods as they are anti-bacterial and have antiseptic properties. A traditional remedy for colds and flu is a soup made with 6 onions, a whole garlic, 1in (2.5cm) of grated fresh ginger, and some cayenne pepper mixed in a vegetable or chicken stock. You could also add lemongrass. For children it is probably preferable to leave out the cayenne pepper –

although it does make the other herbs more effective, it is often too hot.

- Liquorice is a pleasant-tasting food that you can make into tea and eat as confectionery if it is sugar free. It has both anti-viral and anti-bacterial properties and will soothe the throat when it's inflamed.
- Whilst you have a cold or flu try to base your diet on fruits, vegetables and brown rice with a little fish, chicken or pulses. Keep your diet clean. See *General Health Hints*.
- Drink plenty of lemon and ginger herbal tea or make your own by finely chopping a 2.5cm piece of fresh ginger, stand it in boiling water for 15 minutes with a squeeze of lemon juice and freshly chopped spring onions; strain and sip.
- Keep up your fluid intake – tea and coffee dehydrate the body, so drink plenty of water and herbal teas. Pau d'arco or green tea will help boost immune function.

Useful Remedies

- Propolis – from bee hives – has anti-viral and anti-bacterial properties. Taking 1 to 3 grams daily can help reduce the severity of a cold and taken all year round (500mg daily) can help boost immunity.
- Echinacea and Golden Seal, taken either as tincture or tablets every couple of hours, really helps fend off a cold or flu. Echinacea has been shown in a number of studies to shorten the length of a cold from 7 days down to 3–4 if taken regularly, generally 1–4ml every 2–3 hours. A great formula is available from www.holoshealth.com
- I tend to take herbs like Echinacea in the winter when we are more susceptible to colds. It is more effective when taken cyclically. Take for a month, then stop taking for a week. Continue throughout the winter.

- Vitamin C is strongly anti-viral and research has shown that it can shorten the severity and duration of most colds and flu if taken in sufficient amounts. During the winter, take 1 gram daily, but if you feel a cold coming on, increase your intake to 1 gram 3 times daily. Take it with meals in an ascorbate form until the cold has gone.
- Take a multi-vitamin and mineral that contains at least 30–60mg of zinc to boost the immune system while fighting an infection. See Kudos 24 in *General Supplements*, p.160. **KVH**
- If you are suffering from a sore throat try zinc gluconate lozenges that contain 15–25mg of zinc. Take 1 every 3–4 hours. The zinc lozenges help to kill bacteria in the throat.
- Olive leaf extract acts like nature's antibiotic. I take 2 daily to help keep my immune system in shape when I am feeling run down.
- Sambucol is an extract of the European black elderberry plant, which has potent anti-viral properties. If taken at the onset of a cold or flu it can help reduce the severity and length of the illness. Available from all health stores or call 01782 794300 for your nearest stockist.

Helpful Hints

- Homeopathic Aconite 30c can be taken 2 or 3 times daily at the onset of a cold to help stop the cold from developing.
- Ainsworth's famous Anti Cold and Flu Remedy is a homeopathic preventative for colds and flu symptoms, which is tailored to the current strains each year. They also supply a remedy called Anas Barb Co, which is for use at the onset of a cold or flu to prevent symptoms from developing further. Contact Ainsworth Homeopathic Pharmacy at 36 New Cavendish Street, London W1G 8UF. Tel: 020 7935 5330. Website: www.ainsworths.com
- Keep warm and avoid changes in the temperature of your surroundings for at least 48 hours until symptoms subside. Rest is essential if you have a temperature.
- Do not struggle into work if you have a really bad cold – all you do is make it last longer and you pass it on to your colleagues.
- Wash your hands regularly if you are in contact with people who have a cold as viruses can

easily permeate the soft skin on the palms of the hands. Washing hands is especially true for kids whose hygiene levels are often lacking!

- Viruses are airborne and spread quickly at large gatherings. Avoid being in stuffy, smoky rooms for too long. Get plenty of exercise and fresh air.

COLD SORES (see also *Herpes*)

Cold sores are caused by the herpes simplex virus. Once contracted the virus lies dormant in the body and tends to re-activate if you become run down, stressed or after sudden exposure to very hot or cold weather. Some women suffer an attack during menstruation. Others find that if they eat large amounts of nuts or chocolate that contain the amino acid arginine, on which the virus thrives, this can also trigger an attack. There have been a number of studies showing that you can reduce the frequency of attacks by taking vitamin C and the amino acid lysine on a regular basis.

Foods to Avoid

- Foods that are very rich in arginine, an amino acid found commonly in chocolate, lentils, beans and nuts.
- Avoid sugar, refined foods made with white flour and high saturated-fat foods, which again have a negative effect on the immune system.
- Certain people notice when they eat too much dairy produce from cows they suffer an attack.

Friendly Foods

- Eat good-quality protein such as lean meats including turkey, duck (without any skin), lean pork plus fish, corn and soya, all of which are rich in lysine, an amino acid which has been shown to interfere with replication of the virus.
- See *General Health Hints*.

Useful Remedies

- At the onset of an attack take up to 4 grams of lysine daily. Many companies now make lysine and vitamin C together. At the onset take 4 grams of vitamin C daily with food.
- To help prevent attacks take 1 gram of vitamin C daily. Take 3 grams of Propolis capsules and use the cream topically to help shut down an attack and ease the irritation. And then take 500mg of propolis daily to help prevent further attacks. Propolis is strongly anti-viral – and in studies has been proven to be more effective than some anti-viral drugs.
- If you find you or your children regularly suffer cold sores you definitely need to include a good quality multi-vitamin and mineral in your regimen. There are now plenty of sugar- and additive-free chewable vitamins for children (Nature's Plus make great ranges for kids), or add liquid vitamins and minerals to their food.

Helpful Hints

- Make sure you change your toothbrush and face towels regularly as these can harbour the virus.
- Calendula tincture can be dabbed directly onto the sores.
- Homeopathic Rhus Tox 30c helps to eliminate the eruptions. Take as soon as the tingling starts. Take twice daily for 3 days.
- Several people have told me that when they take Bach Rescue Remedy internally and dab it externally onto the cold sores it prevents the cold sore from developing. As Rescue Remedy is also available in a cream this is certainly worth a try.

CONJUNCTIVITIS

(see also *Eye Problems*)

Conjunctivitis is an inflammation of the outer surface membrane that lines the eye. This can be triggered by an external allergen such as perfume or an insect spray in which case the eyes are usually very red, itchy and irritated. But if conjunctivitis is caused by bacteria or a virus this can be accompanied by a yellow or white mucus-type discharge and it should be treated by a doctor. People who suffer chronic conjunctivitis are often deficient in vitamin A.

Foods to Avoid
- All foods and drinks containing sugar which reduces the body's ability to fight an infection.
- Reduce your intake of animal fats, and white-flour-based cakes, breads and biscuits, all of which weaken the immune system.
- See *General Health Hints*.

Friendly Foods
- Bilberries, blueberries, blackberries and all blue and purple coloured fruits are rich in antioxidant nutrients that nourish the eyes.
- Foods rich in vitamin A such as leafy green vegetables, calves' or lambs' liver, cod liver oil, carrots and fish help encourage healthy eyes.
- Natural carotenes found in tomatoes, sweet potatoes, dried apricots, mangoes and raw parsley are all great foods for the eyes.
- Eat more pineapple – rich in the enzyme bromelain, which has anti-inflammatory properties.

Useful Remedies

- Echinacea, eyebright and bilberry tincture; 1–4ml a day.
- Bromelain; 1,000–3,000mcu a day. **FSC**
- When the infection is acute take 20,000iu of vitamin A daily for 14–21 days as some people with conjunctivitis are deficient in vitamin A. But if you are pregnant take no more than 3000iu of vitamin A per day.
- Vitamin C (1000mg, 2–3 times per day) and zinc (30–50mg per day) strengthen your immune system and help you heal faster.

Helpful Hints
- Try using a few drops of liquid colloidal silver solution directly into the eyes to help kill any bacteria or viruses. **HN**
- Conjunctivitis is highly contagious when caused by a viral infection. Be really careful not to use the same handkerchief or tissue to wipe both eyes. Be scrupulous with hygiene and make sure no one else uses your towels, make up or pillow.
- Eyebright tincture plus goldenseal tincture: take 2 drops of each and add to an eye bath full of purified or boiled water and use when cool. Use twice daily. Alternatively try Potter's Allerclear Eyedrops with eyebright.
- Dilute homeopathic Euphrasia mother tincture in an egg-cup full of cooled boiled water and use as an eye bath. Alternatively you can try Visualise Herbal Eye Wash with chamomile and blueberry (herbal eye drops also available). From good health stores or call Sloane Health Shop. **SL**
- Chamomile and calendula herbal teas can be used to make warm compresses to soothe the eye. The heat also helps kill the bacteria that cause the infection.
- Did you know that many eye drops are made from urine! Urea is an important component that helps break down mucus deposits and has anti-microbial actions. Bathing the eyes in fresh urine (which is a sterile liquid) on a cotton wool pad can help alleviate most eye problems.

CONSTIPATION and BLOATING

(see also *Absorption, Candida* and *Leaky Gut)*

Even though government advisors, health magazines and doctors all advise us to eat more fibre, we are one of the most constipated nations on earth. In an ideal world we should have a bowel movement after every meal, but most people in the West are lucky if they have one a day. Having clean bowels in one of the best ways to prevent most diseases in later life. Even if you have a daily bowel movement – you can still be constipated. Over time, we can experience a gradual build-up of matter, which adheres to the walls of the intestines and becomes compacted in certain sections. This build-up is caused by insufficient fibre and too many refined foods, which can eventually inhibit proper assimilation of nutrients from the diet and supplements. It also adds to the weight of the colon, therefore placing more stress on the lower organs like the uterus and bladder.

Millions of men and women have large, protruding abdomens. This means that all the major organs in that area, such as the liver, heart and bowels are surrounded by a layer of deadly fat deposits. They are also likely to be carrying a lot of waste matter. Henry VIII had more than 84lb (38kg) of faeces in his bowel after his death and he had a very big stomach indeed!

When food leaves the small intestine, which is over 20 feet long (almost 7m), it passes into the large intestine or colon where it is gradually compacted into semi-solid faeces. The bowel is a term for the large intestine. Most of the absorption of nutrients from our diet and supplements happens in the small intestine. The large intestine (colon) is primarily involved with the breaking down of foods for elimination.

The more faeces in your bowel the more toxic your entire system becomes. If you are not eliminating properly these toxins are re-absorbed into the bloodstream and can be eventually dumped into the skin resulting in conditions such as acne. People from primitive cultures tend to evacuate twice the amount of faeces that their Western counterparts do due to their higher intake of fibre and raw foods.

Peristalsis is the rhythmic movement of the colon, which helps to move the waste material out of the body. If you tend to eat a poor diet, low in fibre then the muscles in the colon can become lazy which over time can lead to chronic constipation. Also if you over-eat, food putrefies in the bowel, triggering symptoms such as bloating, gas, constipation or diarrhoea, irritable bowel, poor skin, dull hair and so on. Haemorrhoids or piles (varicose veins of the anus) are the result of years of straining to go to the loo and straining also contributes to varicose veins in the legs. If ever you experience blood in your faeces or any changes in bowel habits, it is **vital** that you see a doctor immediately.

Foods to Avoid

- All animal products, especially red meats, which have a long transit time through the bowel and should only be eaten in moderation.
- Many people do not have the enzyme needed to break down lactose, the sugar in milk, which can also lead to putrefaction in the bowel. This is especially common in African and Caribbean people.
- If you tend to be a big dairy fan, try cutting back, as all dairy-based foods are mucus forming, which adds to the plaque in the intestines. However organic rice, oat or goat's milk are generally better tolerated.
- Refined sugars found in cakes, biscuits, desserts and highly processed foods ferment in the gut, causing gas and bloating as healthy bacteria are destroyed. These bacteria help break down digested foods and aid in the manufacture of certain B-group vitamins. If these healthy bacteria

are missing, your digestion and elimination are impaired.

- When you mix flour and water it makes a gooey paste, it does the same in the bowel, therefore cut down on pastries and flour-based foods.
- Low fibre foods such as jelly, ice cream and soft desserts, all white flour products and refined breakfast cereals, which contain virtually no fibre and lots of sugar.
- Also avoid foods to which you have an intolerance, for example cow's milk has been found to be responsible for a lot of infant constipation.
- Cut down on full fat cheeses and don't eat melted cheese over food – it sets like plastic in the bowel.

Friendly Foods

- Bran, as it is an insoluble fibre derived from rice, soya or oats. The insoluble fibre is needed to stimulate the bowel to work properly. Wheat bran is fine as long as you don't have an intolerance to wheat, otherwise this can actually aggravate the problem.
- Try eating more brown rice (or rice bran) plus beans like black-eyed beans, kidney, haricot, butter and cannelloni.
- Linseeds (flax seeds) are a blend of insoluble and soluble fibres, which bulk the stool, encouraging it to move gently through the bowel. I use a tablespoon in a fruit smoothie every day, which breaks up the flax seeds and makes them more effective. You can buy ready cracked flax seeds (which should be kept in the fridge) from all health stores.
- Wholewheat rye bread, Ryvita-type crispbreads, rough oatcakes, or amaranth crackers can be eaten as an alternative to wheat bread.
- Other high fibre foods are fresh and dried figs, blackcurrants, ready to eat dried apricots and prunes, almonds, hazelnuts, fresh coconut and all mixed nuts.
- All lightly cooked or raw vegetables and salads will add more fibre to your diet.
- Eat more live, low-fat yoghurts, which contain healthy bacteria – a lack of which can exacerbate constipation.
- Drink at least 6 glasses of water daily.
- Psyllium husks are a great way to add bulk to the stools. Take a tablespoon of psyllium husks in water before breakfast to help keep things moving. Then make sure you drink plenty of water during the day.

Useful Remedies

- Use 1–2 tsp a day of any good quality organic green powder, such as Dr Gillian McKeith's Living Food Energy Powder. This blend of fibres and nutrients helps improve bowel function and digestion.
- Acidophilus and bifidus are healthy bacteria, which can be taken after a meal, particularly if constipation has started after antibiotics.
- Vitamin C powder with added calcium and magnesium, 1 level tsp 2–3 times a day for a few days, can help soften the stool and increase the frequency of bowel movement; magnesium also helps to tone the bowel muscles.
- One of the best ways I have found to eliminate constipation is to replace one meal a day with a fruit and vegetable blend, whilst eliminating all flour from any source for at least 2 days. I put half a cup of aloe vera juice, a banana, blueberries, an organic apple and any fruit I have to hand, plus a teaspoon of any good green food mix, a tablespoon of sunflower seeds, a dessertspoon of linseeds (flax seeds) and a teaspoon of olive oil into my blender. To this I add half a cup of organic rice milk and blend. It's delicious and packed with fibre. On alternate days I make a vegetable juice to which I still add the aloe vera juice but not the rice milk.
- Aloe Ferox crystals are a type of super-concentrated aloe vera that act as a natural digestive enzyme and also have a pro-biotic effect on the bowel flora, providing the stools with more

mucus which, in turn, encourages regular bowel movements without causing troublesome diarrhoea. Take 1–2 capsules daily before meals. They really do the trick. **NC SL**

- The Herbal Colon Programme – based on Dr Christopher's (he was a brilliant and respected nauropath in the US) herbal cascara formula. For details of The Herbal Colon Programme, call Specialist Herbal Supplies. **SHS**
- Colosan is an oxygenating powder, which helps to cleanse the bowel and detoxify the body. Taken regularly 1 tsp a day normally keeps the bowels open, and this supplement is non-addictive and safe to use in the long term. Because it brings more oxygen into the body it also helps with overall health. For details call The Finchley Clinic on 020 8349 4730. Website: www.thefinchleyclinic.com

Helpful Hints

- Squatting to pass faeces helps to encourage elimination, as it is a more natural position for the colon.
- Over use of laxatives makes the bowel lazy.
- It is very important that you eliminate any underlying causes for your constipation. Visit your GP and make sure there is nothing more serious going on.
- Do not bear down too much when you have a bowel movement as this places a strain on the vascular system and can, over time, lead to varicose veins and haemorrhoids or piles. Remember rather than fall asleep after every meal, go for a leisurely walk. This will make you feel less bloated, aid digestion and encourage healthier bowels.
- In Chinese medicine the best time to walk is between 5am and 7am, which encourages the colon to work more efficiently. I think I'll pass on this one!
- When you feel the need to pass a motion, be sure not to ignore the signal; take the time to read a magazine on the loo.
- For healthy bowel movements you need about a pint of fluid in between each meal to get waste moving through successfully.
- Stress is a major factor as it slows down the peristalsis movements.
- When you add more fibre to your diet and you're not used to it, it is essential that you drink more water. Adding fibre without more fluid can actually aggravate the problem.
- In the elderly a lack of folic acid has sometimes been found to be the cause of constipation, therefore, supplementing with folic acid in the form of a good quality multi-vitamin/mineral should help.
- For severe constipation especially after surgery, and with your doctor's permission, try colonic irrigation. I have a colonic every month. Some people say it's harmful (but there has never been any research or reported cases of colon therapy being harmful when carried out by a properly trained therapist). If done properly it can be a godsend. For details of a practitioner, see *Useful Information*.
- You can also use a warm water enema at home. Available from Best Care Products on 01342 410303. Email: info@bestcare-uk.com.

CONTRACEPTIVE PILL   (see *Infertility* and *Pill, Contraceptive*)

COUGHS   (see also *Bronchitis* and *Colds and Flu*)

Coughs are often due to an infection such as a cold or flu and sometimes asthma. Many people who smoke develop a persistent cough. Sometimes the cough can lead to production of phlegm, if this is yellow or green in colour it is indicates a bacterial infection, in which case you would need to see a doctor. If you have a cough that persists longer than two weeks or produces blood at any stage, it is very important to seek medical attention and have an X-ray. Coughs that produce a lot of catarrh are often helped by mullein and other expectorant herbs. If the cough is dry and tickly, cherry bark is more useful. A persistent cough, especially after eating foods containing wheat or sugar could be linked to candida (see *Candida*).

Foods to Avoid
- For a few days, eliminate all cow's dairy products – even skimmed milk. I also find that if I have a cold I also need to avoid soya milk, which can increase mucus production.
- Cakes, biscuits, sausage rolls, meat pies, burgers and so on should all be avoided for at least 14 days to give your sinuses and throat time to clear all mucus. Also avoid white bread and pasta.
- Most foods containing sugar tend to be high in fat, and sugar lowers immune functioning.

Friendly Foods
- Manuka honey – 1 tsp before each meal helps coat the throat but also has antiseptic properties. The higher the Umf (5+ to 20+), the stronger its antiseptic properties.
- Drink plenty of water to keep the throat well-lubricated.
- Pineapples help loosen up mucus and make breathing easier. Fresh pear juice is also good for easing coughs.
- If the cough is making you feel tight-chested and congested try adding horseradish, cayenne or ginger to meals.
- Liquorice either as a tea or sucked as a pure liquorice juice stick can be very soothing.
- Tea made from fresh thyme can ease the cough and has historically been used for whooping cough.
- Eat plenty of fresh vegetables, chicken, fish, pulses, grains and fresh fruit.
- Drink herbal teas such as lemon and ginger and try organic rice milk as a dairy substitute.
- Live, low-fat plain yoghurts are usually well tolerated and they help to boost friendly bacteria in the gut.

Useful Remedies
- Comvita propolis elixir is a great remedy for coughs. It contains propolis, tea tree and Manuka honey. It is antiseptic, immune boosting, and soothing. From all health shops.
- Mullein Formula; 1–3ml a day. Expectorant and anti-viral herbs combine to make a wonderful cough mixture. **FSC**
- Bioforce Ivy–Thyme Complex Tincture, taken as directed.
- Zinc lozenges. Suck one every 3–4 hours to ease discomfort of sore throats and reduce the tickling of the cough. Ultimate Zinc-C Lozenges from Now contain vitamins A and C, zinc, echinacea, bee propolis and slippery elm.
- Olive leaf extract acts like a natural antibiotic and has been found especially useful for respiratory problems. Take 3 capsules daily while symptoms last. A good olive leaf extract is Eden Extract by Tigon.
- Include a multi-vitamin and mineral in your regimen.
- Colloidal silver can be sprayed straight into the throat or used as a gargle. **HN**

Helpful Hints
- If you begin wheezing after food or when stressed, you may have developed a touch of asthma – see *Asthma* and see a doctor.
- If you find you get tight chested after exercise, 2 grams of vitamin C can often be very helpful.
- Taken at the first sign of a cough, homeopathic Aconite 6c can help prevent the cough developing.

- Keep a food diary and note when symptoms are worse. For example, if your nose runs within a few minutes of eating certain foods, especially cow's milk, wheat- and sugar-based foods, then you may be sensitive to those foods. High-sugar fruits such as grapes can even be a problem for some people.
- Dilute a few drops of essential oil of sweet marjoram and frankincense in a grapeseed oil base and massage into your chest and back to encourage deeper breathing.
- Take 2 tbsp of aloe vera juice every day to soothe your throat and boost your immune system.
- Stop smoking.

CRADLE CAP
(see Dermatitis)

CRAMPS
(see also Circulation)

Most people will experience cramp at some time or other and it's a painful muscular spasm or contraction, often caused by a poor blood supply to the muscles. It can also be triggered by extreme exercise. Unless you live in a very hot country where you are sweating profusely, it is unlikely to be due to a lack of sodium (salt) – that is, dehydration. Chronic depletion of body fluids from diuretics and poor fluid intake predispose seniors to cramps.

Cramp is most commonly caused by poor circulation and lack of magnesium, calcium or potassium. Low levels of calcium and magnesium are common in a normal pregnancy unless these minerals are supplemented to the diet.

Foods to Avoid
- Cut down on white-flour-based foods like white rice, biscuits, cakes, pizza and pasta, and all forms of sugar and coffee.
- Avoid carbonated drinks; they contain phosphoric acid which increases calcium loss from bone.
- All of these foods deplete magnesium and potassium from the body. Some breads now have added calcium – check the labels.

Friendly Foods
- Plenty of fresh fruits and vegetables, especially bananas, raw cauliflower and jacket potatoes, fresh fruit juices, dried apricots and dates, seafood, leafy greens, avocado, lean steak, mackerel and beans in particular are all good sources of magnesium and potassium.
- Eating a banana before going to bed helps reduce cramps, as bananas are rich in potassium and magnesium.
- Snack on almonds, sesame seeds and Brazil nuts – all rich in minerals.
- Calcium foods are dried skimmed milk, sesame seeds, sardines, muesli, Parmesan cheese and curry powder.

Useful Remedies
- Black cohosh and cramp bark; 1–2mls as needed. **FSC**
- Take ginkgo biloba, try a one a day (900mg) from Kudos, as this herb helps to increase circulation. If you are taking drugs such as warfarin – then before taking this herb check with your doctor. **KVH**
- A liquid multi-mineral supplement taken in water daily can help reduce cramps. Trace Minerals. Tel: 01342 824684. Website: www.mineralresourcesint.co.uk
- Concentrace-ionic trace mineral drops from the isolated waters of the north arm of the Great Salt Lake, Utah, USA, by Trace Minerals (details as above).
- Take 500mg of extra magnesium at night, which is often lacking in people who suffer cramps.

Helpful Hints

- If you tend to get cramps at night, try stretching out your calves before going to bed. If you have a friend or a dog you can walk with – have a regular evening walk.
- Exercise regularly, but not to excess and indulge yourself with a massage on a regular basis. Use geranium, ginger and cypress oils in your mix of oils.
- Reflexology helps to improve circulation and reduce cramps if undertaken on a regular basis (see *Useful Information*).

CROHN'S DISEASE   (see also *Absorption, Candida* and *Leaky Gut*)

Crohn's is an inflammatory disease of the small intestine, which can also affect the bowel (large intestine). Up to 6000 new cases of Crohn's are diagnosed each year and sadly as many as 1 in every 400 children suffer this condition – this is a 50% increase in the last 10 years. This condition causes ulcers and scarring to the wall of the intestines and often occurs in patches with healthy tissues in between. It is the scarring that narrows the passages, thus disrupting nutrient absorption and normal bowel function. Blood in the stool, weight loss, loss of appetite, nausea, severe abdominal pain, diarrhoea, fever, chills, weakness and anaemia are all common symptoms of this disease and it is quite often associated with other inflammatory conditions within the body that affect the joints, eyes and skin. Malabsorption of nutrients from the diet is one of the biggest problems with Crohn's and up to 85% of sufferers are known to have deficiencies. There is a known genetic link, but Crohn's has been labelled a modern disease as in 'primitive' cultures it is virtually unknown.

C

Up to 60,000 people in Britain suffer with this painful condition most of whom were born after 1950 when we really began eating a more refined diet. Over-consumption of antibiotics and eating antibiotic- and hormone-fed meat and milk, plus vaccinations are all suggested as possible triggers, as is a possible auto-immune factor – in which the body's own immune system attacks part of the intestines. Children who are breast-fed are less likely to contract Crohn's. Candida is also linked to this disease, as is a leaky gut.

Foods to Avoid

- Sugar has been strongly linked with the development of Crohn's and some people find that avoidance of sugar slows down the rate of progression.
- Tomatoes, raw fruit and nuts are often problematic for some people.
- Yeast and dairy are two food groups that many people find difficult to digest and avoidance of them has helped many sufferers.
- Gluten-rich foods such wheat, rye and oats are often a problem.
- Avoid and reduce foods associated with inflammation – alcohol, simple sugars, refined white rice, bread, cakes and pastries and caffeine
- Foods high in salicylates such as tomatoes, aubergines, peppers, courgettes and berries, such as black- and blueberries, strawberries, and so on may also cause problems for sufferers.

Friendly Foods

- Oily fish, which is a rich source of EPA and DHA, two essential fatty acids, have been found to reduce the severity of Crohn's and the frequency of attacks via their anti-inflammatory action.
- Studies in Japan showed that the type of fibre found in barley was beneficial to sufferers – reducing frequency and quantity of diarrhoea. Add more organic barley to soups, broths, stews, and mix with brown rice.
- It is important to eat unprocessed foods in their fresh state.

- Protein is important for the healing and repair of the intestines. Most sufferers can tolerate meat once or twice a week; if this is a problem lightly steamed fish and grilled chicken are often easier to digest. Eat with plenty of lightly cooked vegetables.
- If raw fruit is a problem, lightly stew or grill fruits which makes them a little easier to digest.
- A couple of teaspoons of apple cider vinegar in a little warm water sipped throughout the morning helps to correct the pH level within the bowel and aid liver function.
- Drink the water that you cook any cabbage in as it helps to heal the digestive lining. If you can't face drinking this, at least make your gravy with cabbage water.

Useful Remedies

- As malabsorption is a big problem, liquid vitamins and minerals are a better choice as they are more easily absorbed. Patrick Holford's Get up and Go contains lots of beneficial fibre, vitamins and minerals – available from www.healthproductsforlife.com
- Quercetin is a type of flavonoid known for its anti-inflammatory action. Take 300mg 1–3 times per day. Allergy Research's Quercetin 300 is available from the Nutri Centre. **NC**
- Make sure you take a high-potency B-complex tablet every day, as low levels of folic acid and B12 are often lacking in Crohn's patients.
- Liquid amino acids aid digestion and healing. Contact www.positivehealthshop.com for Lamberts Protein Build Formula. Take 5 grams once daily, half an hour before a meal. Mix with fruit juice or water rather than with milk.

- Glutamine and butyrate are the primary fuels for the repair of the digestive lining, helping repair and healing. Studies show that both are low in Crohn's patients. Take 4–6 x 500mg of glutamine capsules, split throughout the day, before main meals. Also available in a powder from Higher Nature or Nutri Centre. Whey protein is also useful as it is rich in L-Glutamine and a highly absorbable protein. **HN NC**
- Zinc, 30mg a day, to aid tissue-healing.
- Vitamin A 25,000iu daily for one month (only 3000iu daily if you're pregnant).
- Cod liver oil 1–3 capsules a day or 1 tsp a day as this contains EPA, DHA and vitamin D. EPA and DHA are anti-inflammatory and the vitamin D is needed to maintain healthy bones.
- Take Polyzyme forte, a digestive enzyme needed to help absorption of nutrients with meals – after the first few mouthfuls. If you are having a large or rich meal you may need 2 capsules. **BC**
- Make sure you take friendly bacteria daily – acidophilus and bifidus are available at all good health stores and should be taken after meals. These really help to reduce food sensitivities.

Helpful Hints

- When beginning to use digestive enzymes and other digestive supplements it is best to do this gradually so as not to shock the system. For example, if the directions suggest 1 three times per day, build up to this over a week.
- Evidence that food intolerances trigger Crohn's are thin on the ground but it is widely acknowledged that they may aggravate and irritate the intestines – hence making the condition worse. It may be worth checking for intolerances and avoiding offending foods. Individual Well Being Diagnostic Laboratories offer a FACT food intolerance test and can be contacted on 08704 190 435, or check out their website at www.iwdl.net
- Smoking has been linked with the development of Crohn's disease.
- Lymph drainage massage and skin brushing help to eliminate toxins from the body.
- Buy foods as fresh as possible – this way they will be more nutrient-rich. Everything will taste better and you'll appreciate the effort in the long run.
- Crohn's disease is exacerbated by stress, therefore any techniques known to reduce stress such as yoga, T'ai Chi, meditation, massage or hypnotherapy will help. Spiritual healing has helped many sufferers (see *Healing*).

- Adequate rest is essential for any Crohn's sufferer and gentle exercise, such as walking and swimming, will also help.
- To re-balance your diet and make sure you are taking the right supplements and herbs in the correct amount for your case, I strongly suggest you consult a doctor who is also a nutritionist (see *Useful Information*).
- Avoid wearing tight clothing around the waist as this can make you more uncomfortable.
- If you suffer from Crohn's in the long term your risk of colorectal cancer is increased, therefore if you are over 30 you should have regular check-ups.
- For further help, contact The National Association for Colitis and Crohn's Disease (NACC), 4 Beaumont House, Sutton Road, St Albans, Hertfordshire AL1 5HH. Information Line: 0845 130 2233 (weekdays 10am–1pm). Email: nacc@nacc.org.uk Website: www.nacc.org.uk
- A helpful site for children with Crohn's can be found at www.cicra.org. It includes finding penpals, how to cope at school and what to expect when you go to hospital. They can also be contacted at: Crohn's in Childhood Research Association (CICRA), Parkgate House, 356 West Barnes Lane, Motspur Park, Surrey KT3 6NB. Tel: 020 8949 6209.

CYSTITIS
(see also *Candida* and *Thrush*)

Cystitis is more common in women than men and can also affect children. It is caused by a bacterial infection in the bladder and symptoms include a frequent urge to urinate plus a burning sensation when passing urine. With cystitis or thrush there can be a whitish/yellow discharge – but this is more common with thrush which is a yeast overgrowth. Whatever the cause, the entire outer area can swell which makes sitting extremely uncomfortable indeed. If lymph nodes in the groin begin to swell (near the bikini line) or if you have pain in the loins, blood in your urine, or a fever, this denotes a kidney infection and you must see a doctor. A urine test can confirm which bug is responsible and usually antibiotics are then prescribed. Women who suffer candida and food intolerances regularly suffer thrush or cystitis (see also *Candida*).

These types of infections are more likely to occur in warm, moist, humid atmospheres. If you are run down, you are more prone to an attack. If you suffer thrush regularly you may be diabetic. Have a urine test to eliminate this possibility.

Foods to Avoid
- While symptoms are acute avoid as much as possible all foods and drinks containing sugar and yeast – especially cheeses, malt vinegar, ketchups, soy sauce, miso, pickled foods, breads and cakes containing yeast, mushrooms and alcohol.
- Sugar in any form including honey, maltose and so on as all sugars feed the yeast. For the first week also avoid all cakes, biscuits, pizza or fizzy cola type drinks.
- Avoid junk-type burgers and fried foods which are hard to digest and add to the toxic load.
- Avoid high-sugar fruits, such as grapes, melons and bananas for the first few days.

Friendly Foods
- Eat plenty of live, low-fat yoghurt that contains the friendly bacteria acidophilus and bifidus.
- Cranberry juice without sugar or eat fresh or frozen cranberries – they are rich in hippuric acid which helps prevent bacteria clinging to the bladder walls.
- Drink 8 glasses of water every day.
- To re-alkalise your system, eat plenty of salads and green vegetables.
- Include bananas, apples, cherries, pineapples, papaya and pears for fruits.
- Eat more garlic and onions, which are anti-bacterial.

■ See also *Candida*.

Useful Remedies

■ Bromelain 1000–3000mcu extracted from pineapple for its anti-inflammatory properties.

■ Vitamin A 10,000–15,000iu daily for 2 weeks (only up to 3000iu daily if you are pregnant).

■ Vitamin C and flavonoids help to fight the infection. Take up to 4 grams daily with food for the first week and then reduce to 1 gram daily. When you take large doses of vitamin C make sure it's in an ascorbate form, which is gentle on the stomach.

■ Take 2 acidophilis/bifidus capsules daily with food for at least 6 weeks.

■ Include a high strength multi-vitamin and mineral in this programme.

■ Cran-Max is a supplement made from 100% cranberry fruit solids and is sugar and preservative free. One capsule daily; 500mg will help to fight and prevent urinary tract infections. **BC**

■ Try Higher Nature's very effective Citricidal Grape Seed Extract, which comes in liquid form. Take a few drops in water or juice. **HN**

■ Oregano tincture (Nature's Answer), 4 drops in half cup of water, has powerful anti-bacterial and anti-fungal properties. **SL**

Helpful Hints

■ Make a douche with essential oils of tea tree and camomile – three times daily if you can. For details of pure therapeutic oils call Susie Anthony on 01749 679900

■ Consuming live yoghurt on a daily basis can reduce the incidence of developing cystitis or thrush.

■ Drink organic aloe vera juice containing extract of cranberry and cherries.

■ Drink three to four cups of nettle tea daily. Goldenseal tea may also be helpful, as it contains berberine, an alkaloid that inhibits bacteria from adhering to the wall of the bladder.

■ Drink plenty of water each day to help flush out unhealthy organisms from the bladder.

■ Urinate as soon as possible after having sexual intercourse to stop transmission of bacteria into the bladder. If symptoms are acute, avoid intercourse for at least one week, as you can pass the bacteria from one partner to another.

■ Avoid perfumed soaps and vaginal deodorants at all times.

■ Wear cotton underwear. Avoid tightly fitted jeans, especially in hot weather.

■ As much as possible when you are at home wear a skirt and no underwear to keep the vaginal area cool.

■ If you have to sit all day, get up and walk around regularly.

■ Get plenty of rest.

■ Use a pH-balanced soap.

■ Douche daily with diluted tea tree oil, crushed garlic and lavender oil or add a few drops to your bath.

■ Acupuncture and homeopathic remedies such as Cantharis 30c reduce the burning sensation and have helped many sufferers (see *Useful Information*).

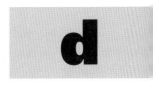

DANDRUFF (see *Scalp Problems*)

DEPRESSION (see also *Stress*)

More than 3 million people suffer depression in the UK, and almost 1 in 10 say they regularly feel depressed and low. But there is a world of difference between having a bad day and suffering full-blown depression. Older people tend to suffer more incidences of depression due to poor nutrition, the loss of a loved one, feelings of no longer being useful and so on. Up to 15% of older adults have clinically significant symptoms of depression and 60% of these adults are not receiving the proper therapy. And persistent mild depression at any age lowers immunity and the ability to fight off disease.

A truly depressed person has an all-pervading feeling of sadness. Other typical symptoms include feeling worthless, inadequate or incompetent. And if you also suffer from loss of interest or pleasure in your job, family life, hobbies or sex; difficulty concentrating or remembering; insomnia, over- or under-eating, unusual irritability, a sense of humour failure, a feeling of being downhearted that just won't go away, frequent unexplained crying spells, recurrent thoughts of death or suicide, then you may be clinically depressed and you should seek help.

Depressed people often isolate themselves by withdrawing from friends and family. Not all symptoms denote clinical depression, for example if you are feeling total apathy, like you just don't want to get up in the morning, then such symptoms can be linked to adrenal exhaustion (see *Stress*). Hormonal imbalances, low blood sugar, and poor thyroid function can also trigger depressive type symptoms (see these specific sections for extra help).

Foods to Avoid
- Avoid or reduce alcohol, it can make depression worse as it lowers levels of the feel good hormone serotonin, plus B-vitamins needed for energy and nerve health in the mind and body.
- If you eat too much refined sugar, your blood sugar levels keep fluctuating, which can greatly affect your mood (see *Insulin Resistance* and *Diabetes*).
- Excessive consumption of refined, processed, fatty foods and caffeine can make your depression worse as they deplete vitamins B and C and the mineral chromium.
- Avoid the sweetener aspartame at all costs, which can have neurological side effects and has been shown to interact negatively with antidepressants. A study looking at whether aspartame would influence mood was halted by psychiatrists because of negative effects to mood. For further information log on to www.dorway.com.
- Which foods do you tend to crave and eat the most? It could be flour based, sugary foods and snacks. If this is the case be aware that the foods you crave are usually the ones that make your symptoms worse. It takes discipline but for 7 days avoid these foods and replace with fresh fruits, vegetables and grains like brown rice and see how much better you feel.
- Lack of iron is also linked to depression, but iron accumulates in the body and is linked to heart

disease. Your doctor can find out if you are deficient.

Friendly Foods

- The brain is made up of around 60% fats, so eat more of the right kind of fats including oily fish, linseeds (flax seeds), soya beans and wheat germ, which are all rich in omega-3 essential fats.
- Walnuts, pecans, Brazil nuts and hazelnuts, plus sunflower and pumpkin seeds are all rich in omega-6 essential fats.
- Use unrefined nut and seed oils for salad dressings (see *Fats You Need to Eat*).
- Increase your intake of fresh fruits, vegetables, whole grains such as brown rice, pastas and lentils.
- To help raise serotonin levels eat more foods containing tryptophan, such as fish, turkey, avocado, cottage cheese, organic meats, beans, lentils, cooked tofu, wheat germ and bananas.
- Foods containing the amino acids phenylalinine and tyrosine can also help to raise mood and boost motivation, these include low-fat meats, fish, eggs, wheat germ, dairy foods, oat flakes, eggs, nuts, avocados, bananas and chocolate. This is why eating chocolate often makes you feel good. If you are a chocoholic try taking 250 to 500mg of DLPA (DL-phenylaline) with 2mg of vitamin B6 and 500mg of vitamin C on an empty stomach before breakfast.
- Spicy foods that contain cayenne pepper produce endorphins that help raise your mood.
- Drink 6 glasses of water daily to help remove toxins.

Useful Remedies

- First begin taking a high strength multi-vitamin and mineral to give you a good nutrient base plus the B-vitamins, a lack of which can trigger depression and low mood. See details of Kudos 24 in *General Supplements*, p.160. **KVH**
- Various B-vitamins play a major role in maintaining proper brain chemistry and deficiencies of B-vitamins are common in depressed people; take a 50mg B-complex in addition to your multi twice daily. B-vitamins turn your urine bright yellow – but this is normal!
- 1gram of vitamin C daily.
- Omega-3 fats are vital for improving depression and have been shown in many cases to be more effective than antidepressant drugs. If you are not eating oily fish 3 times a week then take an omega-3 fish oil capsule that contains 500–1000mg of EPA plus DHA daily.
- 5-Hydroxy Tryptophan (5-HTP) helps raise serotonin levels in the brain. Extracted from the Griffonia plant from Africa, 5-HTP helps balance mood, helps you to fall asleep more easily, reduces aggression, reduces appetite and creates a more relaxed waking state within 45 minutes. Recommended dose: 50mg up to 300mg per day. For best results, start on a low dosage; take at bedtime along with a small carbohydrate snack, such as an oat cake. If you need to, gradually work up to 3000mg. If your mood stabilises, gradually lower the dose until you find how much you need. Taking more than you need will not be helpful in the long run. This supplement is more effective if taken with B-vitamins and 10mg of zinc. Be patient as it can take a few weeks for the full effects of 5-HTP to work.
- Try Patrick Holford's Mood Formula, which contains amino acids, zinc, B-vitamins and 5-HTP. Available from all good health shops or Higher Nature. **HN**
- In a study DHEA hormone supplementation was tested on middle-aged and elderly patients with major depression for 4 weeks. Depression ratings and memory performance significantly improved. DHEA in other human studies significantly elevated mood in elderly people. Recommended dose: 50mg a day for men and 15–20mg per day for women – not available in the UK unless you have a prescription but DHEA can be bought freely in health shops in the US or log on to www.lef.org or www.pharmwest.com. (See also *Menopause*.)

- SAMe (S-Adenosylmethionine) acts as a natural antidepressant. It can give good effects within a week, but should be taken for 5–6 weeks for optimum results. Ask for a good-quality, enteric-coated supplement, which tends to be more stable. 200mg twice daily.
- Ginseng is an adrenal tonic that is useful for people that are depressed as their adrenal glands (see *Stress*) are usually functioning under par. Take two Panax Red Ginseng capsules, one with breakfast and one with lunch; and avoid taking before bed time.
- The herb St John's wort has been proven to help milder forms of depression. In more than 25 double blind studies of more than 1,500 people, St John's wort demonstrated its effectiveness in improving mood, lessening anxiety and reducing sleep disorders. St John's wort helps to reduce the sadness, stress and feelings of helplessness from depression. Recommended dosage: 900mg daily of 0.3 percent hypericin concentration, 600mg with breakfast and 300mg with lunch. Do not take St John's wort if you are pregnant or on the Pill and avoid intense sun exposure while using it, since this herb can make the skin more sensitive to sunlight. Do not take St John's wort with 5-HTP and drugs such as Prozac, Zoloft and Paxil.
- The herb rhodiola, grown in Siberia, has been shown to help protect against the negative affects of the stress hormone cortisol, it increases energy levels and, most importantly for anyone suffering depression, rhodiola helps the brain to make serotonin a key neurotransmitter which makes you feel happier and more positive. Low levels of serotonin trigger depression and low moods. Kudos make a high strength one-a-day rhodiola. **KVH**

Helpful Hints

- Natural sunlight helps to suppress production of the hormone melatonin and improves immune function. This hormone is produced by the pineal gland at night, hence why we tend to feel more depressed and sleepy during the winter months. Melatonin aids sleep and acts as an important antioxidant, but if you are depressed then you need less melatonin. Therefore, get out into daylight as much as you possibly can, especially in the mornings, and if you work in an office without full-spectrum lighting, make sure you use full-spectrum light bulbs at home and where you can at work. They last for ages and use less electricity. Available from most stores or call Higher Nature. **HN**
- Regular exercise is vital in the fight against depression. I know of one New York doctor who asks all his depressed patients to walk for 30 minutes in sunshine and then to tell him how they feel. This is because exercise and sunlight releases endorphins, natural antidepressants, which raise your mood. Regular exercise can help you sleep better, feel better, look better, and provide you with an enhanced self-image. A German study showed a significant reduction in depression when patients walked for 30 minutes a day and other studies show that regular exercise is as effective as antidepressants and more effective against relapse than drugs.
- Studies have shown that having control over roles such as being a parent, grandparent or provider can add value to an elderly person's life. Many companies are at last waking up to the fact that people over 65 are more committed, take less time off sick, and are more experienced workers who tend to be more cost effective than younger people. Take charge of your life!
- Ask your doctor if you can see a counsellor – a problem shared is a problem halved; and counselling is often far more successful than taking antidepressants. Talk your innermost fears through with a friend or relative, they may not even realise you are depressed. For details of your nearest qualified counsellor contact the British Association for Counselling, BACP House, 15 St John's Business Park, Lutterworth LE17 4HB. Tel: 0870 4435252. Website: www.bacp.co.uk
- Do volunteer work as helping others can boost self-esteem.
- Watch videos, DVDs and films that make you laugh. Laughter produces natural mood-boosting chemicals in the body.

- Be sure to get enough quality sleep, but get up after 8 hours or so.
- Blend pure oils of bergamot, clary sage, geranium and neroli in a base of almond oil and ask a friend or relative to give you a massage. These aromatherapy oils help lift your mood. For details of Therapeutic Grade Essential Oils see page 15.
- Hypnotherapy and Neuro Linguistic Programming (NLP) has helped many people (see *Useful Information*).
- For further help read *Optimum Nutrition for the Mind* by Patrick Holford (Piatkus).
- MIND is the leading mental health charity in England and Wales and has lots of local centres throughout the UK. Find them through the MIND information line. Tel: 0845 766 0163, or check out their website at www.mind.org.uk

DERMATITIS – Seborrheic dermatitis (Cradle cap)
(see also *Eczema*)

Seborrheic dermatitis is basically a type of eczema that commonly occurs on children's scalps. This is why it's often known as cradle cap. In most infants it tends to clear up in the first year or so. Symptoms are thick scaly tissue on the scalp in particular and sometimes around the eyes and ears. The problem is linked to a deficiency in essential fatty acids and one of the B-vitamins, biotin. Eliminating allergens from the diet usually helps clear cradle cap. You can also suffer varying degrees of dermatitis in adult years – triggered by exposure to hair colourants, paints, hairsprays and all manner of chemicals in cosmetic products and household cleaners and detergents. Non-specific skin rashes can also be linked to liver toxicity (see *Liver Problems*) and food intolerances (see *Allergies*).

Foods to Avoid
- The most common offending foods for causing cradle cap are cow's milk and produce, wheat and eggs. As with any problem which may be influenced by food intolerances, it is important to identify which are the problematic foods. Generally the child's diet needs to be cleaned up. (See *Allergies*.)
- Avoid mass-produced, refined, white-flour based foods and any foods and drinks that are high in sugar.

Friendly Foods
- Make your child nutrient-rich fruit blends – add any fruit you have to hand such as bananas, kiwi, raspberries etc. and put them in a blender with a tablespoon of sunflower seeds and flax seeds (linseeds; rich in essential fats). Add a low-fat, live fruit yoghurt such as Rachel's (available from most supermarkets) and whiz for 30–40 seconds. This makes a healthy dessert.
- Oils such as Udo's Choice, which is a perfect blend of omega-3 and -6 fats, can be added to food once cooked – a teaspoon a day should be fine. I find that if you cook some sweet potatoes and mash them with a little skimmed milk and then add the oil as they are cooling, the child cannot taste the oil. Otherwise add to thick vegetable soups and stews before serving.
- For adults with dermatitis, eat plenty of fruits, vegetables, whole grains such as brown rice or quinoa, barley and oily fish. See *General Health Hints*.

Useful Remedies
- Many companies make liquid multi-vitamins and minerals for children, which you can add to cold dishes to make sure your child is not malnourished. Nature's Plus makes an excellent children's range. **NP**

- Alternatively you can add organic source green food powders rich in vitamins, minerals and essential fats to breakfast cereals or desserts.
- Biotin, a B vitamin that is often lacking – 6mg daily.
- If the child is being breast fed it is useful for the mother to take 10mg of biotin – which will in turn be delivered through the milk – or eat more biotin rich foods, such as liver and egg yolk.
- Essential fats can be applied directly to the affected areas. It should be applied twice a day for 2–4 weeks. Use either evening primrose or borage oil. You can also take 2000mg of evening primrose oil daily.
- As all the B-vitamins work together in the body, if you are breast-feeding or an adult with this condition, also take 1 high-strength, B-complex daily.
- Adults should take a high strength multi-vitamin and mineral plus an essential-fatty-acid formula daily. See details of Kudos 24 in *General Supplements*, p.160. **KVH**

Helpful Hints

- Note that many toothpastes, shampoos, soaps, detergents, perfumes etc. contain a myriad of chemicals. I have met several dozen hairdressers who suffer this condition caused by all the chemicals they are in contact with daily.
- Apply a little Manuka honey cream from Living Nature or the Organic Skin Rescue Oil from the Organic Pharmacy. Or contact their pharmacist who can suggest a specific remedy for your particular symptoms. **OP**
- Buy products in their most natural and unadulterated state which are gentler on a child's delicate skin. For anyone who suffers dermatitis or skin allergies, The Green People Company makes organic skin, hair, body lotions, sun screens, and toothpaste and also have an advice line. Tel: 01444 401444. Email: organic@greenpeople.co.uk Website: www.greenpeople.co.uk
- Use aloe vera gel topically to help calm the itching.

DEEP VEIN THROMBOSIS   (see *Jet Lag*)

DIABETES – Types I and II
(see also *Circulation, Insulin Resistance* and *Weight Problems*)

The World Health Organisation states that the number of people with diabetes will more than double from 120 million today to 300 million in just over one generation. The tragedy is that 'late-onset' diabetes is now occurring in children as young as 13 who are eating too much junk food, and has become a health time bomb. Make no mistake late-onset diabetes can shorten your life and yet it is totally preventable. A staggering fact that you may like to keep in mind is that the average adult eats 60lbs (27kg) of sugar a year.

Type II Diabetes is also known as late-onset diabetes, and now affects more than 2 million people in the UK alone and accounts for 90% of diabetes cases.

It is the fourth leading cause of death in the UK, which costs the NHS almost £6 billion a year to treat. Three quarters of cases are triggered by being overweight, resulting from our over-consumption of refined, sugar-based carbohydrate foods such as cakes, biscuits and sugar filled fizzy drinks. The rarer Type I Diabetes is a life-long condition, which usually starts during early childhood. Both types of diabetes involve too high a level of sugar in the blood. The hormone insulin is responsible for lowering blood sugar levels. Whereas Type I is caused by the failure of the pancreas to secrete adequate insulin, Type II Diabetes is generally characterised by too much insulin, but the body has become resistant to it and simply doesn't respond to the insulin as it should. Therefore, despite high levels of insulin, glucose is not properly transported into the cells and it increases to unacceptable levels in the blood. Your body tries to get rid of excess sugar in the urine, hence why doctors test for diabetes through urine, although a blood test is more accurate.

Diabetes can trigger heart, brain, eye and arterial problems and the life-expectancy of an individual with diabetes is therefore considerably below what it should be. Also the risk of heart disease in diabetics is up to 3 times greater than in those who do not have the disease. While diabetes can have a hereditary link, your genes interact with your environment (including your diet) to either improve or worsen your health. We can inherit more from our parents than just their genes, their eating habits are often passed on too.

The main symptoms of diabetes are excessive thirst, frequent urination, increased appetite, fatigue and loss of weight. Other symptoms, though less common, include muscle cramps, blurred vision, itchy skin and poor wound-healing. If you are diagnosed as diabetic by your doctor with blood and urine tests, you will very likely be offered various courses of action. In mild cases, late-onset diabetes can be kept in check by diet alone. If severe, the diet is accompanied by oral medication or injections to either increase the production of insulin or improve your sensitivity to insulin. Over the years I have interviewed many elderly diabetics and have been appalled that they have not been offered any advice on diet and yet most cases of late-onset diabetes can be kept in check by eating a healthier diet. It's worth noting that if you suffer thrush regularly – you may be diabetic.

Foods to Avoid

- See also diet in *Insulin Resistance*.
- Avoid sugar and foods containing sugar, such as fizzy drinks, chocolate, desserts and sweets, which release their sugars too quickly into the bloodstream.
- Avoid all refined, mass produced 'white' flour and rice-based foods such as pizza, white rice and pastas, white breads, cakes and biscuits which are usually high in sugar and saturated fats.
- Honey, maltose, dextrose are still sugars and can exacerbate the problem.
- Beware that most foods advertised as being low in fat are often high in sugar.
- Don't drink concentrated shop bought fruit juices. Make fresh juices or dilute no added sugar juices with two parts juice to one part water.
- Reduce saturated fats from animal sources to less than 10% of daily food intake.
- Basically cut out red meats or only eat occasional lean steak and lamb.
- Reduce your use of sodium-based table salts, look for magnesium rich sea salts and only add a little to the food on your plate.
- Too much iron and copper in the body increases the risk of diabetes and heart disease – read labels especially on fortified cereals – and cut right down on red meat. Eat more curcumin (turmeric), which detoxifies the body of these metals.

Friendly Foods

- Eat more unrefined, high-fibre carbohydrates such as wholemeal bread, brown rice, buckwheat, oats (especially porridge), jacket potatoes plus low-fat proteins such as beans, pulses, lentils and barley.
- Fruits and vegetables are high in antioxidants and soluble fibre; eat them raw as much as possible.
- Fish oils have been shown to improve the pre-diabetic condition and insulin resistance, and help to prevent full-blown late-onset diabetes developing, therefore eat more oily fish and fresh fish. But don't fry it – poached or grilled is best.
- Eat more unrefined sunflower, pumpkin, sesame and linseeds (flax seeds) and their unrefined oils, which are rich in omega-3 and -6 essential fats.

- Blend these oils half and half with extra virgin olive oil for salad dressings.
- Vitamin E-rich foods help to lower the risk of many conditions associated with diabetes such as circulation and eye problems. Food sources are soya beans, raw wheat germ, sprouting seeds, avocados, green vegetables, eggs, unrefined and unprocessed nuts especially almonds and hazelnuts. Look for a low-sugar muesli that is rich in nuts, oats and sprinkle raw wheat germ onto the muesli.
- Eat fresh bilberries, blueberries and blackberries when in season, or use frozen, as these fruits help to protect the eyes.
- You need to eat more foods with a low glycaemic index (GI), such as wholemeal breads and pastas, brown rice, rye bread, oats, fresh fruits, kidney beans, dried beans, lentils, chickpeas and green vegatebales (see *Low Blood Sugar* for a larger list).
- Use lots of cinnamon in your foods – as it has been shown to help reduce glucose levels in the blood.

Useful Remedies
- A high-strength, multi-vitamin and mineral complex taken every day provides a good baseline of nutrients. See Kudos 24 in *General Supplements*, p.160. **KVH**
- The mineral chromium (200mcg) is vital for helping to control and prevent late-onset diabetes. Scientists in the US found that taking 200mcg of chromium daily helped reduce the incidence of late-onset diabetes by up to 50%. Chromium also helps to reduce cravings for sweet foods. And in time, chromium should enable you to reduce·your medication, which you would need to discuss with your doctor.
- Vitamin C 1000mg twice daily can lower glucose response.
- Magnesium, which is needed to process insulin, is usually lacking in diabetics. Take a multi-mineral daily that contains 300–450mg of magnesium, 20mg zinc, and a trace of copper.
- Take a B-complex, as diabetic patients are usually deficient in B-vitamins, needed for energy production and nerve health.
- If you don't eat oily fish regularly then take a 1 gram fish-oil capsule daily and make sure it is free from PCBs and dioxins. BioCare, Higher Nature, FSC and Seven Seas all make pure fish oil capsules. **BC HN FSC**
- Alpha lipoic acid has also been shown to improve insulin action. Take 50–60mg daily.
- The hormone DHEA (see *Menopause*) helps to lower insulin levels, and protect vital organs, particularly the kidneys against damage due to high blood glucose. Never take hormones unless you have been shown to need them.
- Aloe vera juice helps to lower blood-sugar levels in non-insulin dependant diabetes.
- **NB:** taking supplements can affect blood sugar levels. Diabetes must be supervised by a medical practitioner, so any supplement regimen should only be undertaken with the help of a medical doctor and/or a nutritionist.
- Nettle tea helps to lower blood sugar.

Helpful Hints
- If you are overweight you greatly increase your risk for diabetes, especially after 50 (see *Weight Problems*).
- Exercise is vital because it reduces the need for insulin, reduces blood cholesterol and prevents obesity. It doesn't have to be intense exercise, but try and walk for at least 30 minutes daily, as regular walking has been shown to improve insulin sensitivity and glucose management. If you have been a "couch potato" for a long time, just start gently, walk for 15 minutes a day and then build up over a month to 30 minutes daily and within another month this can be increased to 45 minutes to an hour. Get a dog! And keep in mind that regularity is crucial.
- Don't go overboard on sweet foods that claim to be suitable for diabetics. It's very likely your

d

attraction to sweets that got you into this mess, so it's time to retrain your taste buds and kick the sweet habit. A little of these foods on occasion is fine, but the 'suitable for diabetics' label is not an open invitation.

- Have regular eye check-ups and see a chiropodist who can keep an eye on your feet, as both can be affected by diabetes.
- Have regular reflexology on your feet, which improves circulation (see *Useful Information*).
- For further help contact Diabetes UK, Macleod House, 10, Parkway, London NW1 7AA. Tel: 020 7424 1000. Website: www.diabetes.org.uk
- Try reading *How To Prevent and Treat Diabetes with Natural Medicine* by Dr Michael Murray. Call the Nutri Centre bookshop on 020 7323 2382, or have a look at the author's website on www.doctormurray.com

DIARRHOEA (see also *IBS*)

Diarrhoea can have several causes including infectious bacteria, food poisoning, food allergy or intolerance, IBS or yeast overgrowth (see also *Candida*). It may also be associated with more serious conditions like Crohn's disease and ulcerative colitis. If it is a chronic problem it is more likely to be associated with a food intolerance or a parasite. Severe diarrhoea, especially in babies and children, must be treated quickly, as the body can rapidly become dehydrated and the person can eventually lose consciousness. Adequate intake of fluids, particularly water, and electrolyte sachet drinks should be given hourly to prevent severe dehydration. Babies and children must see a doctor.

Foods to Avoid
- Certain foods can aggravate the problem, for example, concentrated fruit juices could make the situation worse.
- Avoid sorbitol, which is used as a sweetening agent.
- Lactose, the sugar in milk, is a common cause of chronic diarrhoea.
- If you are a regular coffee-drinker, it's worth giving it up for a few days to see if this helps.
- Many people who have a sensitivity to wheat and gluten suffer chronic diarrhoea. See also *Leaky Gut*.

Friendly Foods
- Although we tend to associate fibre with ensuring adequate bowel movement and frequency, it can also help to control diarrhoea as the fibre will give bulk to the stool. Try soluble fibres like oat or rice bran, linseeds (flax seeds), psyllium husks, and plenty of water or electrolyte drinks.
- Drinking 3–4 cups of camomile or black tea a day has been used for many centuries as a gentle way of dealing with diarrhoea.
- Eating either dried bilberries or bilberry juice can also help (but not fresh bilberries as they can actually aggravate the problem).
- Fresh vegetable soups with a little root ginger, or a small portion of poached fish and brown rice are usually well tolerated. Move onto solids only when symptoms begin to ease as sometimes diarrhoea is your body's digestive system telling you it needs a rest.
- Eat plenty of low-fat, live yoghurt to replenish healthy bacteria in the bowel.
- Drink plenty of cooled, boiled water or ginger ale.
- For acute diarrhoea, grate an apple, let it go brown and then eat it. Greenish bananas are very binding.
- Slippery elm powder can be mashed into a paste with banana and honey.

Useful Remedies

- Whilst symptoms last take 15,000iu of vitamin A daily for one week (but no more than 3000iu if pregnant), as it helps protect the lining of the gut. Plus 30mg of zinc, as lack of zinc has been shown to trigger diarrhoea.
- Thereafter, take a good-quality vitamin/mineral to help prevent malnutrition. See details of Kudos 24 in *General Supplements*, p.160. **KVH**
- The herb pau d'arco or propolis help kill many harmful organisms. Take 2–3ml of tincture 2 or 3 times a day, or 1 gram of capsules 2–3 times a day.
- If you are susceptible to diarrhoea when you travel abroad, taking acidophilus for two weeks prior to your trip can help increase the number of healthy bacteria in the gut which reduces the risk of picking up a tummy bug.
- Floraguard by BioCare contains healthy bacteria plus garlic, oregano oil, clove oil and cinnamon and rosemary. It can be taken daily with food when you are abroad to help kill off any invading bacteria. It can be very handy for holidays, but do not take it if you are pregnant. **BC**
- Bee propolis, grapefruit seed extract and olive leaf extract are all natural anti-bacterials.

Helpful Hints

- Drink water from cooked brown rice or mix 15 grams of carob powder with some apple purée to make it palatable. Carob has a history of helping alleviate diarrhoea.
- Potter's make a Spanish Tummy Mixture containing herbs and tinctures to heal the gut. Available from all good health stores. To find your nearest stockist call Potter's (Herbal Supplies) Ltd Tel: 01942 219960. Website: www.pottersherbal.co.uk
- Stabilised liquid oxygen helps to re-alkalise the body, encourages healthy bacteria in the gut and has been shown to kill bacteria such as E-coli, and some viruses, parasites and fungi.
- Never drink tap water unless you are sure it is safe to do so. Avoid salads and fruit washed in local tap water in places like India, Africa, the Far East and in any country you think the water may be questionable. Avoid ice cubes made from local tap water. Eat only thoroughly cooked foods. Use bottled water and fizzy drinks but only if they have sealed tops.
- If the diarrhoea resembles water coming out of a hose try homeopathic Podophyllum 30c every few hours for a day. Charcoal tablets are also useful for stopping diaorrhea.
- For teething children who have this problem use homeopathic Chamomila 30c, 3 times daily.
- If you suffer persistent diarrhoea, you must see a doctor.

DIVERTICULAR DISEASE or DIVERTICULITIS

Diverticulitis is a disease of modern Western civilization as it rarely occurs in people or cultures that eat a high-fibre diet. It occurs when the mucous membranes lining the colon form small finger-like pouches, known as diverticula, that protrude out of the intestinal wall. 30–40% of people over the age of 60 have diverticular disease and generally these pouches do not cause problems. If, however, they become inflamed and infected diverticulitis results, it causes extreme pain – primarily in the descending colon, which is situated on the left-hand side of the abdomen. Symptoms include pain, bleeding, diarrhoea and fever. Chronic constipation is the most common underlying cause of this condition as a soft, bulky stool is easy to push along the colon and a hard, dry stool makes the muscles of the colon work too hard. Most sufferers tend not to drink sufficient water and ingest insufficient fibre (see also *Constipation*). Occasionally, a pouch may burst, which requires urgent medical attention.

Foods to Avoid

- Foods containing seeds like tomatoes, grapes and strawberries, and poppy, sesame and pumpkin seeds as the seeds can lodge in the pockets and cause a lot of pain.
- Although fibre is necessary for a normal bowel movement the abrasive fibres in wheat bran or high-fibre breakfast cereals such as All Bran can temporarily aggravate the problem.
- For many people wheat found in bread, cakes, biscuits, pizza bases, pasta and so on, can have a constipating effect – try avoiding these foods for 2 weeks to see if it helps.
- Avoid fried or spicy foods.
- Reduce saturated fats such as full-fat milk, cheese and chocolates as these can trigger inflammation, are mucus forming and can make constipation worse.
- Avoid as much as possible white bread and pasta, white rice, cakes, biscuits, take-aways and mass-produced burger-type foods.
- Greatly reduce your intake of red meat, which takes a long time to pass through the bowel.
- Whilst symptoms are acute also avoid all yeast-based foods including Marmite, Bovril, cheese, soy sauce, vinegar and so on.
- Avoid all sweeteners containing fructose, sorbitol and aspartame.
- Carageenan is a milk protein stabilizer often used in ice cream, that causes problems for people with digestive/bowel problems.
- Tea, coffee, fizzy drinks and alcohol all dehydrate the bowel.

Friendly Foods

- When the bowel is inflamed, eat soothing foods such as vegetable soups with cabbage, celery, ginger and whey protein plus lightly stewed apples, apricots, prunes, papaya and porridge made with non-dairy light soya, almond or rice milk.
- Once the inflammation is under control introduce a little steamed or grilled fish and low-fat meat such as skinless poultry.
- Gradually increase your intake of high-fibre foods such as brown rice, bread and wheat free pasta, fresh vegetables, pulses, oat-based cereals and fruit (especially figs). There are many excellent organic high-fibre mueslis and cereals made from ancient grains such as amaranth, kamut and quinoa.
- Live, low-fat yoghurt containing acidophilus and bifidus helps maintain the level of bacteria in the bowel and stool, which encourages regular bowel movement.
- Drink at least 8 glasses of water daily to make sure there is adequate fluid in the bowel.
- Use extra virgin unrefined olive or sunflower oils for your salad dressings.
- Eat garlic for its antiseptic qualities.
- Add ginger to foods and juices, which soothes and heals the gut.
- If you cook cabbage, leave the cooking water to cool and then drink. This is rich in cabigin, a nutrient that helps to heal the bowel.

Useful Remedies

- 2–5 grams of psyllium husks with plenty of water once the inflammation is under control.
- The anti-inflammatory essential oils found in evening primrose oil also promote healing and repair; take 1000–2000mg daily. **BC**
- Add half a cup of aloe vera juice to fresh vegetable juices daily to help heal the gut, soothe the mucous membranes and increase bowel movements.
- Slippery elm is gentle, soothing and nourishing to the digestive lining. Drink as a tea, chew on the bark, or take 2–3 tablets before meals. Contact Specialist Herbal Supplies, who make pure slippery elm tea and they can recommend specific herbs for your particular symptoms. **SHS**
- Good bacteria (acidophilus/bifidus) can help fight infection whilst it is active and help to reduce constipation. During a flare-up take 2 capsules three times per day. To protect for the future,

take 1 capsule twice a day.
- Vitamin A heals soft tissue. Take 10,000iu daily for three weeks (if pregnant only 3,000iu).
- UltraInflamX is a pleasant-tasting easily absorbed liquid multi that is also designed to reduce inflammation in the body. Take 2 scoops in juice or water or add to smoothies. Available from www.positivehealthshop.com
- Calcium fluoride tissue salts help to strengthen the intestinal walls. Take 4 daily.

Helpful Hints
- Exercising regularly – gentle walking and swimming helps to work the stomach muscles and encourages bowel movements.
- Leave time to visit the loo – relax and don't rush.
- Remember to drink plenty of water as this helps to prevent constipation – 6–8 glasses per day. These are best drunk away from meals so that they don't dilute the digestive juices that are needed to thoroughly break down food. See *Constipation*.
- Stress makes any digestive, gut or bowel problem worse. Look at your lifestyle and take time out to practise yoga or T'ai Chi.
- Enemas using either a solution of colloidal silver (from Higher Nature), diluted in lukewarm water, or saline, can help to fast track healing. You can buy home enema kits from all large pharmacies.
- An informative website can be found at www.digestive.niddk.nih.gov
- Lots of useful fact sheets about diverticular disease can be found at www.corecharity.org.uk, or you can contact them at CORE, 3 St Andrews Place, London NW1 4LB. Tel: 020 7486 0341.

DIZZY SPELLS   *(see Low Blood Sugar, Low Blood Pressure and Vertigo)*

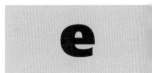

EARACHE   *(see also Glue Ear, Ménière's Syndrome, Tinnitus and Vertigo)*

Most earaches are caused by the build-up of fluid in the middle ear, which can lead to an infection causing pain, fever or loss of hearing. Children under the age of 5 are particularly prone to ear infections, usually triggered by a sensitivity to foods such as corn, eggs, peanuts, cow's milk and wheat. Cow's milk and milk products are without doubt the most likely culprit. I have vivid memories as a child screaming with chronic earache until eventually both my ear drums burst. My poor mother had no idea that it was our diet of milk, cream trifles, cheese, chocolate treats and lots of lard and dripping (solidified beef, lamb and pork fat) sandwiches that caused the problem. I was prescribed almost continuous antibiotics, which undoubtedly contributed to my acne, thrush and chronic fatigue during my teens. So if you have young children, try as much as possible to avoid antibiotics by changing your child's diet and give supplements to boost their immune function.

Cutting sugar also helps, as most foods containing saturated fats also contain sugar, which converts to fat within the body if not used up during exercise. Note that many yoghurts and 'low-fat' foods are high in sugar! If the earache is persistent, many doctors suggest insertion of grommets through minor surgery but in the majority of cases this procedure can be avoided. To make sure your child does not become malnourished, I suggest you consult a qualified nutritionist. (See *Useful Information*.)

Foods to Avoid
- Any food to which there is a sensitivity, particularly dairy from cows plus wheat based foods and eggs.
- Generally whilst symptoms are acute avoid mucus forming foods, such as chocolate, milks, cheese and so on, but note that any foods to which you have an intolerance will trigger mucus production.
- Avoid sugar as it tends to weaken the immune system and leaves children more susceptible to infections. This includes fizzy drinks and desserts, which are often packed with sugar
- Excessive amounts of fruit juice as these are often citrus-based which sometimes adds to the problem. Remember that most canned fizzy drinks contain up to 10 tsp of sugar, and never use drinks containing aspartame as they place too much of a strain on the liver which can further exacerbate the problem.

Friendly Foods
- Once you have identified any problem foods such as cow's milk, look for alternatives such as oat, rice or almond milk. I would not recommend soya milk and foods for any child under the age of 5 years.
- There are plenty of wheat-free pastas now available based on lentils, quinoa, rice, corn and vegetables.
- Bread can be replaced by rye or rice bread, or rice, rye or amaranth crackers, cakes and oatcakes.
- Eat plenty of fruit and vegetables to keep the immune system in good shape, particularly those rich in the carotenoids like sweet potatoes, carrots and spinach. Other useful foods for the immune system are cauliflower, broccoli and Brussels sprouts.

Useful Remedies
- The herb echinacea, if used as a tincture use one drop per 13lbs (6kg) of body-weight. Take 3–4 times a day for up to 3 weeks at any one time.
- To help fight infection and boost immunity, take up to 1 gram of vitamin C with food daily, preferably as a powder dissolved in diluted low-sugar apple juice.
- Children's multi-vitamin and minerals to make sure children are not deficient in any nutrients, which can impair their immune system. Nature's Plus makes an excellent children's range. **NP**
- As antibiotics destroy healthy bacteria, encourage your children to eat non-dairy, low-fat live yoghurts once daily, containing the friendly bacteria acidophilus. If they hate the taste of plain yoghurt, add any fresh fruit you have to hand and whiz in the blender for a few seconds. Make low-sugar jellies with fresh fruit juices and serve with low-fat yoghurt instead of ice cream.

Helpful Hints
- If parents smoke, it is definitely worth them trying to cut back or not smoking near the children as this has been strongly linked to the development of ear infections.
- A warm hot-water bottle wrapped in a towel can be placed by the ear. Or buy a wheat bag – and warm through, then place near the ears.
- Warm an onion and place the core of the onion just inside the affected ear wrapped in muslin, or squeeze a **small** amount of onion water into the ear. Onion and garlic are natural decongestants.
- Homeopathic Pulsatilla 30c or Belladonna 30c every 3–4 hours helps if the earache is in the right ear.
- If in the left ear try Hepar Sulph 30c.

- If there is a sticky discharge try Kali Bic 6x.
- Do not let a child swim under water if their ears become infected.
- Children who are given dummies are more prone to ear infections.
- Consult an allergy specialist who can test for food intolerances, which can exacerbate and trigger this problem.
- See a cranial osteopath or chiropractor to check the alignment of the head and neck, as mis-alignment and poor drainage can cause earache (see *Useful Information*).
- For irritations in the ears and sinuses, mucus and catarrh, use ear candles, which gently remove excess ear wax without pain. Excellent for children as they are fun to use and not painful. Available from all good health stores, or for details call 020 7976 6615 or 01895 629950.

ECZEMA   (see also *Allergies, Asthma, Leaky Gut, Irritable Bowel* and *Liver Problems*)

Eczema affects 6 million people in the UK alone. It is often an inherited condition that is linked to asthma and rhinitis – a blocked or runny nose. During flare-ups the skin can become very inflamed, itchy and sometimes develops into open bleeding sores. It is sometimes triggered by an external irritant, such as perfumes, washing powders, shampoos (how many hairdressers have you seen with eczema on their hands and arms?), paint, house dust mites, or cat hairs; but most commonly it is linked to a food intolerance (as many as 80% of sufferers show a positive reaction to allergy-testing) or a leaky gut.

Eczema can appear at any age seemingly from nowhere. It tends to be aggravated by stress, exhaustion, sometimes by heat and frequently by exercise. Eczema does tend to come and go and people find it difficult to track down the trigger. For most people, symptoms worsen when they are under stress, but others notice that it is aggravated by certain foods especially sugar, wheat, orange juice and cow's milk, or drinking too much tea or coffee. If it starts in early childhood, the most likely culprit is cow's milk and products. Either the child has been fed formula milk or the residues are ingested via the mother's breast milk. The commonest triggers for eczema in babies are dairy products, eggs, citrus and wheat. Avoidance of the offending food often resolves the problem.

It is very important to remember that by the time the eczema shows up on the skin it has worked its way through the body and you really need to address the root cause of the problem. With any skin condition it is a good idea to support the liver, which is the most important cleansing organ of the body. If the liver becomes overloaded with toxins it tends to start dumping them into the skin, so anything you can do to keep your liver functioning more efficiently will in the long term help your skin.

I'm embarrassed to say that I broke out in eczema on my arm when I was under tremendous stress finishing a book! And these days I have learned how to control it, but occasionally if I eat too much wheat or cow's milk **and** become too stressed then one small patch breaks out on my chest. Along the way I met a wonderful dermatologist – Dr Anne Maguire – who told me that in her 50 years experience she has found that people who tend to suffer eczema on their chests have a problem speaking up for themselves, they don't tend to like confrontation, and that the eczema is like the body 'getting its negative stuff out'. Dr Maguire says that eczema is literally 'the skin weeping', and often once you get to the root cause of any emotional blockages, and look after your diet, the eczema will disappear. Interesting – as I do indeed hold anger in, which affects the liver, which in turn affects the skin.

Also, drugs such as Ibuprofen have been known to trigger an attack in some people, as this drug can cause a leaky gut.

Foods to Avoid

- Avoid all dairy products from cows, as well as coffee, tea, chocolate, beef, citrus fruits, eggs, wheat, alcohol, tomatoes and peanuts. This is a long list of foods, but if you have eczema and cut out all of these foods, the eczema is virtually guaranteed to improve.
- It is important to note that even decaffeinated coffee causes problems in people who are sensitive to coffee – it's not just the caffeine. The solvent used to extract the caffeine can affect a number of skin conditions.
- As much as possible, avoid preservatives, additives, pesticides, food colourings (such as in the bright red glacé cherries on fancy cakes) and refined sugar-based, mass-produced cakes, biscuits and pies (see also *Allergies*).

Friendly Foods

- Wherever possible go organic and eat plenty of fresh fruits and vegetables.
- Include lots of cabbage in your diet – and drink any water the cabbage has been cooked in. It contains L-glutamine, which helps to heal a leaky gut.
- Beetroot, artichokes, celeriac, celery and radicchio are foods that cleanse the liver. If you cannot bear to eat freshly picked dandelions from your local fields then it is easily available in a tincture.
- Pear juice is a good alternative to orange juice.
- If you react to cow's milk, there are plenty of alternatives such as low-fat soya, rice, oat and buffalo milk all of which have a much lower incidence of reaction, taste good and mostly work fine in cooking.
- Sugar-free, live sheep's or soya yoghurt will help digestion and reduce the risk of a leaky gut.
- Oily fish can be particularly beneficial as the essential fatty acids in fish are anti-inflammatory and have been shown to improve eczema conditions. Eat 3 times weekly as long as you are not intolerant to it.
- Try eating plenty of seeds – sunflower seeds, sesame seeds, linseeds (flax seeds) and pumpkin seeds – and nuts with the exception of peanuts. The fatty acids and high levels of zinc and protein in these foods will help nourish the skin and speed up the healing process.
- Wheat germ (not the same as refined wheat) and avocados are rich in vitamin E, which also aids healing.
- Use extra virgin olive oil, plus unrefined walnut and sunflower oil in salad dressings.
- Use non-hydrogenated spreads such as Biona and Vitaquell in preference to mass produced hard fats (see also *Fats You Need To Eat*).
- Fill up your plate with colour – orangey-coloured fruit and veg contain beta carotene the vegetable source of vitamin A, known to be beneficial to skin health. Try squashes, sweet potatoes, pumpkin, cantaloupe melon, peppers, carrots and apricots

Useful Remedies

- There is now good research showing that people who take healthy bacteria (probiotics) regularly are less likely to suffer eczema, as healthy bacteria help improve digestion and reduce any immune response. Have a word with the nutritionist at BioCare or at your local health store to find which pro-biotic would suit you best. **BC**
- Evening primrose oil 1–4 grams a day. This is the one supplement with the most research showing benefits in eczema – it is also available on prescription.
- Also take 400iu of full-spectrum, natural-source vitamin E daily. The vitamin E will also help prevent scarring and itching.
- The mineral zinc is needed to ensure adequate absorption of fatty acids, and it's invariably deficient in eczema sufferers. It also speeds skin-healing – 30mg twice daily for a couple of months then reduce to 20mg per day.
- Research shows selenium levels are low in people with inflammatory conditions such as eczema.

Make sure your multi provides 200mcg as it works well with vitamin E.

- Vitamin A is really important for skin-healing – once a month for a week if you are not pregnant or planning a pregnancy, take 20,000iu of vitamin A daily to boost levels in the body. If pregnant then 3000iu is fine daily.
- Include a high-strength multi-vitamin and mineral that includes a full spectrum of B-vitamins, which help reduce stress, and improve digestion and the absorption of fatty acids. Try Kudos 24 (details in *General Supplements*; p.160), which comes as a highly absorbable powder.
- Burdock and nettle tincture; take 10–20 drops 3–4 times a day. This tincture should help to reduce the itching and help cleanse the liver. Burdock could appear initially to make the condition worse as it encourages the eczema to leave the body. If this happens, reduce the dose dramatically and start gently, maybe just taking it once a day and gradually pick it up until you are comfortable with the rate of progress. **FSC**
- Nettle works as a mild antihistamine, which can reduce the itching. This tincture can be applied both externally and taken internally. Ideally, do not apply to broken skin as the small amount of alcohol would sting the skin. For young children use 1 drop per 13lbs (6kg) of body weight – this will ensure you don't give them too much.
- The herb milk thistle has been shown to help regenerate and support liver function. Either take 500mg twice daily with meals; or Kudos make a 900mg one-a-day capsule. **KVH**
- Omega 7 fats extracted from sea buckthorn berries are highly effective at relieving dry skin. Made by Pharma Nord. Their advice line is freephone 0800 591756. **PN**

Helpful Hints

- Many people have found that aloe vera juice taken internally and the gel used topically has proved helpful for eczema.
- Allergenics cream is available from Health Imports. This cream soothes the majority of cases and some people have said it has actually cleared their eczema up. For details, call Wellbeing 08707 479131.
- Do something positive to help relieve the stress that may aggravating the eczema. Try meditation, yoga, T'ai Chi, or some other means of relaxation. If you can, get away and bask in some sunshine – and salt water, which usually aids eczema.
- If you have access to and can afford a reflexology treatment or aromatherapy massage, not only will the oils improve the condition but they are also incredibly relaxing. A few drops of essential oils of lavender, Roman camomile, geranium, rose and cedarwood mixed in a good base carrier oil such as calendula can be applied to the affected areas.
- Exercise is generally beneficial for both reducing stress and improving the condition, however, wear lightweight, cotton, loose fitting clothing, as if you get too hot and sweaty this may aggravate the condition.
- Relief Cream, made from calendula, manuka honey, aloe vera and gotu kola, works really well on eczema and psoriasis and is great for babies. For details visit www.planetblueshop.com. One of the finest eczema creams I have come across is the Ultra Dry Skin Cream by the Organic Pharmacy. **OP**
- Constipation and a liver under stress from too many toxins is also associated with eczema, as toxins cannot be broken down and removed from the body efficiently (see also *Constipation* and *Liver Problems*).
- If a sensitivity to certain foods is suspected, then avoid the offending food (see *Allergies*).
- Avoid mass-produced soaps and soap powders. Ask at your health store for pH-balanced soaps – or natural soaps that contain say olive oil or vitamins A and E.
- Chinese herbs have proved helpful in many cases but you need to see a qualified Chinese herbalist and may need to have your liver function checked before and during treatment. Others report great success through homeopathy (see *Useful Information*).

- Reduce your exposure to house dust mites by using a vacuum cleaner with an allergy filter, and vacuum mattresses once a week.
- Putting duvets and pillows out in bright sunlight for a few hours a month will help to kill off the mites.
- For further help, contact the National Eczema Society, Hill house, Highgate Hill, London N19 5NA. Tel: 020 7281 3553. Helpline: 0870 241 3604 (Monday to Friday, 8am–8pm). Website: www.eczema.org

ELECTRICAL POLLUTION and ELECTRICAL HEALING

Electrical pollution from computers, mobile phones, satellite receivers, transmitters and other electronic devices are becoming a major health hazard. Roger Coghill, a bio-electromagnetics research scientist who is one of the UK's leading authorities on this subject, based in Torfaen in Wales says "Firstly, people need to understand that we are electrical beings in a physical shell and electricity can be used to harm or to heal us. Every cell in the human body emits its own unique range of frequencies. These frequencies are as unique to us as our DNA. When functioning properly, our cells or groups of cells such as our liver or kidneys emit a harmonic signal (denoting that the organ is healthy), which can clearly be seen on specialist scanners. If we become ill, cells begin emitting a disharmonic set of frequencies, which again can be detected. Every food you eat also emits a specific range of frequencies, as does every nutrient and everything on the planet – even rocks. This is how scientists measure what other planets and stars are made of, by measuring their spectral frequencies. But electrical pollution from external sources is now without doubt a major contributing factor to many illnesses. A UK Government sponsored study in 2005 found that children living near power lines are almost twice as likely to contract cancer. Another study in Maila in Germany, found that out of 1000 patients living within 400 metres of cell phone masts, were 3 times as likely to get cancer. Appliances in the home and outside are undoubtedly contributing to illnesses such as ME (chronic fatigue), cancers, depression, migraines and insomnia. Depressive illness has now been shown to be linked to electrical pollution – and more than half of the exposure is from appliances and wiring within the home."

Sixty years or so ago a few households enjoyed the luxury of a radio set but today we are all being bombarded by a dangerous enemy. As I write (November 2005) there are more than 52 million mobile-phone subscribers in the UK alone and 1.3 billion worldwide. Five years ago this was 500 million.

Studies now show that excessive use of mobile phones triggers solid cancerous tumours, brain tumours and lymphomas. The hands-free kits are also linked with health problems and if you use these phones for more than 20 minutes at a time you are at a much greater risk. We are living in a sea of artificial frequencies and because animals, especially whales, dolphins, insects and birds, are more sensitive to these manmade emissions, their sensory abilities are being greatly affected – hence why so many whales are beaching themselves. Humans are also becoming more electro-sensitive and there are even societies which help people who are either affected by, or whose fields affect electrical equipment. Approximately 7% of the population is now electro-sensitive. Also if you have subterranean flowing water under your home or office, this often compounds health problems, as the water can create an inharmonious electromagnetic field. Hundreds of years ago, builders would watch carefully where sheep settled at night and would not build in places where sheep refused to sleep. Studies show rats also avoid areas of high electromagnetic fields. Every time you turn on a light switch or any electrical equipment, your brain's rhythms change immediately. Spending too much time under fluorescent lighting or in front of a computer screen can suppress the brain chemical melatonin. This can have negative effects as diverse as infertility, depression and insomnia, and can increase the risk of cancer.

Foods to Avoid
- Junk foods have a dull energy field frequency – which will eventually trigger negative symptoms if you eat junk foods to excess. But it is important to note that as all foods emit their own frequency and if you eat certain foods, whether considered healthy or not, which emit a frequency that is incompatible with your own frequency range, this too can trigger symptoms in sensitive individuals.

Friendly Foods
- Foods in as near a natural state as possible. For example, if you look at the energy field of a raw cabbage it has a really bright energy field – but once cooked the energy field is greatly reduced. See *General Health Hints*.

Useful Remedies
- One of the best ways to help protect yourself is the hormone melatonin. Roger Coghill has developed a supplement called Asphalia, which is taken under the tongue at night before bed and which maintains melatonin levels. Roger has permission from the MHRA (Medical Healthcare Regulatory Authority) to sell this supplement in the UK. Take at night. For more details log on to www.cogreslab.co.uk; or tel: 01495 752122.
- The Bicom machine developed in Germany picks up the electromagnetic frequencies emanating from the body, which an experienced practitioner can interpret and then determine which frequencies should be amplified back into the patients energy field, to enable the body to heal itself. There are details of how this works under the *Healing* section. Cells carry a memory of certain diseases that you thought long ago had left your body. For example when I was tested with the Bicom (at the Hale Clinic in London, see page 361 for contact details) my cells showed a positive reading for the memory of glandular fever, which I suffered during my teens – so the therapist inverted the frequency of the Epstein Barr virus (from a tiny phial containing Epstein Barr) back into my body to neutralise any remaining memory. The Bicom is brilliant for helping people eliminate allergies, chronic fatigue, endometriosis, treating intestinal parasites and eczema. For more details contact Peter Smith at the Hale Clinic (see page 361 for contact details).
- Electro-crystal healing, invented by scientist Harry Oldfield, works on similar principles except that the therapist pulses the calming or stimulating frequencies through crystals that are held in a saline solution. I have interviewed dozens of people who have been crippled with arthritis and other conditions who have been greatly helped by this type of therapy. Harry has trained hundreds of therapists worldwide. For details of your nearest therapist log on to www.electrocrystal.com. This is more fully explained in the *Healing* section.

Helpful Hints
- The subject of energy medicine is now becoming a mainstream subject and for those who want to know more, I recommend you read *Virtual Medicine* by Keith Scott-Mumby, who is the Professor of Medical Bio-Physics at the Capital University of Integrative Medicine in Washington DC (Timpangos Publishers). To order call the Nutri Centre on 020 7323 2382 or log on to Keith's website: www.alternative-doctor.com
- The basic rule is that moving electric fields are harmful – that is, mobile phones or power lines – and static magnetic fields, like the earth on which we all evolved, are beneficial to health.

- Avoid using a mobile phone inside a car, building or any enclosed space, because the phone is forced to increase its output power, which can affect health more quickly. Never use a mobile for more than 20 minutes at a time.
- When you attach a phone ear piece directly into your ear, Roger says that you risk pulsing radio waves straight into the brain, and you need to look for sets that have ferrite components, which block radiation from travelling up the wire.
- There are many companies manufacturing protection chips and Roger says research is ongoing, but if you have access to the Internet look at Techno AO, Talk Safe, Q Link or Pamex on www.pamex.com
- Keep electrical appliances in the bedroom to a minimum. Turn off all mains switches in the bedroom at night. If you live near an electrical power station, put large copper jugs or ornaments in the windows. Avoid placing 'touch lamps' with thyrister dimmers anywhere near your bed. Also turn off computers and TVs at the mains at night. Leaving TVs and so on on 'standby' wastes huge amounts of energy.
- Avoid sleeping with an electric blanket on, warm the bed thoroughly before you get into bed and then switch it off for the night. However, if you are over 60 and have poor circulation and have been specifically told to sleep with it on, for goodness sake don't get too cold!
- Studies show that microwave ovens alter the chemistry of food. Irradiating (x-raying) food could, in the long run, prove very dangerous. If any foods like strawberries are still healthy looking after being in your fridge for a few days, then they have most likely been irradiated.
- The Coghill Research Laboratories will either rent or sell you an ELF Meter to tell you the field strengths in your home. For details Tel: 01495 752122. Or read Roger's book *Something in the Air*. To order or for more information, log on to www.cogreslab.co.uk
- For the latest updates on electrical pollution, log onto www.em-hazard-therapy.com, which is the site for *The Electromagnetic News Report*, which publishes a newsletter. Or call Electro Magnetic Hazard and Therapy Helpline on 0906 4010237.
- Have your home dowsed by an expert if you are worried about suffering from overexposure from electricity, then contact The British Society of Dowsers. Tel/fax: 01684 576969. Website: www.britishdowsers.org

EMPHYSEMA

Emphysema is a condition that usually occurs in middle and old age, which affects the lungs reducing their capacity to absorb oxygen and causing difficulty in expelling air. Normally, sufferers complain about increasing breathlessness, which is exacerbated by exercise. Other symptoms include skipped breaths, insomnia, fatigue, swelling of feet, ankles or legs, and irritability. It is nearly always triggered by smoking – 80% of cases – or exposure to other atmospheric pollutants and chemicals; aerosol sprays, non-tobacco smoke, and exhaust fumes. As asthma can cause a stretching of the alveoli (the place where carbon dioxide is exchanged for oxygen, which is the main job of the lungs), this can also be a contributory factor. Low levels of protective antioxidants (such as vitamin C, E and so on) and high levels of oxidative stress caused by damaging free radicals (from burnt food, pollution, chemicals and so on) are also seen in people suffering from emphysema. Emphysema patients have an increased risk of contracting pneumonia so keeping the immune system strong is essential. See *Immune Function*. Heart disease is another risk factor as the heart has to work extra hard to make up for the lungs.

Foods to Avoid

- Avoid foods that contain hydrogenated/trans fats and oils, found in many pre-packaged and processed foods, which can trigger inflammation and compete with the good fats that help keep the alveoli in the lungs supple so that they can do their job more easily.
- Any foods to which you have an intolerance – the most common being wheat and dairy from cows.
- If you find you are making too much phlegm, this is almost always linked to high-fat foods, including full-fat cheese, chocolate, milk, eggs, white bread, croissants and bananas, and for some people soya products.
- Fried and barbecued foods as they have high levels of damaging free radicals.
- Generally cut down your intake of red meat and if you choose to eat meat always cut off the fat first.
- Eggs are hard to digest for some people and it's well worth being tested to see if they are a problem. See *Allergies*.
- Sugary foods and drinks suppress immune function, which leaves you more susceptible to infections. Also, most foods high in sugar are also high in fat. And keep in mind that many low-fat foods are high in sugar, which unless burnt during exercise will be converted to fat within the body.

Friendly Foods

- People who eat fruit and vegetables on a regular basis seem less likely to develop emphysema, focus on foods rich in natural sources of carotenes, which help to protect mucous membranes in the lungs. Go for apricots, mangoes, green vegetables, watercress, parsley, red peppers, spinach, sweet potatoes, watercress and cantaloupe melon.
- Vine-ripened tomatoes are rich in the carotene lycopene, this helps to support the lungs. Cook in a little olive oil to help release the lycopene. Guava and pink grapefruit also contain a fair amount of lycopene.
- Go for organic whenever possible as fruit like apples are great for lung health but can be covered in up to six pesticides – you need the apple but not the pesticide!
- Quercetins – flavonoids found in apples, pears, cherries, grapes, onion, kale, broccoli, garlic, green tea and red wine – help protect the lungs from the harmful effect of pollutants and cigarette smoke. Eat more fresh pineapple.
- Use organic rice or almond milk as non-dairy alternatives. Some people find low-fat goat's or sheep's milk better.
- Choose low-fat dishes including cottage cheese and replace too much butter with healthier spreads such as Biona, Vitaquel or Benecol.
- Use olive oil for salad dressings and eat plenty of brown rice, lentils, barley, oat-based dishes, wheat-free breakfast cereals – Nature's Path make a great range. There are also plenty of wheat-free pastas available such as lentil, rice, corn and potato pasta and flour.
- Liver, kidney, butter, and skimmed milk contain retinol, the animal form of vitamin A, which is good for tissue-healing. Don't go mad on the butter – and make it organic.
- Eat more garlic and onions as these help to fend off infection and clear the lungs.
- Fenugreek or liquorice tea can help to soothe the lungs.
- See *General Health Hints*.

Useful Remedies

- N-Acetyl Cysteine (NAC) 500mg 1–2 times a day. This amino acid is one of the best-researched nutrients for emphysema, as it helps protect lung tissue and improve breathing.
- Vitamin C. Take 1–2 grams daily with food in an ascorbate form to help clear mucus and improve respiratory ailments – works well with NAC (above).
- L-carnitine, 2 grams daily, if breathing is made worse by exercise.
- Mullein formula, 2–3ml a day, contains a blend of herbs, including mullein, that are anti-viral

and expectorant and help to ease breathing and congestion. **FSC**

- Microcell Nutri Guard Plus contains high potency lycopene, selenium, zinc, alpha lipoic acid vitamins A, C, E, which all help to support lung tissue. **BC**
- Include a high-potency multi-vitamin and mineral in your regimen.
- Bromelain extracted from pineapples is great for helping to break up mucus. If symptoms are acute take 1000mcu daily.
- Co-enzyme Q10 is a powerful antioxidant that helps the lungs. Take 100mg, twice daily but not at night as CoQ10 also increases energy levels.
- Magnesium helps to relax bronchial muscles for easier breathing. Take 500mg twice a day. www.positivehealthshop.com
- The amino acid taurine can help to improve breathlessness. Take 1000mg twice a day before meals.

Helpful Hints

- Don't smoke, and if you do smoke – quit. Avoid smoke-filled rooms and sources of second hand cigarette smoke
- To help break up any thick mucus that may collect in the lungs drink plenty of fluid.
- Avoid air pollutants such as dust, aerosol sprays, herbicides, pesticides, fumes from fuel and exhausts, smoke from bonfires and barbecues, and dust stirred up by house-cleaning.
- Stabilised liquid oxygen helps to re-alkalise the body and gets more oxygen into the system. Available from all good health stores or call Waters For Life on 020 7483 1991, or check out their website at www.watersforlife.co.uk

- Use an Ultrabreathe – a small, inexpensive device that helps to exercise the lungs. For details call 0870 608 9019, or visit their website at www.ultrabreathe.com
- Gentle exercise can help relieve the symptoms of this condition by building lung capacity and cleansing the lungs of stale air. Start slowly and build up gradually. Choose walking, swimming or cycling.
- Reflexology has proved successful with some sufferers. Yoga can also be beneficial as this therapy will teach you relaxation techniques and how to breathe properly (see *Useful Information*).
- Aromatherapy has also been of benefit to some sufferers. Fill a basin with boiling water and add three drops of eucalyptus essential oil. Put your head over the basin with a towel over and inhale the steam.
- Be careful about visiting high altitudes as this makes it harder to breathe.
- An ioniser in the home may be useful for lowering levels of dust in the house. www.healthprod-uctsforlife.com has a range to suit all needs and budgets.
- Sing when you can which helps increase lung capacity. Take deep breaths regularly. You can increase the efficiency of your lungs a thousandfold by increasing your air intake by 5% on each breath.
- Environmentally friendly cleaning products are kinder to your lungs as they don't contain harsh chemicals that can be breathed in. Try Ecover products – available in health stores and super-markets.
- www.lef.org – a US research site (The Life Extension Foundation) – offers a wealth of informa-tion for people with emphysema.

ENDOMETRIOSIS

Endometriosis is a condition where tissue that normally lines the womb, grows outside the womb. The endometrial tissue can be found in places such as the ovaries, fallopian tubes or pelvis. It is not certain what causes this condition, but some doctors theorise that during menstruation womb tissue flows not only down to the vagina but up through the fallopian tubes eventually sticking to other structures. The displaced tissue acts in the same way it would if it had stayed in the womb and has a monthly bleed. In mild cases the blood is reabsorbed but in more severe cases cysts can form and irritate the pelvis. It can be very painful particularly during ovulation, menstruation and sexual intercourse. Pain can also be triggered by a bowel movement or emptying the bladder. Internal examinations are necessary to diagnose the condition, but sometimes these can aggravate the condition. Nevertheless they are necessary to rule out anything more serious. Endometriosis is one of the more common causes of infertility. Some doctors recognize that excess oestrogen can exacerbate symptoms. The chemical dioxin (from vinyl, plastics and produced during incineration and forest fires) and numerous other toxic chemicals found in our air and water have also been linked to this condition – dioxins can interfere with the metabolism of B-vitamins, which are needed for liver function, which in turn is needed to break down excess oestrogen. Most nutritional practitioners also believe there is a strong link between endometriosis and candida overgrowth (see *Candida*), which when treated greatly alleviates symptoms. Many of the women suffering this condition note that symptoms are definitely worse when they are stressed or really tired.

Foods to Avoid
- Avoid alcohol and saturated animal fats found in red meat and dairy these can elevate oestrogen levels and place a strain on the liver, which in turn can increase the pain and inflammation.
- Sugar and sugary foods trigger inflammation in the body, so sweets, puddings, cakes, sugary fizzy drinks, and pastries are best avoided.
- Caffeine reduces the body's ability to cope with pain and blocks absorption of some minerals.
- If you suspect candida – symptoms include bloating, constipation and/or diarrhoea, thrush, food cravings and chronic fatigue – then avoid sugar, refined carbohydrates, cheese, mushrooms, concentrated fruit juice and yeasted breads for a couple of weeks to see if this helps.
- As with so many other conditions, if there is a food intolerance it will almost certainly aggravate the problem. Avoid wheat and dairy for at least one cycle.
- Peel all fruit and vegetables if they are not organic as this is where the pesticides and herbicides that disrupt hormones are more concentrated
- Reduce wheat and wheat bran in the diet as they contain phytic acid which binds to essential minerals, such as zinc and magnesium, which are needed for hormone balance and muscle relaxation.

Friendly Foods
- Fermented soya-based foods have an ability to control excessive oestrogen levels; as do beans, lentils, chickpeas, cauliflower, Brussels sprouts and broccoli.
- Add sunflower, pumpkin, sesame and linseeds (flax seeds) to your breakfast cereal, which provide essential fatty acids and zinc that are vital for soft tissue healing. Nuts, with the exception of peanuts, are a good source of fatty acids and zinc.
- Eat more oily fish – wild salmon, mackerel, fresh tuna, and sardines and anchovies – along with nuts and seeds for their anti-inflammatory properties.
- Pineapple is rich in bromelain, which has a potent anti-inflammatory affect.

- Ginger and turmeric (curcumin) are also anti-inflammatory, and ginger is very soothing within the gut.
- Eat foods high in natural carotenes – spinach, carrots, apricots, pumpkin, parsley, mangoes, cantaloupe melons and sweet potatoes.
- Natural wheat germ and avocados are rich in vitamin E, which is known to help reduce scar tissue associated with endometriosis.
- Eat more magnesium-rich foods – cashew nuts, almonds, broccoli, bananas and prunes – as these will help to reduce cramping.
- Brown rice, millet and oats contain lots of fibre, which binds to excess oestrogen so that it can be removed from the body.
- Milled linseeds (flax seeds) are high in lignans, which have a stabilising effect on hormones. High in fibre, linseeds also help to eliminate any excess oestrogens from the body.
- Dandelion coffee helps to support the liver so that it can remove excess hormones more easily.
- Add fresh coriander to your diet as it helps remove toxic metals from the body.

Useful Remedies

- Take 3 grams of evening primrose oil, as the fatty acids help regulate hormones and reduce discomfort.
- Most sufferers are lacking in the mineral magnesium. Take 200–600mg daily.
- Zinc, 30mg per day, as most sufferers are deficient and zinc, which ensures proper absorption of fatty acids and aids hormone balance.
- A strong B-complex will help absorption of fatty acids and support liver enzymes in the breakdown of excess oestrogen.
- Soya isoflavones, 50–100mg, a day to help regulate hormone levels.
- Wild yam 1–3ml of tincture or 1–3 grams a day of tablets, has been shown to reduce the discomfort of endometriosis and help reduce excessive bleeding.
- Take 500mg of the amino acid L-methionine, which helps detoxify oestrogen in the liver.
- Include a high-strength multi-vitamin and mineral in your regimen, such as Kudos 24 (see *General Supplements*; p.160), which contains a full spectrum of the B-complex vitamins, with zinc, magnesium and essential fats.
- The amino acid DLPA can help reduce endometrial pain. Take up to 2000mg. **NB: do not take DLPA if you are on antidepressant medication.**

Helpful Hints

- Anthony Porter, a reflexologist since 1972, went to China and the Far East to teach reflexology during the 80s and found that their methods combined with his own gave even better results. He has taught his advanced techniques to thousands of reflexologists internationally and says "With ART we can not only balance various parts of the body (which is what happens with normal reflexology), but we can also feel more subtle changes within the 7000 nerve-endings or reflex areas of the feet, and after working on them this has a profound therapeutic affect. Medical research with a leading gynecologist has shown huge success with easing the pain and distress in these types of conditions. To find an ART therapist in your area log on to www.artreflex.com
- Naturopathy and Chinese medicine have proven beneficial to many sufferers. If you decide to try Chinese herbs make sure your doctor keeps an eye on your liver function. (See *Useful Information*.)
- Epsom salts added to the hot bath relaxes and soothes; add a drop of lavender oil to relax.
- Remove chemicals from your home as many have hormone disrupting action, and use biodegradable products whenever possible. Look out for Ecover products available in most supermarkets and health food stores.
- Use a hot water bottle or alternatively a heat pad, available from www.conformuk.com, or call

0870 762 4841, to help relax cramping muscles.

- Massage your abdomen with gentle strokes using lavender and neroli essential oils as they both have a calming and antispasmodic effect so will help cramping. To find out more about pure-healing, therapeutic Young Living essential oils, see details on page 15.
- Acupressure: you may be able to alleviate cramping by applying pressure to Spleen 6, located on the inside of the leg 2in (5cm) above the centre of the ankle bone. Do not use this point if you are pregnant.
- Always use pure cotton towels that are guaranteed free from dioxin. Beware of tampons as they can exacerbate symptoms.
- Light exercise will help to raise levels of endorphins, which make you feel good and help pain relief. In winter double the benefit by walking in daylight as this can also lift your spirits.
- To reduce tension, drink soothing herbal teas made with herbs such as hops and valerian.
- Hypnotherapy can be an effective way to manage pain. To find a qualified practitioner visit The National Council of Hypnotherapists at www.hypnotherapists.org.uk. Write to PO Box 421, Charwelton, Daventry, NN11 1AS, or call 0800 952 0545.
- If excess oestrogen is a problem, Natural Progesterone cream may help to address the hormone imbalance. For an information pack contact the Natural Progesterone Information Service, PO Box 24, Buxton SK17 9FB. Tel: 07000 784849. Also see details of Natural Progesterone under *Menopause*.
- Contact the Women's Nutrition clinic, Mon–Fri 9am–5.30pm. Tel: 01273 487366.
- Further help is available from The National Endometriosis Society, 50 Westminster Palace Gardens, Artillery Row, London SW1P 1RL; or call their help line on 0808 808 2227 which is open every day, 365 days a year. Website: www.endo.org.uk

EXHAUSTION (see also *ME* and *Stress*)

Being 'Tired All The Time' has become like a mantra for so many people. In fact there are several books with this title – and which also include *Tired Or Toxic*, and many other variations. Out of the 50,000 letters I have answered during my 13 years as a health journalist, the most common without doubt have been from people, particularly women, who feel tired all the time. Being tired much of the time is often linked to toxicity in the body (see *Liver Problems*), stress (see *Stress*), and/or being overweight (see *Weight Problems*). However, the list of possible causes is fairly extensive, and you may also need to have your thyroid checked as chronic exhaustion is also linked to an underactive thyroid. One of the most common causes of constant tiredness may simply be lack of sleep. When you are under pressure you have more difficulty getting to sleep and then you have to get up for work feeling almost as tired as you did the night before. There is no right or wrong amount of sleep, we are all unique; Margaret Thatcher could manage on 4 hours, but I need 8. Everyone knows how much sleep they need to be fully functioning the next day.

Obviously there are varying levels of exhaustion, but if you find you suffer from palpitations regularly during the day, or chronic headaches, have an urgency to keep going to the loo or experience a red flushing in your upper chest and throat area, this is most likely your adrenal glands telling you that your body is on limits. And if you start crying without cause and begin to suffer a total sense of humour failure, you urgently need to listen and take note of the signals – or worse is to come. Your immune system is lowered and you are more likely to pick up anything that's going. Rest is your best option at this point. Know when to walk away. It's not worth dying for – literally.

Foods to Avoid

- Unfortunately, stimulants like coffee, tea, alcohol and sugar give a short-term energy boost, but this soon wears off, leaving you craving more sugary, refined foods. Therefore greatly reduce your intake of colas and fizzy drinks, black tea, chocolates, biscuits, cakes, snacks, croissants and mass-produced refined foods. Not only do they leave us feeling tired, but they also deplete important nutrients like magnesium, chromium and the B-vitamins, and we become even more exhausted.
- Don't eat heavy protein meals late at night as they take a long time to digest.

Friendly Foods

- Eat more high-energy foods such as alfalfa or aduki bean sprouts, wheat grass and fresh fruits and vegetables.
- Include more whole-grains like brown rice, oat-based cereals and millet, which are packed with B-vitamins and so help support your nerves.
- Magnesium and calcium are known as nature's tranquillisers so eat more green vegetables like kale, cabbage and broccoli, as well as almonds, Brazil nuts, sesame seeds, pineapple, papaya, Parmesan cheese, fish, dried apricots, pilchards and skimmed milk. Chocolate is also high in calcium, but the benefits are offset by the caffeine content. Just eat it in moderation; and make it dark and organic.
- At night, eat wholewheat pastas, and jacket potatoes, which are more calming. Make thick vegetable soups, which are easier on the digestion.

- Generally control your blood sugar levels – eating small meals regularly instead of bingeing on junk foods will help to reduce the constant exhaustion. See *Low Blood Sugar*.
- Drink herbal teas throughout the day, which are free from caffeine, and choose a calming blend such as liquorice, yerba mate or camomile.
- As your digestive system is bound to be stressed, eat a low-fat, live yoghurt with meals.

Useful Remedies

- Take a high-strength B-complex to help calm your nerves and aid digestion, plus 500mg of pantothenic acid (B5), which helps support adrenal function. If you wake regularly between 3 and 5am, this can be linked to adrenal exhaustion; also if you find you need to urinate regularly but don't have a bladder infection, this can also denote that your adrenals are on limits.
- As the digestive system begins malfunctioning when we are really tired, take a digestive enzyme or betaine hydrochloride (stomach acid) with meals to improve the absorption of nutrients. Do not take the betaine if you have active stomach ulcers, instead take a digestive enzyme capsule with main meals.
- Co-enzyme Q10 is a supplement well proven to improve energy levels. The body produces CoQ10 naturally, but as we age or when stressed we produce less. And as most people no longer eat organ meats, rich in Co-enzyme Q10, it is best taken as a supplement of 100mg daily.
- Calcium and magnesium are often depleted – take 500mg of calcium with 300–400mg of magnesium an hour before going to bed. Stress and exhaustion make the body more acid and these minerals help to realkalise your system. Most companies sell calcium and magnesium in one formula.
- Siberian ginseng is useful as a general tonic that helps to support adrenal function. There are plenty of liquid formulas and this can be taken for a month. Holos Health makes an advanced stress formula containing Siberian ginseng, ashawagandha and gotu kola, which help regulate cortisol levels. Website: www.holoshealth.com
- L-carnitine – an amino acid helps to improve energy levels; 1 gram a day before meals for a month.

■ Try using Oxygen Elements Plus a liquid oxygen supplement that also contains minerals, enzymes and amino acids, which all help to boost energy and detoxify the body. For details call The Finchley Clinic on 020 8349 4730. Website: www.thefinchleyclinic.com

Helpful Hints

■ If you are at rock bottom, a few vitamin pills and a couple of nights sleep will help, but are not the long-term solution. You must try to address the root cause of your exhaustion.

■ Generally try to take at least 1 day a week for yourself and make dates in your diary for exercise or time simply to call your own.

■ Breathe deeply into your tummy every hour. Get up, walk around, have a stretch.

■ If your exhaustion is linked to personal problems, ask your doctor to refer you to a counsellor. Talking problems through gives you a better perspective. See also *Depression*.

■ Homeopathic Phos Ac 30c twice daily for 3 days helps restore energy levels.

■ Never take work to bed and always finish work at least one hour before going to bed – otherwise your mind simply keeps churning your thoughts over and over.

■ Gentle exercise like yoga, T'ai Chi, qigong, or walking at leisure in nature helps to make you feel more positive and re-build energy levels.

■ Find a practitioner who can really sort out your diet, such as a nutritionist or naturopath, and make a determined effort to improve your food intake (see *Useful Information*).

■ If at all practical treat yourself to three days at a health spa to rejuvenate and rest.

EYE PROBLEMS (see also *Cataracts*, *Conjunctivitis*, and *Macular Degeneration*)

Blepharitis

If red eyes are accompanied by a burning sensation, excessive tearing, itching, sensitivity to light, swollen eyelids, blurred vision, frothy tears, dry eyes or crusting of the eyelashes on awakening, then Blepharitis (inflammation of the eyelid caused by an infection) should be considered. Visit an eye-care specialist to check this out (see also *Red-rimmed Eyes*).

Foods to Avoid

■ Avoid saturated fats found in red meat and dairy foods, and sugar, as these foods create inflammation in the body, and can block the essential lubricating fats found in oily fish, nuts and seeds from doing their job.

Friendly Foods

■ Eat plenty of dark-purple fruits like bilberries, blueberries, blackberries and cherries, as they are rich in bioflavonoids, which protect and strengthen the eyes and help reduce the risk of eye damage from other diseases.

■ Eat more green vegetables especially raw spinach, cabbage, kale and watercress, plus sweet potatoes and carrots, which are all rich in carotenes that nourish the eyes.

■ Eat more oily fish – salmon, mackerel, tuna, sardines and anchovies – along with nuts and seeds. These are rich in essential fats, which help to lubricate the eyes from the inside out.

■ Immune-boosting foods rich in vitamin C and zinc are essential, as these will help the body to fight of any infection. Eat more red and yellow peppers, kiwi fruit, green leafy vegetables, whole grains, nuts and seeds.

Useful remedies

- Higher Nature's Essential Oil Balance contains a good combination of the essential fats needed to lubricate the eyes. Take 3 per day. **HN**
- If the blepharitis is severe, an eye-care professional may prescribe antibiotics. Healthy bacteria found in the gut need to be taken alongside the antibiotics. Take 1 BioCare bio-acidophillus as far away from the antibiotics as possible. See *Antibiotics*. **BC**

Helpful Hints

- Castor oil has been used traditionally as an anti-inflammatory remedy for treatment of blepharitis. Eyelid inflammation may initially increase after starting treatment, but with repeated use over a week, the inflammation should be reduced. Refresh Endura contains castor oil and is available from most health stores. Use 1–2 drops a few times a day.
- Gently massage the eyelids through a clean, warm steamy flannel (change each time) for 5 minutes 2–4 times daily. Wipe all debris off the lids with cotton wool soaked in warm, salty water.
- Note that many eye drops are on based on urine (urea). Therefore, if you can stand it, use fresh urine – which is a sterile liquid – and dab it around the eyes.

Dark circles under the eyes   (see also *Hayfever*)

The obvious culprit for dark circles is lack of sleep, and if you are chronically short of sleep, then the adrenal glands become exhausted which will make your eyes even darker. Dark circles can be triggered by allergies either to products (creams, hair sprays and so on) that you are using, or by foods to which you have an intolerance. And if you suffer from hayfever, then rubbing your itchy eyes can make dark circles worse. If you have truly 'black', panda-like eyes, ask your doctor to check for an underactive thyroid or low iron levels. Food intolerances are one of the most common causes of dark circles and wheat is usually the main culprit. In a few cases it may be hereditary. Pregnancy and menstruation can cause skin under the eyes to become more pale which allows underlying veins to show through, thus making the circles look darker, as can certain medications used to dilate blood vessels, which cause circles under the eyes to darken. Too much ultraviolet light – from the sun or sunbeds – and smoking can also make dark circles worse, as can water retention caused by kidney problems (in Chinese medicine the eyes directly relate to the kidneys) or PMT (see *Pre-menstrual Tension*). If you have a tendency for dark circles under your eyes, as you grow older, they are likely to become more noticeable and permanent. Excess folds of skin under the eyes will also make dark circles more pronounced. Therefore it makes sense to first make sure you are getting enough sleep, and if you are, but still suffer dark circles, try eliminating wheat for 4 days. I'll bet you will be amazed at the difference.

Foods to Avoid

- Cut down on alcohol and salt and drink plenty of water to flush toxins from the body.
- Processed foods, packet sauces and ketchup-style foods often contain huge amounts of hidden salt so are best avoided.
- If you are sleeping well but still have circles after 3 or 4 good nights' sleep, then eliminate wheat for a week and see if this helps. If there is no change, then try eliminating cow's milk. These are the most common triggers.

Friendly Foods

- Drink plenty of water to eliminate toxins and generally eat a clean diet, avoiding too much refined food and sugar. See *General Health Hints*.
- Green leafy vegetables, seaweeds, kelp, lentils and peas are all rich in vitamin K, which has been

shown to help with bruising and under eye circles.

- Natural source carotenes especially lutein, plus vitamin C, are great eye nutrients – eat more strawberries, kiwi fruit, red, yellow and green peppers, squashes, sweet potatoes, oily fish, spinach, watercress, mangoes, and green leafy vegetables.

Useful Remedies

- If you are totally exhausted see *Useful Remedies* under *Exhaustion*.
- Eyecare contains bilberry extract, antioxidants (vitamins A, E and C, plus selenium) potassium, grapeseed extract, ginkgo biloba, lycopene and chromium. **BC**; otherwise all companies mentioned on pages 13–15 make good eye complex formulas.
- Dr Haushka's organic and environmentally friendly Daily Revitalising Eye Cream is composed of nourishing plant oils and medicinal herb extracts that provide a calming, soothing, and fortifying care to the skin around the eye area. Available from all health stores and good pharmacies.

Helpful Hints

- Do not drag or rub the delicate skin under the eyes when using cleansers and make up.
- Use specific skin-care products especially made for the eyes, as regular moisturisers can be too heavy and lead to puffy dark circles.
- Beware of using concealers as many are too heavy for this delicate area and actually make the problem worse. However, one of best I have found is Jane Iredale's mineral make up. Available at good pharmacies and the Organic Pharmacy. **OP**

Itchy eyes

(see also Conjunctivitis and Hayfever)

Itching of the eyes can be due to an infection like conjunctivitis, allergies or hayfever, or exposure to a smoky or polluted atmosphere. It can also be due to over-exposure to computer screens – as well I know as I sit typing this book! Eyes also become irritated on long-haul flights and when they are tired. If you suffer dry, itching eyes after a long flight, then use Natural Tears Eye Drops regularly and take more essential fats, which help nourish your eyes from the inside out. (See *Fats You Need to Eat*.)

  If the problem is linked to your PC, then take regular breaks, get out in the sunshine and get some rest.

Foods to Avoid

- Avoid dehydrating beverages, such as caffeine and alcohol. Just like every other part of the body the eyes need plenty of fluid intake to keep them in good shape – drink more water.
- Avoid saturated fats, found in red meat and dairy foods, as these create inflammation in the body, and can block the essential lubricating fats found in oily fish, nuts and seeds from doing their job.

Friendly Foods

- Eat plenty of dark-purple fruits like bilberries, blueberries, blackberries and cherries, as the bioflavonoids in these fruits not only protect and strengthen the eyes but they help reduce the risk of eye damage from other diseases.
- Eat more green vegetables, sweet potatoes and carrots all rich in the carotenes that nourish the eyes.
- Eat more oily fish, which are rich in essential fats which help prevent the eyes from drying out.
- Eat more unsalted nuts (not peanuts) and seeds, which are high in zinc and selenium.

Useful Remedies

- Vitamin A, 25,000iu a day for 1 month. If you are pregnant limit to 3000iu per day.

- Zinc, 30mg a day, is essential for enhancing vitamin-A absorption.
- A strong B-complex: B-vitamins – in particular B2 – are necessary for the prevention of dry eyes.
- Take a high-strength multi-vitamin, mineral and EFA formula; see Kudos 24 in *General Supplements* (see p.160).

Helpful Hints

- Eyebright, raspberry and pau d'arco can be made into an infusion, strained and, when cooled, applied to each eye using an eye bath. Make sure you sterilize the eye-baths before use. The infusion has anti-inflammatory, astringent, antiseptic and anti-catarrhal properties. **SHS**
- I often find that if I sleep in an air-conditioned room this can make my eyes very sore; similarly in rooms that are too hot. In winter keep a small bowl of water near radiators to keep the air in the rooms moist.
- The homeopathic version of eyebright, euphrasia, can be used for bathing the eyes and is very soothing. Use Euphrasia Mother Tincture about 4 times a day using a disposable eye-bath. Most good health stores should stock this.
- Heel Homeopathics makes disposable remedies in single phials – order through your local pharmacy or any homeopathic pharmacy. They are excellent for any eye problems.
- Another way to relieve itchy eyes is to brew a pot of camomile tea and lay the tea bags, when they've cooled, on the eyelid. Ideally, leave on the eye for about 15 minutes.
- Don't use anyone else's face cloth or towel just in case the problem is infectious. If your eyes are inflamed, Chloride Compound is useful to reduce redness around the eyes. **BLK**
- Traynore Pinhole Glasses help to take the strain off the eyes and help your eyes to focus properly. Sold at all good health stores, or visit the Body and Mind Shop online store at www.bodyandmindshop.com, or call 01237 472064.
- If you suspect allergies are the problem keep your home free from pet dander and house dust, and stay inside when a lot of pollen is in the air. Air ionizers can help to keep the air clean. Find one at www.healthproductsforlife.com (see also *Allergies*).

Macular degeneration (see *page 235*)

Optic neuritis

This is an inflammation of the optic nerve, which carries information from the seeing part of the eye, the retina, towards the brain. It can cause partial or complete loss of vision, which comes on over a few hours or days and may be accompanied by pain in the eye. Optic neuritis can be one of the symptoms of multiple sclerosis but can also be triggered by sinus problems, severe high blood pressure, post-viral and post-meningitis infections or more serious problems – so always check out symptoms with your doctor.

Foods to Avoid

- Foods that would aggravate inflammation, including red meat and dairy foods (butter, cheese, cream and milk).
- Try to avoid alcohol and caffeine, which can interfere with blood circulation to the eyes.
- Cut down on sugar in any form, as sugar triggers inflammation in the body. All the usual suspects I'm afraid: cakes, biscuits, sweets, puddings and fizzy drinks.

Friendly Foods

- Pineapple is a rich source of bromelain, an anti-inflammatory enzyme.
- Oily fish is rich in essential fats, which are anti-inflammatory. Eat more mackerel, sardines,

anchovies, wild salmon, fresh tuna and herrings.
- Spices such as ginger, turmeric and cayenne, are all great at reducing inflammation as well as improving circulation to the eye.
- Bilberries, blueberries, blackberries, and all blue and orange fruits will help to nourish the eyes.
- Resveratrol is an anti-inflammatory compound that helps to relieve pain associated with inflammation. You can find it in red grapes – enjoy a glass of red grape juice daily, or an occasional glass of red wine (preferably organic).

Useful Remedies
- Bromelain, 2,000–3,000mcu a day, can reduce the inflammation and improve circulation.
- The herb ginkgo biloba helps to strengthen the capillaries in the eye and improve the circulation; 120–240mg of standardised extract a day.
- Vitamin A – 10,000–25,000 units a day, for one month (only 3000iu if you are pregnant).
- The antioxidant astaxanthin has been shown to support eye tissue. It is found in marine algae, which pink-coloured birds such as flamingos feed on. Astaxanthin can cross the blood-brain barrier as well as the brain-eye barrier. Higher Nature makes a high-strength astaxanthin complex. Take 1 capsule daily. **HN**

Puffy eyes

Puffiness and bags under the eyes can denote kidney problems and a build-up of toxins within the body. The condition also signifies that the sodium and potassium levels within the body are out of balance. In this case take 100mg of potassium daily for a week or so, and reduce your intake of sodium-based salts. Puffiness can also be associated with food intolerances and conditions such as hayfever (see *Hayfever*). Drink more water to flush the kidneys and for at least three days, avoid wheat and dairy products and note if your eyes go down. Puffy eyes can also indicate an underactive thyroid, therefore if the problem continues after making these changes, have a check up with your doctor.

Foods to Avoid
- If underneath the eyes is both puffy and dark, it is very likely that you have food intolerances, so it is important to identify these. The most common intolerances are dairy from cows, and wheat, citrus fruits, eggs and nuts.
- Salt is a major trigger, and definitely exacerbates any water retention and increases swelling in all parts of the body.
- Mass-produced breakfast cereals often contain more salt than the average bag of crisps.
- Dairy products from cows, cheese and cottage cheese are high in sodium.
- Most pre-packaged, refined foods will have additional salt and a lot of foods which are naturally sweet have salt added partly as a preservative, but also to take the edge off the sweeteners.
- Look out for hidden sources of salt/sodium found in high quantities in ketchups, pickles and relishes, olives, and frankfurters from such things as sodium benzoate E211 – a preservative – and monosodium glutamate (MSG), also known as E621
- Cut down on all foods and drinks containing caffeine and alcohol, which further dehydrate the body.
- Reduce heavy red meat to reduce the burden on the kidneys.

Friendly Foods
- Water is really important, drink 6–8 glasses a day.
- Eat lots of fruit and green vegetables – especially celery and dark green leafy vegetables, dried fruits, nuts, sunflower seeds, and seafood. These are all rich in potassium, which can improve

the balance of minerals in the body, particularly if your salt intake is high.

- Eat more artichokes, beetroot, celeriac, celery and fennel.
- If you are not a big fan of fruit and vegetables, at least try drinking a couple of glasses of fruit juice or freshly made vegetable juice daily. Don't use oranges for the juice, as orange juice is a common trigger for puffy eyes.

Useful Remedies

- Dandelion tea or tincture taken with every meal; total 5ml daily.
- Take a digestive enzyme with all main meals. Try Supergest by Higher Nature. **HN**
- A good multi-vitamin and mineral. Try Solgar VM75 available from most good health food shops and online at www.positivehealthshop.com.
- Vitamin C, 1 gram daily as potassium ascorbate to encourage lymph drainage. **BC**
- Celery seed extract; 500mg twice daily to aid drainage. **BC**

Helpful Hints

- One of the most effective ways of getting rid of puffy eyes (as well as the enclosed hints) is to have regular acupuncture – which can help tone up the kidney meridians, which in turn should reduce the swelling. Facial acupuncture is great for reducing eye problems. (See *Useful Information*.)
- Manual lymph drainage (MLD) can also aid this condition (see *Useful Information*).
- Dry skin brushing will help to break up toxins stored under the skin, so that the body can eliminate them. Combine the skin brushing with an Epsom salt bath to really help flush out toxins. Use 1 cup per every 60lbs of body weight and add to a warm bath. Soak for 15 to 20 minutes and rub your skin all over with a flannel. Don't rinse off before getting out of the bath; just dry off and retire for the evening. Keep some drinking water handy by the tub as a warm bath can make you thirsty.
- Make an infusion with camomile tea bags and, when cool, apply to the eyes.
- Take the homeopathic remedies Apis and Kali Carb which are excellent for reducing puffy eyes.
- Bach flower remedies have been found very useful for this condition, as has reflexology and facial acupuncture (see *Useful Information*).
- Lymph drainage done mechanically either through massage, reflexology or even bouncing up and down on a rebounder can be quite helpful.
- If you suspect a food intolerance get this checked out through York Laboratories. They offer a home test kit called The Food Intolerance Indicator for £19.99. This checks for the most common culprits and gives you the option of going onto a more thorough test should you have a positive result. Contact them at www.homeinonhealth.com or call 0800 458 2052.
- The puffy eyes may be related to an underactive thyroid so it is worth checking with your GP and getting a thyroid test.

Red-rimmed eyes

Consistently red-rimmed eyes can be a sign of malnutrition or lack of B-vitamins. It can also be a sign of malabsorption of nutrients within the gut from your diet (see also *Absorption* and *Leaky Gut*). It can also be associated with hayfever or hangovers – and if symptoms also include a burning sensation, excessive tearing, itching, sensitivity to light, swollen eyelids, blurred vision, frothy tears, dry eyes, or crusting of the eyelashes on awakening, then blepharitis – inflammation of the eye lid – should be considered. Visit an eyecare specialist to rule this out. Red-rimmed eyes can also of course simply denote extreme tiredness; get some rest.

Foods to Avoid

- Refined carbohydrates, such as biscuits, cakes, white bread, pizza and pasta, which all deplete the B-vitamins you need for good eye health.

■ Avoid caffeine in foods and drinks, as these tend to over-stimulate the system and deplete B-vitamins still further.

Friendly Foods

■ Brown rice, wholemeal bread and pastas, lentils, barley, oat-based cereals, nuts and seeds, and green leafy vegetables, bananas, avocados and mushrooms are all rich in B-vitamins, which help maintain healthy eyes.

■ See also *Friendly Foods* under *Itchy Eyes*.

Useful Remedies

■ A high-strength B-complex.

■ Dandelion and burdock tincture, 1–3ml a day. If the red-rimmed eyes are due to a build up of toxins, these herbs can help eliminate them from the body as well as improving liver function and digestion. **FSC**

■ Always include a high-strength, multi-vitamin and mineral and essential fats formula in your daily regimen.

Helpful Hints

■ Bathe the eyes in cooled camomile tea bags, which are very soothing, or apply cooled slices of cucumber.

■ Soak some pads in witch hazel and rose water and lay them on the eyes for 10 minutes. Use a soothing eye balm made from cucumber extract.

■ If the condition is linked to blepharitis, then massage the lids through a clean, warm, steamy flannel (change each time) for 60 seconds, and wipe all debris off the lids with cotton wool soaked in warm salty water. If the blepharitis is severe, an eyecare professional may also prescribe antibiotics or steroid eyedrops, which need to be followed by a course of healthy bacteria – take BioCare bio-acidophillus forte for a month. **BC**

General hints for eye problems

■ If the whites of your eyes are dull or yellowish in colour – this indicates that your liver is struggling. Eat more green vegetables, fruits and whole grains, try dandelion coffee, and take the herb milk thistle to help cleanse the liver. Eat fewer saturated fats, and less sugar, alcohol and coffee. See also *Liver Problems*.

■ Trayner Pinhole Glasses help strengthen weak eye muscles. Available from the Body and Mind Shop Ltd at www.bodyandmindshop.com, or call 01237 472064

■ Dr. Hauschka's Eye Solace is an organic and environmentally friendly solution that you can add to cotton wool pads, lie back and enjoy. It contains eyebright, anthyllis and camomile extracts, which soothe and refresh sore, reddened, overtired eyes. Available from many good beauty salons and online at www.drhauschka.co.uk

■ For people like me who spend a lot of time reading and working in front of a computer screen, take breaks as often as you can. Whilst sitting at your desk, look into the distance to stretch your eye muscles, and get out in the fresh air and natural sunlight as often as possible.

■ Get plenty of sleep.

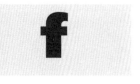

FATIGUE

(see *Exhaustion, ME* and *Stress*)

FATS YOU NEED TO EAT

For more than 13 years I have been telling people about the health benefits of essential fats – as have many other health writers, doctors, scientists and nutritionists – and at long last the message is finally filtering through. It needs to.

After all, your brain is almost 60% fat, but it needs more of the right type of fats to function effectively. Essential fats (EFAs) are essential to life, hence their name, and as we cannot manufacture them in the body we must take them in from external sources through our diet. Most people consume approximately 42% of their calories from fat, but unfortunately it's usually the wrong type of fat.

Dr Udo Erasmus, a Canadian-based bio-chemist, and world renowned authority on fats and oils, says "A huge proportion of degenerative health conditions are triggered not only by eating excessive animal fats, but also over-consumption of mass-produced fats and oils. The majority of vegetable oils found in supermarkets have been refined, bleached and deodorized and then used for frying, which introduces huge amounts of ageing free radicals into the body." To compound the negative health affects, a commercial practice called hydrogenation, in which liquid oils are turned into spreadable fats called trans-fatty acids, found in most margarines, mass-produced cakes, biscuits, cereal bars, flapjacks, chocolates, crisps and so on, are also unhealthy fats. Erasmus adds to this list sweet and starchy foods: desserts, high-sugar fizzy drinks, filled pastries, chocolates and so on, which tend to be high not only in sugar but also saturated fats. If it is not used up during exercise, sugar coverts to fat in the body and sits on your hips, thighs and stomach.

But before sugar turns into fat, it triggers cross-linking in the skin, which means you develop wrinkles faster; bacteria thrive on sugar, which will impair your immune system; and sugar increases inflammation in the body, and inflammation can trigger practically every disease from arthritis to Alzheimer's, cancers to Parkinson's.

Having said this, some children, especially young girls, are becoming obsessed with eliminating all fat from their diets – this is really dangerous. If the body becomes too low in fat, then chronic depression and a host of skin disorders, such as eczema, can result. Children (and adults) need fats for vital functions, such as the manufacture of hormones and energy. That said, I would not encourage really overweight children, who do little or no exercise, to eat lots of junk-fatty foods; but I would never recommend that normal-weight children give up all fats. We all need treats, but we do need to stop living on them. The body also needs essential fats to encourage weight loss, as EFAs help to burn stored fat.

There are two main types of EFAs, omega-3 (alpha-linolenic acid) and omega-6, which comes in two forms, linoleic acid and gamma-linolenic acid (GLA). There is more about GLA under *Useful Supplements*. The best source of omega-3 is oily fish, which contains EPA and DHA (easily utilised types of omega-3 fats). Eating lots of oily fish is why Eskimos rarely suffered heart disease – until they began eating a Western diet. Linseeds (flax seeds), walnuts, hemp seeds and pumpkin seeds also contain omega-3 fats, which the body then converts into the useful EPA and DHA forms; in fish oil this has already been done by nature. There are a few people who cannot easily convert the essential fats in seeds and nuts into EPA and DHA, which is known as atopic tendency, and common characteristics of this condition are asthma, eczema and hayfever. Therefore if you suffer these conditions take fish oils as your first line of defence. Omega-3 fats helps to transfer oxygen around the body, relax blood vessels, and are vital for hormone production, healthy eyes, gut function, weight loss, reducing inflammation, speeding wound-healing, and so on. Unfortunately because we eat 80% less oily fish now than we did in the 1940s, 60% of people are now deficient in omega-3 EFAs.

The second type of EFAs, omega-6, are found in evening primrose, starflower, blackcurrant, walnut and sesame oils. Walnuts, Brazil nuts, pecans, almonds, and sunflower, pumpkin and sesame seeds are also rich in omega-6 EFAs. These fats help to lower blood pressure, thin the blood, and help insulin to work, which keeps blood sugar levels in balance and helps reduce the cravings for sweet foods.

Most people ingest some omega-6s from nuts and non-hydrogenated vegetable oils and margarines, but very few omega-3s – therefore, to address our modern dietary deficiencies Dr Erasmus suggests an intake of two parts omega-3 to one part omega-6.

Another beneficial fat, omega-9, is found in unrefined extra virgin olive oil, a monosaturated fat, which is far more stable for cooking (but never heat until it spits and produces smoke). A lesser-known EFA is omega-7 – also known as palmitoleic acid. This polyunsaturated fatty acid is found in the sea buckthorn berry. It is useful for dry skin and dry eyes, and for mouth and vaginal dryness. (For more help with omega-7 call Pharma Nord on 0800 591756.)

Polyunsaturated fats (also found in seeds, nuts and their oils) are healthy in their cold, unrefined form, and they are rich in omega-6 EFAs. So if you use sunflower, walnut, sesame seed or grape seed oils in their unrefined forms in salad dressings they are healthy. However, once the polyunsaturated oils that you find in most biscuits, flapjacks, margarines, and mass-produced vegetable oils are heated, they become unhealthy.

Many people cook (mostly frying) with oils and margarines labelled 'polyunsaturated' believing them to be healthier, but it is not so. If the oils that you buy are mass-produced, all the processes I mentioned earlier will have long ago destroyed the majority of any health benefits. Butter is actually better for cooking at low temperatures, as it does not turn rancid like the essential fats. Butter contains vitamin A and butyric acid, which has anti-cancer properties, and a little butter, preferably organic is OK, **if** you have sufficient EFAs in the body.

All essential fats need to be kept cool and never heated, as the heat destroys the delicate EFAs – this includes all oil-based supplements that should be kept in the fridge. Having said this, there is now an EFA-based oil made with a blend of avocado, olive, oleic sunflower and toasted sesame seed oil – which remains stable when used for stir-fries. Called simply '3', it is now available in health stores, or call the Nutri Centre on 020 7436 5122.

Typical symptoms of insufficient EFAs are dry skin and eyes, cracked lips, water retention, increased thirst, physical and mental exhaustion, mood swings, inflammatory conditions such as eczema and arthritis, frequent infections, hayfever, allergies, mental health problems, poor memory and learning difficulties, and cardiovascular disease. Most of these conditions we tend to accept as we age, but if you take sufficient EFAs then you should avoid such symptoms for many more years.

Foods to Avoid
- If you like red meat, just eat lean organic meats once a week. Generally you need to cut down on all meats, meat pies, sausages and so on, and if you do eat meat choose a lean cut. With

chicken, turkey, duck, quail, or other game, cut off the skin. If you eat bacon, make it only a once-a-week treat, then grill it and cut off the fat.

- Reduce your intake of full fat milk, cheeses, chocolates, crisps and refined mass-produced cakes and biscuits, which are usually high in hydrogenated or trans fats and which are not good for your health.
- Avoid as much as possible all refined vegetable oils typically found in margarines, biscuits and cakes, and of course mass-produced vegetable oils.
- Eliminate or greatly reduce the amount of fried foods you eat.
- Remember sugar, if not used up during exercise, converts to fat inside the body and many foods advertised as being low in fat are usually packed with sugar!

Friendly Foods

- Look for non-hydrogenated spreads such as Vitaquell, Biona and Benecol.
- If you need to shallow fry use a little olive oil or butter, although butter is a saturated fat, it does not turn rancid like vegetable oils when heated. I also use a little butter for baking cakes. For biscuits and flapjacks I use extra virgin olive oil.
- Nutritionist Gareth Zeal recommends blending extra virgin olive oil with butter to use as a healthier alternative to hydrogenated-trans-fat-based margarines, also for spreads and making cakes and biscuits.
- If you like stir-fries, use a little olive, canola, ground nut (peanut) oil or grapeseed oil. Heat through but not until 'spitting or smoking' then add vegetables and so on and stir for a minute. Then add a little water and 'steam fry' for a couple more minutes. This helps to reduce the amount of free radicals that are produced when you fry food.

- Oily fish, such as mackerel, wild salmon, sardines, tuna and herrings, are all rich in omega-3 fats.
- Soya and kidney beans also contain some omega-3 fats, but try to use only GM-free and organic soya beans.
- Walnuts, pecans, almonds, but not peanuts, are all rich in omega-6 fats.
- If you use linseeds (flax seeds) to increase your omega-3 intake, buy them ready cracked (available from most supermarkets). Keep cracked linseeds in the fridge. Or, grind them first. Use a coffee grinder, which breaks them up in seconds, or simply crush them with a pestle and mortar. Otherwise chew linseeds really well or they will mainly pass through your system whole and you miss out on the omega-3 health benefits.
- Seeds such as sunflower and pumpkin can be eaten as a snack or sprinkled on soups or salads, and added to meals.
- Hemp seed is now readily available and is a good blend of omega-3 and -6 fatty acids.
- Eat more (but not to excess) mono-unsaturated fats, such as those found in avocados and olive oil.
- Eat more raw wheat germ and rice bran, rich in vitamin E, which helps you to absorb the EFAs more effectively.
- Buy good-quality, unrefined and preferably organic sunflower, walnut and sesame oils and mix them half and half with olive oil to make delicious salad dressings, or drizzle them over cooked foods (once they are on your plate). Keep them in the fridge to protect the EFAs.
- Once a week I pop a tablespoon each of sunflower, pumpkin, sesame seeds and linseeds (flax seeds), walnuts, almonds, and Brazil and hazel nuts, into a food mixer and pulse for a few seconds. I then place them in a glass jar in the fridge and use them over breakfast cereals, yoghurts, desserts, fruit salads and so on. This is a great way to get more EFAs.
- See details of '3' above – a new EFA blend that remains stable when used for cooking. For details contact the Nutri Centre. Tel 020 7436 5122.

Useful Remedies

- If you are not vegetarian, then take 1–3 grams of fish oil capsules daily. Many people no longer take fish oils as they worry about the concentrations of toxins, such as PCBs and dioxins, but Higher Nature, BioCare, FSC and Seven Seas One-a-Day fish oils are all guaranteed to be free from toxins. **HN BC FSC** Eskimo 3 stable fish oil capsules are the best and are distributed by PPC Galway Ltd, Mulvoy Business Park, Sean Mulvoy Road, Galway, Ireland. Tel: 00353 91 753222, or email ppc@iol.ie
- GLA is an omega-6 EFA and can be found in evening primrose oil, blackcurrant oil and borage oil. It has anti-inflammatory properties and helps increase your metabolic rate, and reduces symptoms of PMT. Most supplement companies sell GLA and you can take around 250mg daily.
- If you want pure linseed (flax seed) oil try Omega Nutrition from Higher Nature. **HN**
- Udo's Choice Oil is made from organic flax, sunflower and sesame seeds, plus rice and oat germ oils, in the perfect ratio for good health. Dr Udo Erasmus says we need approximately 1 tbsp for every 50lbs (23kg) of body weight, and we need more EFAs in winter than in summer. It is available as an oil, which either can be blended with other oils for salad dressings, or a little can be drizzled over cooked dishes. It is also available in capsules. These oils are highly unstable, should never be heated, and need to be kept in the fridge. Udo's Choice is available from health stores worldwide, or to find your nearest stockist in the UK contact Savant Distribution Limited, Quarry House, Clayton Wood Close, Leeds LS16 6QE, or call 0845 0606070. Website: www.savant-health.com, or email: info@savant-health.com
- Another good blend of omega-3 and -6 oils in capsule form is Efalex from Efamol.
- When supplementing with fatty acids, either in capsule or liquid form, it is very important to take extra vitamin E at least 100iu a day
- For anyone who has had their gall bladder removed, suffers Crohn's disease or colitis, or has a sensitive gut or irritable bowel and cannot tolerate too much oil (as the liver has to metabolise **all** fats and oils) use Dri-Celle Omega Plex essential fatty acid powder by BioCare. **BC** The EFAs have been micro-encapsulated into water-soluble fibre and then freeze-dried using no oxygen or heat. This powdered formula is therefore totally stable, which increases absorption dramatically. It bypasses the liver and is 100% absorbed in the intestines.
- For those who want to know more about this subject Dr Udo Erasmus has written *The Fats That Heal and Fats That Kill* (Alive Books). He has also written an EFA cookbook. To order call 0845 060 6070, or log on to www.savant-health.com

FIBROIDS

A fibroid is a benign tumour made up of muscle and fibrous tissue that grows in the muscular wall of the womb. Fibroids often produce no symptoms at all but they are known to cause heavy menstrual bleeding and may contribute to infertility. The growth of fibroids seems to be related to a hormone imbalance, especially an excess of the hormone oestrogen. If you are on the combined pill or HRT, both of which contain oestrogen, you may wish to discuss coming off these drugs with your GP in order to prevent further growth. If you suffer heavy periods over several months please have this checked out. With any condition that is linked to hormones you really need to detoxify and support the liver – see *Liver problems*.

Foods to Avoid

- Any foods that can cause elevated oestrogen levels or will recycle oestrogen into its aggressive form. These include alcohol, animal fats such as cheese, milk other than fully skimmed, cream, ice cream, butter, chocolates and most meat.

- Don't heat ready-made meals in plastic containers as the plastic residues leach into the food, which again has an oestrogen affect.
- Avoid as much as possible non-organic foods that are often high in pesticides and herbicides – which migrate to fatty tissue and increase oestrogen activity in the body.

Friendly Foods
- Fermented soya-based foods, such as tempeh, have a regulating effect on oestrogen levels and are protective against aggressive oestrogens.
- Chickpeas, broccoli, cabbage, Brussels sprouts and cauliflower are all beneficial foods.
- Linseeds (flax seeds) contain lignan which also helps to balance hormones naturally – I add a tablespoon of Linusit Gold, available from most supermarkets and health stores, to my breakfast cereals and vegetable juices.
- Don't overcook your vegetables and make fresh vegetable juices every day; drink immediately after juicing.
- Eat plenty of foods containing natural carotenes such as cantaloupe melons, apricots, sweet potatoes, parsley, carrots, spring greens, watercress and spinach. Eat more almonds, cod liver oil, avocados, wheat germ and hazelnuts, which are all rich in vitamin E.
- You need plenty of essential fats, which play a vital role in hormone production. Either add Udo's Choice Oil to cooked food or take capsules daily (see under *Fat You Need to Eat*).

Useful Remedies

- Soya isoflavones, 50–100mg, for regulation of hormone levels, and wild yam to help curb excessive bleeding, 1–3ml of tincture or 1–3 grams of tablets.
- Agnus castus – 1–3ml in tincture or 1–3 grams of tablets daily – a herb traditionally used to balance hormones. Use Bioforce agnus castus tincture.
- A high-strength multi-vitamin and mineral for women. **BC HN S FSC**
- Some women stop ovulating at some point between their 35th and 40th birthdays and therefore no longer make progesterone, but continue to make oestrogen. Talk to your GP about using natural progesterone cream, which can help reverse fibroids. This cream is freely available to buy outside the UK, and you can order it for your own use. **PW** Within the UK you need a prescription. For a list of doctors who work with natural progesterone send a large SAE with £1 in stamps to NPIS, P.O. Box 24, Buxton SK17 9FB. Call them on 07000 784849 www.npis.info/contactus.htm
- Silica and calcium fluoride tissue salts can help to break down the fibroids. Take 4 of each daily.

Helpful Hints
- Once you go through menopause the fibroids should shrink naturally.
- Homeopathic Aur-mur-nat 6x taken 3 times daily can help if there are no actual physical symptoms.

FIBROMYALGIA
see *Polymyalgia Rheumatica*

FLATULENCE
(see also *Candida, Constipation* and *IBS*)

Flatulence, wind and bloating is, to say the least, very unsociable and sometimes extremely uncomfortable. It can be due to partly digested foods being fermented in the gut and/or from an imbalance of the organisms that reside in the bowel. The yeast fungal overgrowth candida is often the root cause, as unhealthy bacteria thrive on less healthy foods, particularly sugar, but also the biproducts of partial digestion. It is very important that you chew your food properly as the digestive process begins in the mouth. Almost 60% of carbohydrate digestion is done in the mouth if foods are properly chewed. The majority of protein digestion is done in the stomach, so it is crucial that we have adequate levels of stomach acids and enzymes to break down the foods. Various factors can weaken our ability to digest foods properly: smoking is notorious, but alcohol, sugary foods, high-fat foods, caffeinated beverages, and prolonged stress can all progressively weaken the digestion.

Foods to Avoid

- Beans such as cannellini, kidney, black-eyed and so on, plus lentils, artichokes, broccoli, Brussels sprouts, fizzy drinks and beer are all famous for causing wind. Some people have problems with cabbage and onions.
- Also avoid any food to which you have an allergy or intolerance, the most common being dairy products from cows.
- Try to note any foods that make you feel bloated or cause a lot of wind and see if there is a common denominator.
- If you have eaten a large meal, don't eat large amounts of fruit directly after the meal, as the fruit will ferment in the gut as it becomes stuck behind the other food, and fruit likes a fast passage through the gut. Eat fruit before or in-between meals.
- I often begin a meal with a few chunks of fresh pineapple or papaya, which aid digestion.

Friendly Foods

- Certain foods help to improve digestion, noticeably fennel, celeriac, radicchio, young green celery, and watercress help to stimulate gastric juices and aid digestion.
- Drinking peppermint, fennel or camomile teas, or a combination of them, after meals can often make digestion easier and make you feel more comfortable.
- Add a strip of dried Kombu seaweed when cooking any bean dishes, this helps to predigest the enzymes that cause the wind and bloating. Throw away after cooking.
- Include more fresh root ginger in your cooking, which aids digestion.
- Eat more low-fat, live yoghurts.

Useful Remedies

- Peppermint formula, a blend of herbs that help to stimulate digestion. Take 1–2ml before meals. This is also very useful if you have simply overeaten and feel uncomfortable – 1–2ml generally alleviates the discomfort. **FSC**
- Betain Hydrochloride; 1 capsule taken prior to meals with a glass of water. This helps improve digestion, which tends to weaken as we get older. If you have active stomach ulcers do not take this remedy – take the digestive enzyme instead. Protazyme is an excellent digestive enzyme formula – from health shops, made by BioCare. **BC**
- Acidophilus and bifidus; 1–2 capsules, taken at the end of a meal helps replace healthy gut flora, which in turn helps manufacture gastric enzymes and helps to keep candida under control if this is the root cause of the problem.
- Lepicol contains FOS (a type of sugar that feeds the friendly bacteria) and acidophilus makes an excellent cleanser and bowel regulator.

Helpful Hints

- Try to eat smaller meals, which place less strain on the digestive tract and liver.
- Many people have benefitted from following the principle of food combining, separating carbohydrates and proteins.
- Chronic flatulence can also be a symptom of food intolerance, irritable bowel syndrome, candida, or gut infections. If you are concerned, see a qualified nutritionist (see *Useful Information*).

FLU
(see *Colds and Flu*)

FLUID RETENTION
(see *Water Retention*)

FLUORIDE
(see also *Bleeding Gums*)

Calcium fluoride occurs naturally in most drinking water and in small quantities is relatively harmless. However, artificial fluoride – hexaflurosilicilic acid – is toxic. Added to drinking water in areas such as Birmingham and Newcastle, it is a waste product from phosphate fertiliser plants, brick works and aluminium smelters. Fluoride is used to make pesticides and rat poisons, it is also found in low concentrations in Californian table wines. Fluoride accumulates in bone and soft tissue and can have a devastating affect on the brain, bones and teeth.

Dental fluorosis or mottling teeth is common in areas where the water is fluoridated. Since 1997 the FDA in the US has required a poison label on all toothpastes containing fluoride, but in Britain there is currently no such requirement. Both the American and British Dental Associations make considerable amounts of money by endorsing fluoride toothpastes and mouthwashes. The problem today is that so many products contain fluoride including toothpastes, mouthwashes, medicines (Prozac is fluoxetine), anaesthetics and pesticides, and that it is in our polluted air – and it is the accumulation of this toxin that is causing so many health problems. Currently no testing facilities to determine existing levels are available under the NHS. If you have thyroid problems be aware that fluoride can compete for iodine – needed for thyroid function in receptor sites in the body.

In July 1997 the Union of 1,500 government scientists working at the US Environmental Protection Agency issued a statement saying: "Our review of eleven years' evidence including animal and human studies indicates a causal link between fluoride/fluoridation and cancer, genetic damage and neurological impairment." In 1994 the World Health Organisation warned "Dental and public health administrators should be aware of the total fluoride exposure in the population before introducing any additional fluoride programmes." As a result of new research 11 unions working for the Environmental Protection Agency in the US declared in July 2005 that fluoride is a carcinogen and that fluoridation should be stopped. The research from Harvard University found links between fluoride in tap water (at levels most Americans drink) to osteosarcoma, a rare form of bone cancer. Unsurprisingly a prominent researcher at the Harvard School of Dental Medicine faced charges of misconduct for failing to report these findings in their true light. Most European countries have now banned fluoride and I believe that the UK should do the same.

Apart from the horrendous health concerns associated with fluoride, the National Pure Water Association has estimated that the cost of building plants to enable fluoridation of water will be an estimated £85 million in Yorkshire alone. The health service would need to foot the bill, yet many of our hospitals are under-funded …

Foods to Avoid
■ Read labels carefully and note that tea, salmon and sardines are rich in fluorides. As much as possible avoid non-organic foods that have more than likely been sprayed with pesticides containing fluoride. If you live in a fluoridated area, as much as possible drink bottled, distilled or reverse osmosis de-ionised water. Contact www.purewater.co.uk

Friendly Foods
- Organic foods that are free of harmful pesticides and herbicides. Drink plenty of fluoride-free water in-between meals.
- See *General Health Hints*.

Helpful Hints
- If you drink fluoridated tap water, do not use fluoridated toothpastes or mouthwashes.
- Buy fluoride-free toothpastes – I found one in my local health store called Aloe Dent, containing aloe vera, co-enzyme Q10, tea tree oil, silica and so on, which all promote healthy gums and teeth. They also make a brilliant mouthwash. For your nearest stockist log on to www.optimahealthcare.co.uk. Otherwise ask at your local health store as there are several good natural brands available.
- Young children tend to swallow toothpaste – therefore, make sure it is fluoride free. To avoid fillings greatly limit your child's intake of sugary foods and drinks.
- Consider having a fluoride-removing water filter fitted at home. The Fresh Water Filter Company Ltd offers a broad range of water filters. Call them on 0870 442 3633, or visit their website at www.freshwaterfilter.com
- The Doctors' Laboratory will test for levels of fluoride in the body. You do need a referral from a health professional, such as a doctor or nutritionist. The Laboratory can be contacted at 60 Whitfield Street, London W1T 4EU. Tel: 020 7307 7373. Website: www.tdlplc.co.uk
- For further information and the latest updates on the dangers of fluoride, log on to the National Pure Water Association website on: www.npwa.freeserve.co.uk
- To find out more read *The Fluoride Deception* by Christopher Bryson (Seven Stories Press).

FOOD POISONING (see also *Diarrhoea, IBS and Vomiting*)

Each year an estimated 5.5 million people in the UK suffer from some kind of food poisoning. And this figure is on the low side, as many mild cases go unreported. Food poisoning is mainly caused by various bacteria found in food, but can also be caused by viruses, parasites and toxins in foods, such as those common in many wild field mushrooms. These bacteria and so on are often hard to detect, as they don't usually affect the taste, appearance or smell of food. Food poisoning is more likely to affect people with lowered resistance to disease such as the elderly or sick, babies, young children, and pregnant women. Symptoms of food poisoning are nausea, vomiting, diarrhoea, abdominal pain, headache, and low-grade fever.

The most serious types of food poisoning are due to bacteria, which can cause poisoning in two different ways. Some bacteria infect the intestines, causing inflammation and problems with the normal absorption of nutrients and water, which lead to diarrhoea. Other bacteria produce toxins on the food that are poisonous to the human digestive system. When eaten, these chemicals trigger nausea and vomiting, kidney failure, and in extreme cases even death. The most common and widely known bacteria are salmonella, campylobacter, E-coli, staphylococcus, shigella, and botulism. The more bacteria present on a food, the more likely you are to become ill. Bacteria multiply very fast especially in warm, moist conditions. The presence or absence of oxygen, salt, sugar and the acidity of the surroundings are also important factors. In the right conditions one bacterium can multiply to more than 4 million in just 8 hours.

Bacteria generally like temperatures between 5°C (41°F) and 63°C (145°F) where they can multiply easily. They are killed at temperatures of 70°C (158°F). Most bacteria multiply very slowly at temperatures below 5°C (41°F) and some bacteria die at very low temperatures. Unfortunately, many can survive these low temperatures and can start to multiply again if warm conditions return. This is why proper handling and storage of food, plus sensible hygiene precautions are of utmost importance in preventing food poisoning.

Foods to Avoid

- To help prevent an attack avoid food that has been reheated more than once
- Avoid eating any foods that have been left standing in warm conditions such as at garden fêtes and buffets – and which you know have been there a while.
- Food that is not piping hot – especially warm chicken dishes.
- Food that has come into contact with raw meat or poultry.
- If you are in any country that has poor-quality drinking water, take the following precautions:
  - Drink only bottled water, and also avoid salads at all costs, as the salad has likely been washed in local water. The worst case of food poisoning I ever had was in India, because I thought, "Oh, raw food is fine." Big mistake! Hot food that has been well-cooked is best.
  - Similarly, if you are offered bottles of water or other drinks that are not properly sealed, say no thanks.
  - It may sound ridiculous, but if cutlery has been washed in local streams in, say, India, you would be wise to take your own cutlery.
  - Peel fruit.
  - Beware of ice cubes unless made with bottled water.
  - Do not eat any of the following under-cooked or rare: poultry, burgers, sausages, chicken nuggets, rolled joints, kebabs.

- If you are unfortunate enough to get a bout of food poisoning, short episodes of vomiting and small amounts of diarrhoea lasting less than 24 hours can usually be cared for at home. When a bout of food poisoning is underway, it is best to rest and starve yourself of solid food for 24 hours as this will also starve the bacteria. But if you are not holding down any fluids, you must seek medical help, as dehydration can kill you. This is especially true for young children and babies.

Friendly Foods

- During an attack drink plenty of boiled or bottled water, or sip ginger ale to avoid dehydration.
- After 24 hours of starvation and when you are successfully tolerating fluids, start eating small amounts of brown rice, plain yoghurts, soups, and dry toast or crackers and see how you go. Don't try to eat anything heavy for the first couple of days – be kind to your system.

Useful Remedies

- One or two drops of liquid grapefruit-seed extract can be added to water and sipped throughout the day, as it has strong anti-bacterial action. **HN** or contact www.positivehealthshop.com
- Whenever you have had an episode of food poisoning, probiotics – healthy bacteria found in the bowel – are really essential. They help re-populate the bowel and help protect against further growth of the offending bugs. *Lactobacillus Bulgaricus* has been shown to help reduce diarrhoea. Take one twice a day during the initial phase of food poisoning. **BC**
- Homeopathic Arsen Alb is good for reducing stomach cramps, Nux Vomica helps reduce feelings of nausea and Mag Phos is also great for cramps.
- Once symptoms have begun to settle and nausea and vomiting have ceased you can try the following: Goldenseal is a useful herb once initial symptoms have subsided. It helps to increase appetite and reduce nausea and vomiting. It also has strong properties for fighting off bad bacteria and it also has a soothing effect on the mucous membranes in the gut. Solgar's Goldenseal Root Complex provides 500mg. Available from all health stores. Initially, take 1 a day with food and then increase to 1, 3 times day for two weeks.

- Charcoal capsules or tablets may help in the case of diarrhoea. The charcoal will help bind on to the toxins that will be produced from the bug and will be excreted through the bowel. These are available at most health food stores and some chemists.
- In studies, people experiencing food poisoning in Egypt found that the duration and intensity of symptoms were hugely reduced when using probiotics – healthy bacteria necessary for gut health. BioCare do an excellent probiotic coupled with some natural anti-bacterial agents. It is called Travelguard. Take 1 a day with food when travelling abroad to help prevent the onset of food poisoning. **BC**

Helpful Hints

- Most cases of food poisoning clear up on their own after a few days but you should visit a doctor if the symptoms of food poisoning last for more than 2 or 3 days. Also, if there is a fever and the diarrhoea is very watery, or there is blood, pus or mucus mixed in with the stools, please get medical help.
- Signs of dehydration are intense thirst, dry lips and tongue, increased heart rate, and weakness.
- Bacteria thrive on dirty, damp cloths. So it's very important to wash kitchen cloths, tea towels and sponges regularly. Choose the hottest wash that your washing machine permits to make sure all bacteria are killed.
- Bacteria love to travel and will hitch a ride on anything they can – hands, chopping boards, knives or tongs – and find their way on to foods such as bread or salad. Make sure you thoroughly wash hands and utensils in warm soapy water after touching raw meat and poultry, going to the toilet, touching the bin, and touching pets.
- Don't forget to dry your hands thoroughly, because if they are wet they will spread bacteria more easily.
- Cook meats thoroughly – especially poultry. If you are serving poultry cold, make sure it's kept really cool; and if re-heating, make sure it's hot right through. Chickens need to be roasted at 200°C (400°F), or gas mark 6, for 20 minutes per pound (450g), plus an extra 20 minutes.
- Citricidal – grapefruit-seed extract – has wonderful anti-bacterial and antiparasitic actions and has been proven in laboratory tests to be 10 times more effective as a disinfectant than chlorine. Available from health stores. Use it in the following ways:
  - Anti-bacterial handwash. Ten–15 drops added to an 8oz- (225-gram) pump container of hand soap makes an anti-bacterial soap.
  - Vegetable wash. Add 30 or more drops to a sink full of cold water and briefly soak any vegetables and fruit.
  - Dish- and utensil-cleaning additive. Add 15–30 drops to sink dishwashing water or to final rinse. Add 15–30 drops to an automatic dishwasher with detergent or to a final rinse.
  - Cutting-board cleaner. Apply 10–20 drops of the citricidal to cutting boards and work into the entire board with a wet sponge or dish cloth. Leave on for at least 30 minutes. Rinse with water.
- If you have cooked food that you aren't going to eat straight away, cool it as quickly as possible (ideally within 1–2 hours) and then store it in the fridge. Do not cool it down in the fridge as this can raise the overall temperature in the fridge, which will enable bacteria on food already stored in the fridge to grow.
- Don't store leftovers for longer than 2 days.
- Never use cracked raw eggs.
- Don't put raw chicken or meat next to cooked food on the grill or barbecue.
- Don't add sauce or marinade to cooked food if it has been used to baste raw chicken or meat.
- Store raw chicken and meat on the bottom shelf of the fridge where it can't touch or drip onto other foods.

- Use separate tongs and utensils for raw chicken and meat and for cooked chicken and meat.
- Keep raw meat and ready-to-eat food separate in the fridge and also in the kitchen area. This is especially important regarding raw meat and ready-to-eat foods, such as salad, fruit and bread. As these foods won't be cooked before you eat them, any bacteria that get onto them won't be killed.

FOOT PROBLEMS

All too many of us spend far too long on our feet. A typical person walks 71,000 miles (about 116,500km) during their lifetime. Our often-neglected feet contain 26 bones, 56 ligaments and 38 muscles so there is an awful lot that can go wrong with them. Wearing shoes that are too high can trigger back problems, and if your shoes are too tight they will restrict circulation, triggering problems such as blisters, corns and chilblains. One of the best ways to keep your feet pain-free is to visit a chiropodist regularly.

Cold feet

Cold feet usually relate to poor circulation (see *Circulation*), but can also be associated with low thyroid function (see *Thyroid*). If your feet are chronically cold, even when the weather is warm, ask your doctor to check you for an under-active thyroid or for Raynaud's Syndrome (see *Raynaud's Disease*).

Regular exercise, massage with essential oil of black pepper (mixed with a base oil), acupuncture, and reflexology will all help alleviate cold feet. Wearing bed socks helps – and keeping a magnet in your shoes encourages better circulation to the feet. For all foods and supplements – see *Circulation* and *Raynaud's Disease*. One very useful herb for cold feet is gotu kola, as it increases circulation in the lower limbs. You can also include more fresh root ginger in your diet, or take ginger capsules as they bring more warmth to the body.

Cracked heels   (see also *Thyroid*)

Also referred to as fissures, for most people cracked heels just look unsightly, but for others they can become quite painful. Cracked heels are mainly due to excessively dry skin on the outside of the heels but can also be due to a thyroid problem, prolonged standing, inactive sweat glands, obesity, wearing of flip flops or open backed shoes, flat feet (see *Fallen Arches*, below), use of excessively hot water, walking abnormally, eczema and psoriosis.

Foods to Avoid
- Avoid alcohol and caffeine found in coffee, tea, power drinks and some painkillers, as these dehydrate the body.
- Reduce saturated fats found in red meat and dairy – trim all fat from the meat, and grill rather than fry your food. These 'bad' fats prevent the good fats from doing their job (see also *Fats You Need To Eat*).

Friendly Foods
- Aim to drink plenty of water per day, building up to this gradually, to help rehydrate your skin.
- Zinc-rich foods, such as brown rice, lentils, and pumpkin, sunflower and sesame seeds, plus almonds, are rich in minerals and essential fats that nourish your skin from the inside out.
- Use more organic olive, walnut, sesame and avocado oils in salad dressings or drizzle over

cooked foods.

- Magnesium-rich foods are dark green leafy vegetables, cashew nuts, broccoli, bananas and prunes; whilst selenium-rich foods are Brazil nuts, oats, and brown rice.

Useful Remedies

- The herb ginkgo biloba helps circulation, which in turn helps to get the nutrients to where they are needed. Take 15 drops 3 times a day.
- A good all-round multi, such as Solgar's VM75 x 1 per day.
- Higher Nature's Essential Balance Oil contains all of the necessary essential oils, and will help to lubricate the skin. It comes in capsules – take 3 per day or buy a bottle of the oil and drizzle it over cooked vegetables or baked potatoes, or it use for salad dressings.

Helpful Hints

- Find a really good cream for extra-dry skin. The Organic Pharmacy makes several. Apply twice daily especially before going to bed, and then put on an old cotton sock so that the cream can really soak into the dry areas. **OP**
- Soak your feet daily in warm soapy water for 15 minutes and use a good pumice stone or foot scrub on the thick skin on your heels and then thickly apply a moisturizing cream, sit back, and let it soak in. Avoid open-backed or thin-soled shoes and buy shoes with a good shock-absorbing sole. Never try to cut back the hard skin yourself with a razor blade or a pair of scissors – see a chiropodist. Ask in any large Boots the Chemists, or call the Institute of Chiropodists and Podiatrists on 08700 110 305 to find a qualified chiropodist in your area. Website: www.inst-chiropodist.org.uk

Fallen arches

Most people when standing have a gap between the inner side of the foot and the ground they are standing on – this is called the arch. Fallen arches – also known as flat feet – happen when there is a flat arch and the foot rolls over so there is little or no gap. Symptoms depend on the severity of the condition, but corns, hard skin under the sole of the foot, and a tender arch area are common and shoes will tend to wear out quickly. In severe cases calf, knee, hip or back pain can be experienced. Fallen arches may be hereditary, but in most cases it is caused by abnormal walking where the joints in the foot roll in too much. A ruptured tendon can also lead to a flat foot, as can cerebral palsy, spina bifida and muscular dystrophy.

Helpful Hints

- Find a good local health clinic that deals with sports injuries. If they have an in-house chiropodist or podiatrist you can be fitted for individual orthotics – inserts made specifically for your feet, these give your foot all the support it needs. Otherwise large chemists and foot specialists like Scholl offer a variety of orthotic inserts especially to support the arches. One of the best inserts I have found is Orthaheel, which is available worldwide. Log on to www.orthaheel.com. To find a qualified chiropodist in your area, ask in any large pharmacy or chemist, or contact the Institute of Chiropodists and Podiatrists at www.inst-chiropodist.org.uk, or call them on 08700 110 305.
- MBT shoes (Masai Barefoot Technology) are state-of-the-art shoes that support the feet really well. These shoes greatly alleviate many structural problems including back, knee and joint pain. Have a look at www.mbt-info.com

Hot, burning feet

Poor circulation is often the cause of this problem (see *Circulation*). It is also common in people suffering from diabetes who frequently have problems with nerves within the feet. Other than diabetes, circulation can be affected by eating too many of the wrong type of fats, which tend to clog up the system. Dehydration can compound the problem as it makes it harder for fluid and nutrients to move around the body. Improving circulation to the feet can often relieve symptoms.

Foods to Avoid
■ Avoid saturated animal fats found in red meat and dairy, plus hydrogenated and trans fats rich in processed foods – especially burger-type foods, and cakes and pastries. See *Fats You Need To Eat*.
■ Reduce or avoid alcohol as this is dehydrating .

Friendly Foods
■ The essential fats found in oily fish such as mackerel, sardines, fresh tuna, anchovies, and salmon plus nuts and seeds.
■ Blueberries and cherries. These contain beneficial properties that help to keep the walls of blood vessels strong so that they can carry fluid and nutrients around the body more easily and efficiently.

Useful Remedies
■ Take a high-potency B-complex daily – aiming for 50mg of the majority of B-vitamins.
■ Higher Nature's Essential Oil Balance contains the correct ratio of the essential oils. Take 3 capsules daily, or buy the oil and drizzle it over cooked vegetables, or rice dishes, or use it for salad dressings.

Helpful Hints
■ Acupuncture and reflexology are also very useful for alleviating this condition (see Useful Information).
■ Try using an 'energy roller' (£23.50 including p&p) – a wooden spiked roller developed over 10 years by a reflexologist. It may hurt a little initially, but it stimulates pressure points and many people, especially diabetics, have said that it has proven to be very helpful. For details send an SAE to Acumag Ltd, 106 West Street, Erith, Kent DA8 1AQ. Tel 01322 447610. Website: www.acumag.co.uk
■ Exercise is great for stimulating the circulation. Take a regular 30-minute walk each day. Any exercise that gently pounds the bottom of the feet will help to improve circulation. Try, dancing, skipping or rebounding.

Numb and tingling feet

It is very important if you have this problem for more than a few days that you see your GP to find out if there is anything more serious going on, as numb or tingling feet can be due to peripheral neuropathy, which can denote late-onset diabetes. A simple urine test is all that's needed to clarify if this is the case. A lack of calcium may also cause this problem. Try taking 1000mg of calcium daily for a couple of weeks.

■ If you have numb and tingling feet, take the supplements suggested under *Circulation*, get plenty of exercise such as walking, skipping or rebounding, which really help bring more blood to the feet.
■ Consult a chiropractor – who can check for trapped nerves and any misalignments that may be triggering this problem. See *Useful Information*.

■ Try reflexology and acupuncture to further improve circulation.

Smelly feet
(see also *Athlete's foot*, *Candida* and *Body odour*)

Smelly feet can be highly embarrassing and in most cases are easily prevented. Initially wash your feet a couple of times a day with warm water with a little added tea tree oil, and then use natural talcum powder to help keep them drier. Always wear 100% cotton socks and leather shoes, as synthetic fibres lead to increased sweating and it is the bacteria in the sweat that create the unpleasant smell. Change your shoes often – alternating pairs daily would help as this gives your shoes a chance to breathe. Going without shoes whenever possible is also a good idea, as the fresh air will help reduce sweating. Some people find that if they put their shoes in a freezer overnight it helps to kill off the bacteria responsible for the odour.

Swollen feet and ankles
(see also *Water Retention*)

As we age the ratio of water found inside and outside our cells changes and we find it harder to properly absorb water into the cells. This extra fluid triggers oedema (collection of water in the body's tissues), which with gravity heads south toward our feet! This problem is common in middle-aged and older ladies, and can also happen during pregnancy. Again, this is mainly linked to circulation and the body's ability to remove excess fluid (see *Circulation*). Any injury of the feet, ankles or legs can also contribute to swelling in this area.

Foods to Avoid
■ Avoid all foods high in salt and sodium, such as preserved meats and fish, crisps, processed foods, packet sauces and ketchup-style foods, which often contain huge amounts of hidden salt. Salt exacerbates any water retention and increases swelling in all parts of the body if you suffer fluid retention.
■ Check the salt-content of breakfast cereals and cereal bars – look for low salt/sodium ones.
■ Look out for hidden sources of salt/sodium. It is found in high quantities in ketchups, pickles and relishes and olives, and in sodium benzoate E211 – a preservative – and monosodium glutamate (MSG), also known as E621. Cut out adding salt to your food and cooking.
■ Avoid burger-type meals that are high in salt and fat; also avoid sausages, and mass-produced pies, cakes and biscuits.
■ Avoid caffeine in any form (watch out for it hidden in energy drinks and some painkillers), plus tea and alcohol, as these will dehydrate the body.
■ Cut back on saturated fats found in red meat and dairy produce. These clog up the lymphatic system, which is responsible for removing excess fluid. See *Fats You Need To Eat*.
■ See also *General Health Hints*.

Friendly Foods
■ Eat foods rich in potassium, such as green vegetables, fresh fruit, dried fruits, unsalted nuts (not peanuts), seafoods, bananas, potatoes, and unsalted sunflower and pumpkin seeds.
■ Eat more oily fish and use unrefined walnut, olive, hemp and sunflower oils for your salad dressings.
■ Try a little magnesium-rich Solo Salt – easily available and found in the majority of supermarkets and all good health food stores.

Useful Remedies
■ Celery seed extract acts like a diuretic. Take 2 capsules twice daily until symptoms ease.
■ Also take 1 gram of vitamin C as potassium ascorbate to improve lymph drainage. This should

help to remove excess fluid. **BC**

- Silica and sulphur compound for three months will help to improve tissue tone. **BLK**
- On days when your ankles are very swollen, take 15 drops of dandelion tincture 3 times a day before meals. Dandelion leaves are a potassium-rich diuretic, which also help to cleanse the liver. Bioforce makes a good one. Tel: 0800 085 0820
- As lack of B-vitamins are linked to this problem take a B-complex daily and look for one that contains 50mg of B6.

Helpful Hints

- Sit with your feet at hip level for at least 15 minutes every day, moving your feet back and forth to improve circulation.
- Rebounding (mini-trampolining) is especially good for boosting lymphatic drainage. Deep-tissue lymphatic drainage can help if the problem is one of a stagnant lymph system.
- Dry skin brushing helps remove excess fluid. Buy a natural (not synthetic), long-handled brush which shouldn't scratch the skin. Begin by brushing the soles of the feet as the 7,000 nerve endings there affect the whole body; next brush the ankles, calves and thighs, then brush across your stomach and buttocks, and lastly brush your hands and up your arms. Follow this with a warm bath or shower and complete the process with a cool rinse to really invigorate circulation. I find this a great way to wake up every morning and it really helps my skin to stay soft and in good condition.
- Call at a homeopathic pharmacy, which can suggest a remedy to suit your particular symptoms. Or call the Organic Pharmacy. **OP**

- If the symptoms persist after following the advice given here, for more than six weeks, ask your GP for a thorough check-up, as occasionally swollen feet and ankles may be a sign of heart, liver or kidney problems.

FROZEN SHOULDER

This condition is often characterised by pain and limited movement in one and very rarely both shoulders. It is owing to the inflammation of the muscles, ligaments or tendons around the shoulders. Exercise is often very painful; however, gentle exercise that encourages blood-flow and does not overstrain the joint or tendons is often helpful. It is common between the ages of 40 and 60, and affects between 2 and 5% of the population.

Foods to Avoid

- Avoid any foods and drinks containing caffeine, which greatly reduces our body's ability to make painkilling endorphins.
- Animal fats from meat, butter, cheese and milk will tend to increase inflammation in the body, as they are acid-forming – see *Acid–Alkaline balance*.

Friendly Foods

- Oily fish contain anti-inflammatory essential fatty acids – especially wild salmon, mackerel, sardines, cod, or red snapper.
- Cherries are high in bioflavonoids, which are mildly anti-inflammatory. Eat more pineapple for its bromelain content, which is also anti-inflammatory.
- Ginger, turmeric, and cayenne pepper are all spices that, used liberally, can help decrease pain.

Useful Remedies

- Ginger, curcumin and boswelia; take up to 4 tablets a day, which should help reduce the inflammation. **FSC**

- Magnesium helps to relax the muscles – while symptoms are acute take 1000mg per day.

Helpful Hints
- Creams made with cayenne pepper can bring rapid pain relief.
- Glucosamine gels with capsicum and MSM can also be applied daily.
- Bags of cherry stones or wheat can be either heated or frozen and then applied to the affected area for 10 minutes at a time to ease pain and inflammation.
- Traditionally, frozen shoulder is treated with physiotherapy. Alternatives are chiropractic and osteopathy, which are available on the NHS in some areas.
- Use your local swimming pool, as gentle movement in warm water loosens the shoulder.
- Acupuncture is great for reducing the acute pain, and aromatherapy massage with the essential oils of eucalyptus, ginger and juniper are all helpful (see *Useful Information*).
- Magnets make powerful pain-relievers – they encourage oxygenated blood to the painful area, which speeds the healing process. Many companies now make magnetic shoulder holders that can really help.

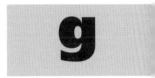

GALL-BLADDER PROBLEMS

(see also *Gall Stones* and *Liver Problems*)

The gall bladder is a small pear-shaped organ (sac), which sits underneath and is connected to the liver. The gall bladder's main function is to store bile, which is made in the liver. The gall bladder passes bile into the small bowel, where the bile helps to break down fat during digestion. If the liver is overloaded, toxins tend to get dumped in the gall bladder, a major cause of gall-bladder disease. The gall bladder can be affected by gall stones, inflammation, and infection. Each of the problems may produce pain on the right side encasing the centre of the abdomen. In some cases the pain can be so severe that the patient feels nauseous and faint.

Foods to Avoid
- High-fat and fried foods put an extra load on the gall bladder and its ability to digest fats.
- Alcohol, coffee and chocolate place an extra strain on the liver, which can make the problem worse. Many people who have gall-bladder problems are overweight and tend to love creamy, naughty foods – you know what I mean! Cut these out, and generally eat less, otherwise you end up having your gall bladder removed and then your body finds it difficult to metabolise fats and you will put on even more weight.
- See also *General Health Hints* and the dietary advice in *Liver Problems*.

Friendly Foods
- People who eat more beans and lentils are less likely to end up with gall-bladder or liver problems. Foods such as celeriac, artichokes, beetroot and celery are all good for liver and gall-bladder function.
- Try making fresh vegetable juices daily with celery, artichoke, parsley, raw beetroot, apples, carrots, and any green vegetables you have in your fridge. Add this to half a cup of organic aloe vera and drink daily to help detoxify your liver and gall bladder.
- Use unrefined extra virgin olive, walnut or linseed (flax seed) oil in small amounts in salad

dressings, all of which help to diminish the risk of developing problems.

■ Drink at least 6 glasses of water daily.

Useful Remedies

■ Milk thistle and dandelion are very effective for maintaining a healthy gall bladder. They both have the ability to enhance bile production, flow and activity. Use the tincture daily; available from good health stores. Otherwise Kudos makes a One-a-Day milk thistle of 900mg. **KVH**

■ Sprinkle 1 tbsp of lecithin granules over breakfast cereals, fruit whips or yoghurts, which helps to emulsify the bad fats within the body.

■ Swedish Bitters is a bitter tonic that aids the liver by enhancing the flow of bile. A few drops in a little water before main meals.

■ Sodiphos contains sodium sulphate and sodium phosphate, which helps the flow of bile; 3 tablets daily. **BLK**

■ See also *Useful Remedies* under *Gall Stones*.

Helpful Hints

■ Generally, to avoid gall-bladder problems you need to control your LDL cholesterol levels, and levels of stress. See also *Cholesterol* and *Stress*.

GALL STONES

Although up to 25% of the population have gall stones, only 15–20% eventually develop symptoms. Gall stones are twice as common in women especially after 40. People who tend to eat high saturated-fat and sugary diets that do not include sufficient fibre, or those who are obese, constantly dieting but rapidly gain weight, or suffer Crohn's disease are at a higher risk. Multiple pregnancies, the Pill and HRT are other factors, as is a high stress level. The gall bladder gets rid of unwanted substances such as cholesterol and bilirubin into the bile duct, which in turn drains into the intestine.

Most gall stones consist of a sediment made up primarily of cholesterol, bilirubin and bile salts, and occur in individuals with excess cholesterol in the bloodstream or as a result of stagnation of bile flow in the gall bladder.

Small gall stones often produce no symptoms, but if they become large enough to obstruct the bile duct they can cause jaundice, inflammation, intense pain and vomiting. Symptoms tend to be much worse after high-fat meals or after foods to which the individual has a sensitivity, such as eggs. Constipation can be linked to the risk of gall stones so it is very important that adequate fibre is eaten to reduce the likelihood of constipation and thereby reduce the risk of developing gallstones.

Foods to Avoid

■ To avoid gall-bladder attacks and gall stones, you really do have to stick to a low-fat diet by greatly reducing your intake of animal fats from any source.

■ Low-fibre foods, such as white bread, cakes, biscuits, ice cream, most puddings, and prepackaged meals should be avoided as much as possible.

■ Foods like eggs, pork, onions, pickles, spicy foods, peanuts, citrus fruits and sometimes coffee are likely triggers.

■ Regular coffee-drinkers (that's real coffee, not decaffeinated) have a much lower risk of developing gall stones, but if you have a sensitivity to coffee then you do need to avoid it.

Friendly Foods

■ Drink plenty of water to prevent the bile from becoming too concentrated – around 8 glasses daily.

- Small amounts of lamb, plus brown rice, and peas, pears and broccoli are usually no problem.
- Keep a food diary and eliminate any foods to which you have a reaction within an hour of eating them.
- Other foods that help the function of the gall bladder include beetroot, artichoke, dandelion, dried beans (aduki, kidney, pinto, haricot and so on), linseeds (flax seeds), and oat or rice bran – all of which are high-fibre foods to reduce constipation.
- Sprinkle a tablespoonful of lecithin granules over a low-sugar, oat-based muesli or cereal, as soya lecithin helps to break down the fat in foods.
- Use wholemeal bread, and pasta made from corn, lentil, rice and potato flour. Include fresh fish, a little chicken without the skin, plenty of salads and fresh fruit in your diet.
- Replace full-fat milks with skimmed and try more herbal teas. Use organic rice milk.
- Enjoy one glass of white wine daily – but if you drink to excess especially on long flights – again you could be in trouble!
- Use organic extra virgin olive, sunflower and walnut oils for salad dressings – these are all rich in essential fats, which help to dissolve stones.
- Freshly made carrot, beetroot and cucumber juices help support better gall-bladder function.

Useful Remedies
- Milk thistle and dandelion in combination as tablets or capsules, or dandelion formula. Take 1 or 2 tablets with every meal, or a measure 10–20 drops of tincture with every meal.
- People with gall stones tend to be deficient in vitamins C and E. Take 1 gram of C daily with food, which is needed for the conversion of cholesterol to bile acids. Take 200–400iu of full-spectrum vitamin E.
- Take Betaine Hydrochloride (stomach acid) – 1 capsule with meals – as many people with gall stones have food intolerances and digestive problems. Many practitioners find that gall-stone sufferers are deficient in stomach acid. Don't take this remedy if you have active stomach ulcers – instead take a digestive enzyme capsule with main meals. **BC** See also *Low Stomach Acid*.
- New Era silica and calcium fluoride tissue salts can help to break down and expel the stones. Four of each daily.

Helpful Hints
- As multiple food sensitivities are linked to gall-bladder problems, it is well worth your while to consult a qualified nutritionist or naturopath who can sort out your diet. The initial few weeks may be hard but there are plenty of foods you can eat. See *Useful Information* for details.

GENERAL HEALTH HINTS

- Make time for breakfast, which is the most important meal of the day. You are literally breaking a fast and to keep your blood sugar on an even keel you need to eat, or you will end up craving sugary snacks by mid-morning. Oat, spelt, quinoa, kamut, amaranth and low-sugar-based cereals or sugar-free muesli makes an ideal breakfast for most people. Eat them with skimmed milk or try organic oat, rice, almond, sheep's or goat's milk. Protein helps to wake up your brain, hence eggs, grilled fish or lean meat also make great breakfasts. Look for 'healthier' eggs – rich in omega-3 fats – meaning that the chickens have been fed a healthier diet. Otherwise wholemeal bread toasted with a non-hydrogenated spread such as Vitaquell, Biona or Benecol and a little honey or low-sugar jam is fine. If you cannot face breakfast, at least take with you an apple or a couple of bananas and a low-fat, live yoghurt to eat later.
- Eat as great a variety of foods as possible, preferably locally grown and organic, which contain higher levels of nutrients than foods flown thousands of miles. Buy fruit and vegetables that are

grown locally and allowed to ripen naturally. Unripe fruits and vegetables do not contain as many nutrients from the soil as those that have been allowed to ripen naturally on the vine. The price of organic foods is coming down and I believe that 100% organic food will help reduce many cancers and greatly alleviate the toxic load on the planet and its inhabitants. Many pesticides, especially the organophosphates (OPs), seep right through the vegetables and fruit and cannot be washed off. They are now linked with many cancers and lowered sperm counts.

- Use only organic products on your skin and hair – we ingest several kilos of chemicals annually through our skin alone. Also try to eliminate chemical-based cleaners and so on from your home.
- In winter, eat heart-warming cooked foods and in summer choose lighter meals with plenty of raw foods and fresh fruit. In winter, I make fruit compotes or I lightly grill fruits – which are more warming – especially with added freshly grated root ginger to aid circulation and boost immune function.
- Drink at least 6 glasses of filtered, bottled or distilled water daily. If you suffer from digestive problems, avoid drinking too much fluid with food because it dilutes the digestive juices, which can lead to poor digestion of food and reduced absorption of nutrients.
- Cut down on coffee, alcohol and caffeinated soft drinks, which dehydrate the body. For every caffeinated or alcoholic drink, you need 8oz (250ml) of water.

- The additives, artificial sweeteners (especially aspartame) and sugar in soft drinks and foods can trigger hyperactivity and mood swings. Sugar depletes the body of vital minerals such as chromium. Forget low-calorie drinks, they place a strain on your liver, which slows weight loss. If you find yourself craving sweet foods take 150mcg of chromium daily. After a few days it will kick in and you will notice that you crave sugar less. A fair amount of self-discipline is also needed.
- Remember it's often the foods and drinks you crave the most that are causing most of your health problems.
- Drink more herbal teas, especially organic green tea, plus dandelion coffee and low-sugar barley drinks.
- Try to eat at least five pieces of fresh, whole fruit and five portions of vegetables daily. Aim to have one salad a day in summer that includes some fresh, steamed or raw vegetables. Otherwise lightly roast the veg, and allow to cool and serve in the salad. The darker green the leaves, the more nourishing they are. Three portions of cabbage a week can reduce the incidence of colon cancer by as much as 60%.
- Steam or lightly stir-fry vegetables when possible, as boiling destroys vitamins.
- Keep food simple – say no to rich foods with rich sauces and to fried, barbecued and burnt foods which are carcinogenic. See also *Cancer*.
- Avoid pre-packaged, take-away and tinned foods whenever possible, as they are often packed with fat, salt, sugar and additives. Also a great majority of these foods are packed in aluminium containers, and aluminium is linked to Alzheimer's and senile dementia.
- Do not add sodium-based salt to your food as it can aggravate water retention and cause blood pressure to rise. Our typical diet contains 9 grams of salt a day and it has been estimated that if we can reduce salt consumption to 3 grams per person per day it would save 70,000 deaths in the UK each year. There are plenty of magnesium- and potassium-based sea salts freely available from supermarkets and health stores.
- Do not become fanatical about fad diets. Everything in moderation and keep a balance of foods at all times for good nutrition. I love cakes but I try to bake them only once a week! I bake cakes with butter, which does not become rancid like some hard margarines when cooked. Use a little organic rice syrup, honey or fresh fruit instead of sugar. Or soak some dried fruits in warm water, drain, chop and add to the cake mix.

- Use extra virgin, cold-pressed olive oil in cooking and try walnut or cold-pressed sunflower or sesame oils for salad dressings. These oils have many health benefits from lowering cholesterol to keeping your skin looking younger. There is also an EFA-based oil that you can now use for cooking (see *Fats You Need To Eat*).

- Eat your meals sitting down – or at least standing still. Chew your food thoroughly; if you bolt down your food your body will tell you. Aid digestion by eating fruit between meals and not as a dessert. Fruit can ferment when eaten after a large meal causing wind and bloating.

- Cow's milk is often a problem for many people. Skimmed milk is higher in sugar (lactose) and many people are intolerant to this. Try organic oat, almond or rice milk which are non-dairy. Also use sheep's or goat's products and eat plenty of live, low-fat yoghurt, which contain beneficial gut bacteria and are rich sources of calcium.

- Avoid any foods and oils that contain hydrogenated or trans fats – these are the bad guys.

- Wheat-based cereals, especially wheat bran, trigger bowel problems for many people. Use oat-based cereals, or oat, soya and rice bran or wheat germ instead. Try lentil-, rice-, spelt-, corn-, spinach- and potato-based flours and pastas.

- Try to avoid red meat, which can putrefy in the gut and may contain antibiotic, hormone and chemical residues. If you adore meat: gentlemen, please don't eat more than 3½ oz (100 grams) at one meal and ladies keep it to 1¾–2½oz (50–75 grams). Go for organic whenever you can to avoid the extra chemicals non-organic meat contains. Other great proteins are fish, free-range eggs, low-fat cheese, chicken, turkey, tempeh, beans, and lentils.

- Avoid smoking and smoky atmospheres.

- Make time to relax. When we are stressed the body starts pumping the hormones adrenaline and cortisol ready for the fight-or-flight response. Eventually this can cause us to blow a fuse. It can be a gastric fuse, leading to ulcers, or a heart fuse causing heart attacks, and so on. The body and mind are one. If you are stressed, something has got to give in the end. Vitamins, minerals and diet alone will not keep you healthy. Stress is a major factor in many of today's health problems. Remember you are special, give yourself the odd treat and make space in your diary for yourself.

- Get plenty of fresh air and learn to breathe deeply; this aids relaxation. Deep breathing also helps to alkalise the body. Stress makes it too acid.

- Sunlight is great for your health and without it you can become very ill indeed. Moderate sunbathing is fine with sun screens; just stay out of the midday sun. As a general rule never let your skin go red.

- Learn to have a good laugh regularly and don't be afraid to laugh at yourself – lighten up.

- Take regular, sensible exercise, which is one of the best favours you can do for your health. Try brisk walking, cycling, light jogging, swimming, skipping, aerobics and/or aqua aerobics, as these exercises have the most health-related benefits. You will be amazed at the difference regular exercise can make to your overall wellbeing. If you do nothing else, try to walk for 30 minutes daily, preferably away from main roads.

- Gradual lifestyle changes are of much greater benefits than 2–4-day fad diets.

- Over time your taste buds will come to love healthier foods.

- Generally eat smaller meals more regularly rather than eating 2 or 3 huge meals a day. Large meals place a strain on the liver and digestive system. Losing weight is easier if you practice this way of eating, which also keeps blood sugar on an even keel thus preventing mood swings.

- Get into blending and juicing. This is a fantastic way to ingest large amounts of nutrients quickly. Buy yourself a blender and twice a week make the following cocktail: 1 tbsp of sunflower seeds, 1 tbsp of linseeds (flax seeds), 1 tsp of any organic green powder mix, a teaspoon of raw wheat germ, 2 ready-to-eat prunes or apricots, 1 box of blueberries, a chopped apple (minus the pips but with the skin), a banana or any fruit you love. To this add a tablespoon of aloe vera juice and half a cup of organic rice milk. If you are worried about your protein intake then also add a dessertspoon of a good-quality whey powder. I use Solgar's Whey To Go. Blend the lot for 30 seconds and drink (or if it's thick, eat with a spoon) as a meal replacement. It's neat fibre, vitamins, minerals and essential fats.

■ With a juicer, on alternate days, make yourself fresh raw vegetable juices, again adding any extras such as the aloe, fresh root ginger, a few drops of any herbal tinctures you like, especially dandelion and burdock, to cleanse the liver, and drink immediately after juicing, whilst the beneficial enzymes are still active.

GENERAL SUPPLEMENTS – Supplements that I take every day

1. KUDOS 24 – Multi-active Age-management Complex.

For years I took up to 30 separate nutrients a day to help boost my immune system, nourish my skin, and protect my bones, eyes, heart, circulation, brain and so on, which in turn helped to keep me healthier and slow the ageing process. But eventually I got tired of swallowing so many pills, which are often not absorbed as well as they might be, especially for anyone who is stressed or suffers from gut problems. And so with nutritionists and bio-chemists from Kudos Vitamins and Herbals, I helped develop a multi-nutrient formula, containing food-state, organic-source, GM-free, highly absorbable nutrients that both men and women could take once daily and which offers 24-hour protection to help keep us healthier and slow ageing at every level. *Multi-active Age-management Complex is suitable for vegetarians, pregnant women and for men and women of all ages.*

■ **Directions:** Use one sachet a day and stir into smoothies, low-sugar juices, vegetable juices, yoghurts, and so on, or over cereals. This formula contains:

* **Organic artichoke** – to help cleanse and support the liver.

* **Organic aloe vera extract** – which contains mannose, the essential sugar that boosts immune function.

* **Antioxidants** – a full spectrum of high-strength antioxidants, including 500mg of vitamin C, selenium, grape seed extract, organic broccoli and pine bark extract. Other antioxidants are listed below.

* **B-vitamins** – a full spectrum of all the B-group, including folic acid, B1, B3, B6, B12 and biotin; all needed to support your nervous system, your hair, skin and nails, and to help in the control of cholesterol. Please note that the B-vitamins turn your urine bright yellow or orange when they are excreted, this is normal.

* **Boron** – an essential mineral for healthy bones and vital for people with inflammatory conditions such as arthritis.

* **Calcium** – for healthy bones and teeth. A natural tranquilliser, also involved in nerve and muscle control.

* **Broccoli extract** – which is packed with antioxidants and helps re-alkalise the body. (See *Acid–Alkaline Balance*.)

* **Bromelain** – extracted from pineapples, this is anti-inflammatory, reduces bruising, and aids digestion and absorption of nutrients from your diet.

* **Natural-source carotenes** – vital for a healthy immune system and for healthy eyes and skin, which convert to vitamin A in the body.

* **Co-Enzyme Q10** – which helps to support your heart and breasts, and increases energy levels. This vitamin-like substance is made naturally in the body, but production is slowed as we age. Anyone taking cholesterol-lowering statin drugs needs to take CoQ10 daily.
* **Carnosine** – helps regenerate ageing cells and skin, improves muscle tone, reduces arterial plaque, and is an important antioxidant. (See *Ageing*.)
* **Chromium** – a mineral greatly lacking in our diets that helps reduce the cravings for sugar and reduces the likelihood of developing late-onset diabetes.
* **Copper** – which helps in the manufacture of neurotransmitters in the brain.
* **Vitamin D** – which is needed to promote healthy bones.
* **Essential Fats** – which are extracted from hemp seed, a great source of omega-3 and -6 essential fats. EFAs are great for your skin, hair, for the brain, for hormone production and weight loss.
* **Vitamin E** – full-spectrum vitamin E, vital for healthy skin, an antioxidant, which also helps keep your blood and circulation healthy.
* **Glutiathione** – is an important anti-ageing brain nutrient, which aids brain function and detoxifies the liver. (See *Liver Problems*.)
* **Iron** – traces of iron from organic asparagus, safe and will not accumulate in the body.
* **Manganese** – involved in reproduction processes and sex hormone formation.
* **Magnesium** – equally as important as calcium for healthy bones; also promotes lung health, reduces stress and keeps the body more alkaline.
* **Molybdenum** – an anti-ageing enzyme that helps maintain DNA.
* **Phosphatidyl Serine** – a vital 'good-mood' brain nutrient that aids memory and learning (see *Memory*).
* **Selenium** – an antioxidant that helps protect against cancers and degenerative disease.
* **Soya Isoflavones** – known to help protect against hormone-disrupting chemicals found in pesticides and herbicides. Regulates hormones in both sexes and helps protect against cancer. Helps keep calcium in the bones and out of the arteries.
* **Soya isolate** – a complete protein that helps to slow ageing.
* **Stomach Acid** (Betain HCl) – to aid digestion and increase absorption of nutrients from your diet.
* **Turmeric** –the yellow spice that you see in curries. It has anti-cancerous and anti-inflamma-tory properties, and helps keep Alzheimer's at bay.
* **Zinc** – essential for healthy skin, wound-healing, fertility and a healthy sex life.

If you were to buy all these nutrients separately, at similar levels, it would cost at least £250.00. For more information, or to order, call 0800 389 5476 or log on to www.kudosvitamins.com. Kudos 24 is also sold at all good health stores and pharmacies.

I'm not claiming that K24 is the be-all-and-end-all for every health condition, as one 'pill' or formula could never make such a claim. Therefore, if for example I were to be suffering from say an infection such as cystitis, I would also take cranberry complex on top of the K24.

2. HEALTHY SMOOTHIE

Every morning in summer I make a smoothie that contains one small box of organic blueberries, one chopped organic apple, a banana and a slice of fresh pineapple. To this I add 1 teaspoon of rice or oat bran; and a few sunflower seeds or linseeds – or a few pumpkin and seasame (about a tablespoon of each but adjust to your individual needs); and a few raisins or a couple of organic dried apricots. I also put in a teaspoon of good-quality green powder – my current favourite is Nature's Living, containing organic whole leaf barley grass, wheat grass, nettle leaf, spinach, kale, ginger root, and so on (for stockists call Kiki Health on 08450 60 10 60. Website: www.kiki-health.com). I also add a spoon of whey protein and the K24, and I blend all this with a small cup of organic rice, oat or almond milk. It's a quick and easy way to ingest lots of nurtients in the mornings and this mix re-alkalises the body. Use fruits that you love and ring the changes by swapping the apple for a kiwi or the pineapple for a papaya and so on. You definitely won't need mid-morning snacks on this drink – it's very filling! Please note that most green food powders are naturally high in iron, so if you are over 50, unless you have a medical condition requiring more iron, use only a teaspoon daily, as you don't want your iron levels to go too high.

3. HEALTHY BACTERIA (PROBIOTICS)
As so many people are now worried about super-bugs and food poisoning, or perhaps you already suffer gut problems, I also take one acidophilus and bifidus capsule daily. This replenishes the healthy bacteria in the gut and helps prevent many problems such as candida, yeast overgrowth, constipation and an over-acid system, triggered not only by our diet but also the chemicals we inhale from the air. Available from all good health stores.

GLANDULAR FEVER   *(see also Candida, Immune Function and ME)*

Glandular fever is caused by the Epstein Barr virus. It is most common in younger people, between the ages of 15 and 25, when the immune system is developing, hence the nickname of the 'kissing virus'. Symptoms include a severe sore throat, fever, swollen glands in the neck, and a feeling of overwhelming exhaustion. Initially it can appear similar to a bad dose of flu, but after a few days it becomes obvious that it is not flu and symptoms can continue for several months. The liver can be affected and some sufferers develop a mild hepatitis caused by the virus. (See also *Hepatitis* and *Liver Problems*.)

Antibiotics are inappropriate because it is a viral infection and certain strengths of antibiotics can actually make this illness much worse. Bed rest and good nutrition are essential to help prevent a relapse, but unfortunately the illness often coincides with stressful academic studies making life rather difficult. It is one of those diseases where you can appear to make a recovery then a month later experience a relapse. For some individuals this can lead to chronic fatigue syndrome or ME. The more you rest when the problem is first diagnosed the more likely you are to make a complete recovery. The yeast fungal overgrowth candida often occurs with glandular fever (see *Candida*), because the immune system is compromised from lymphatic congestion.

Foods to Avoid
- I'm afraid it's a question of really cleaning up the diet by avoiding all pre-packaged, ready-made meals unless they are freshly prepared.
- Try to eliminate hamburgers and eating sugary snacks.
- Colas and fizzy drinks often contain up to 10 tsp of sugar, and sugar in any form will greatly deplete immune function.
- White bread, croissants, Danish pastries, cakes, chocolate snacks, crisps, pork and sausage pies, and all these instant-type foods should be avoided for a few weeks.
- If you know you have a problem with certain foods, the most common being wheat and dairy from cow's milk, eliminate them for two weeks.
- Stimulants such as caffeine and alcohol can overload the body giving brief bursts of energy, but actually reducing it in the long-term.

Friendly Foods
- Try to eat plenty of fresh fruit and vegetables that are rich in magnesium and natural-source carotenes, such as spring greens, cabbage, kale, sweet potatoes, dried apricots, parsley, broccoli, spinach, and all orange fruits.
- If you have a juicer, try a mixture of carrots, raw beetroot, tomatoes, a green pepper, and small amounts of garlic and onion.
- Cook with garlic and onions.
- Make rich soups and stews with added fresh ginger.
- If you prefer fruit juices, try lemon, orange, kiwi, banana and pineapple to which you could add a teaspoon of dried wheat grass powder. (One of the best I have come across is Nature's Living from Kiki Health. Tel: 08450 601060. Website: www.kiki-health.com)
- Plenty of good-quality, high-protein foods, such as fresh fish, chicken, tempeh, beans and lentils, plus free-range eggs, all help to support the immune system. If you are really low then add whey protein powders to breakfast cereals.
- Eat more wholemeal breads and pastas, and jacket potatoes, brown rice, porridge made with rice, almonds, and goat's, sheep's or low-fat soya milk, and low-sugar cereals.
- Eat more low-fat, live yoghurts to help replenish healthy bacteria in the gut.
- Drink at least 6 glasses of water daily.
- Coriander and parsley are packed with nutrients.
- Drink liquorice tea to help support your adrenal glands, which are usually exhausted.

Useful Remedies
- Vitamin C is anti-viral and anti-bacterial. While symptoms are acute take 5–6 grams daily with food in an ascorbate form and after a couple of weeks reduce this to 1 gram daily for several months. If this causes loose bowels reduce dose to just below bowel tolerance.
- A high-strength multi-mineral and vitamin, as when we're fighting an infection we are often depleted in minerals especially calcium, magnesium and zinc. See *Kudos 24*; p.160.
- Vitamin A 25,000iu can be taken daily for one month to help fight the infection. Take only 3,000iu if you are pregnant.
- Anti-viral herbs, such echinacea, golden rod, astragalus, wild indigo, goldenseal and Siberian ginseng are all anti-viral. 3 grams daily of either the single herbs or a combination formula.
- Propolis has been shown to be highly anti-viral; try taking 1–3 grams daily for the duration of your illness.
- If for any reason you end up taking antibiotics, then take some probiotic capsules for a month.
BC

Helpful Hints
- A **gradual** return to normal life is necessary because over-activity too soon can cause a relapse.
- Homeopathic Ailanthus Glandulosa 6c, or Gelsemium 6c, 3 times daily for 10 days should help reduce symptoms dramatically.
- Check for possible iron deficiency with your doctor and take iron if necessary (see under *Anaemia*).
- You should also ask your doctor to check for parasites (see under IBS). If, after two months, your energy and appetite have not returned, contact a qualified nutritionist (see *Useful Information*).

GLUE EAR

(see also *Earache*)

The Eustachian tube is a pathway that allows the equalisation of air pressure between the middle ear and the back of the throat, through which bacteria can enter the middle ear. Ear infections are one of the most common childhood ailments. They are also likely to re-occur over a relatively short space of time. These infections can be very painful. It is understandable that parents would want to give the child immediate relief, the normal treatment being either antibiotics or the insertion of a grommet in the ear drum. Neither of these treatments is particularly effective. In fact almost 90% of children with glue ear have food allergies (see *Allergies*). Identifying allergies is often very difficult and it's also very important you don't suddenly eliminate a whole group of foods and leave the child malnourished. The most common culprits are wheat and dairy from cows. Children who are breast-fed are less likely to develop ear infections. One other odd thing that seems to increase the risk of inner-ear infections is the use of dummies when children are very young.

Foods to Avoid
- Sugar is top of the list, as it weakens the immune system leaving people more prone to infections. Other than sugar it is very important that the food intolerances or allergies are identified as these are likely to be the primary cause. Typically they would include dairy from cows, and eggs, wheat and citrus fruits such as oranges, grapefruit, lemons and limes; but it could be any one of a number of other food groups.

- Keep your child off mucus-forming food, such as full-fat cheeses, pizzas, Greek yoghurts, white breads and cakes, full-fat milk, chocolates and so on. Mucus will also be formed as a reaction to any foods to which the child has a sensitivity.
- Remember that many canned drinks and mass-produced desserts and jams can contain up to 10 teaspoonfuls of sugar, and artificial sweeteners are often a problem for individuals with allergies.
- Try to avoid preservatives and additives.

Friendly Foods
- Fresh fruit and vegetables are rich in vitamin C, which will boost the immune system.
- Garlic helps to fight infections – but note that garlic is a common allergen, so keep a food diary and note reactions.
- Chewing gum made with xylitol seems beneficial as children who chew xylitol-sweetened chewing gum have a much lower rate of inner ear infections. You can also buy xylitol as a sweetener.
- Introduce your child to foods lower in saturated fats, but highly nutritious, such as brown rice, barley, lentils and pulses, and as a treat give them rice or oat cakes. Amaranth crackers are also OK.
- There are numerous health cookery books giving great recipes for cookies, biscuits and cakes that are low in fat and sugar.
- There are plenty of low-fat, live fruit yoghurts freely available that replenish healthy bacteria in the gut, which helps fight infection.
- Use rice, almond or oat milk and bake cakes with barley, buckwheat, rice, potato or spelt flours.
- Use non-hydrogenated spreads such as Vitaquell, Benecol or Biona.

Useful Remedies
- Echinacea either as tincture or tablets. An alcohol-free tincture is often easier for children as it can be added to fruit juice or yoghurt. If the child is very small use 1 drop per 3lbs (6kg) of body weight. It can be used several times a day whilst symptoms last. For more help call the Organic Pharmacy. **OP**

- Vitamin C – for children 250–500mg daily. For adults 1–2 grams daily. Again, as a lot of children don't like tablets, vitamin C is often available as a powder, some of them fairly pleasant-tasting, or you can find ones that can be added to fruit juice and the flavour of the fruit juice is what the child will taste. Alternatively use a vitamin crusher. Available from Orange Burst on 01273 558 112. Website: www.lemonburst.net
- Zinc lozenges and zinc supplements can be given to a child. 1–2 lozenges a day while the child has an infection. Zinc boosts the immune function and helps to fight the infection. 25mg daily for adults and 10–15mg daily for a child over 8.
- A child's chewable multi-vitamin and mineral. For details call Nature's Plus. **NP**
- The celloid potassium chloride helps to unblock the Eustachian tube – 100mg daily. **BLK**; or you can buy Ionic Potassium Chloride by Metabolics from the Nutri Centre. **NC**

Helpful Hints
- A humidifier placed in the main living room or the child's bedroom has been found to reduce the risk of inner-ear infections.
- Many nutritional doctors advocate that your child should not be subjected to vaccinations until the cycle of ear infections is cleared, as vaccines place a strain on the child's immune system.
- Use mullein flower oil as ear drops – available from health stores.
- Use Hopi ear candles to remove excess wax. This is a pain-free way to reduce some of the aching and must be done by a responsible or qualified adult. Available from most health stores.
- Cranial osteopathy helps as it encourages lymph drainage. See *Useful Information*.
- Do not let the child be exposed to cigarette smoke – it increases the incidence of glue ear by 80%.

GOUT
(see also *Acid–Alkaline Balance* and *Arthritis*)

In the 18th century you were considered fortunate to develop gout as they thought this prevented you from contracting fatal diseases. It was seen as a rich person's disease because only those who could afford large amounts of meat, cheese and wine were likely to suffer. Gout is a form of joint inflammation, which is caused by high levels of uric acid in the blood causing crystal deposits in the joints. It is very common in the big toe but can also affect other joints, and the kidneys. The vast majority of gout sufferers are men but more and more women are beginning to suffer gout. An attack can be triggered by ingesting overly rich food and drink, typically this would include shellfish; cheeses such as Stilton; port; red meat; and red wine. Most people who suffer gout tend to drink a lot anyway – especially champagne. Occasionally an accident or trauma to the body can also precipitate an attack.

Foods to Avoid
- Meat, beer and cheese are your main problems in gout.
- Any foods which are rich in purines, found in high-protein foods, such as offal, oily fish including anchovies, herrings, cod and mackerel, plus chicken, caffeine, shellfish (including crab, lobster, scallops and mussels), roe, kidney beans, lima beans, navy beans, yeast-based drinks such as Marmite and Bovril, oatmeal porridge, and lentils.
- Avoid full-fat cheeses, especially Stilton and Brie.
- Most forms of arthritis usually benefit from taking cod liver oil or eating oily fish, however, with gout these foods would almost certainly make it worse.

Friendly Foods
- Cherries and pineapple should be eaten on a daily basis, cherries in particular. They are one of

the easiest ways of keeping gout under control and to prevent it, as they increase excretion of uric acid from the body.

- If you are not a fan of cherries, try eating blueberries, blackberries or bilberries. These are very rich in bioflavonoids, which help reduce uric acid levels in the body.
- A macrobiotic diet, although hard to follow, would almost certainly eliminate the gout.
- Eat plenty of fruit and vegetables especially celery, quinoa, millet, brown rice, and pastas made from corn, rice, amaranth, potato or buckwheat flours.
- Free-range or organic eggs, cooked soya tofu, and lamb should not cause any problems.
- Make a healthy drink containing a small boxful of blueberries, some pineapple, frozen or fresh pipped cherries, a pear, an apple and a banana. Add a teaspoon of any good organic green food powder (see *General Supplements*), and a tiny piece of fresh root ginger. Put in a blender with half a cup of rice or almond milk, whiz for one minute and drink immediately.
- Drink at least 6 glasses of water every day, to encourage excretion of the uric acid.

Useful Remedies
- Vitamin C, 1–2 grams a day taken with food will gradually help lower uric acid levels.
- Bromelain 2,000–4,000mcu a day; this is a very powerful anti-inflammatory.
- Ginger, curcumin and boswelia 4 capsules, or more, a day. These herbs in combination provide relief from any type of inflammation discomfort. **FSC**
- Cat's claw, 400mg 3 times a day for 3 months or more. This herb can gradually help lower uric acid levels, as well as improving bowel function. This herb can help protect your gut lining against the negative side effects of anti-inflammatory painkillers – known as NSAIDs.

Helpful Hints

- Lose weight as this is quite often part of the problem. Remember the gout is pretty much self-inflicted and almost entirely brought on by a rich diet. Be prepared to make some changes.
- Nettle tea will also aid with excretion of uric acid.
- Massage the painful joint with essential oil of Roman camomile, juniper, wintergreen and ginger to help reduce the pain and inflammation. Some of the finest and most effective essential pain-relieving oils I have ever come across are from Young Living in the US. In the UK for help as to which oil you need for your specific condition, call Susie Anthony on 01749 679900, or log on to her website on www.psalifemastery.com and look for the Resources pages.
- Homeopathic Ledum 30c twice daily for 2–3 days will reduce symptoms.
- Do not take aspirin if taking anti-gout drugs.

GUMS

(see Bleeding Gums)

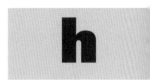

HAEMORRHOIDS

(see *Constipation* and *Piles*)

HAIR LOSS

(see also *Absorption, Circulation* and *Stress*)

The health of your hair depends upon the circulation to the root of the hair and the amount of nutrients present in the blood. Hair is composed of a protein-like substance called keratin, and requires a healthy balanced diet for proper nourishment. Many drugs are claimed to increase hair growth, but some have negative side effects, which include an inability for men to maintain an erection. So, before trying any of these drugs always discuss any implications with your doctor or trichologist.

The average person loses between 70 and 100 hairs a day, and as we age our hair becomes finer and/or thinner. Most of us tend to associate balding and thinning hair with men, and yet many women experience thinning hair too. In fact many trichologists, who 10 years ago tended to see more men than women experiencing hair loss problems, are now seeing just as many women suffering hair loss – even Asian and Caribbean women who traditionally have beautiful, thick hair. Our Western lifestyle seems to be a major factor.

Another important factor is the male hormone testosterone, which is also found in women. Although this hormone is responsible for making men hairy during puberty, it also has a large role to play in hair loss in later life, in both men and women. Some women have too much testosterone, which shows up in excess facial hair and can trigger male-type thinning. In this case taking the herbs vitex, agnus castus, or saw palmetto helps to reduce testosterone levels. Hereditary factors are also important. The more hair loss there is/was in your father, uncles and grandfathers, the more likely you are to lose your own hair. However, dietary supplements and regular daily firm-scalp massage can help slow down hair loss. Hair loss in much younger people is also becoming extremely common, showing that stress is definitely a trigger. Stress and a toxic bowel prevent production of some of the B-vitamins that are necessary for maintaining hair colour and healthy hair.

Hair loss in women is common after childbirth and the menopause, and a lack of protein can trigger thinning hair or even cause it to fall out. Hair loss is also linked to heavy metal toxicity. I have seen several cases of alopecia in young women due to stress, which triggered a leaky gut, and when they started taking a digestive enzyme with an easily absorbed multi-nutrient with meals – the hair grew back.

The health of your hair depends on the circulation to the scalp and the amount of nutrients present in your blood. It is thought that men lose hair on the tops of their heads rather than the backs and sides because the blood-flow to the top of the scalp is reduced in comparison to the sides. When a person is very stressed the scalp becomes tight, which restricts circulation; the hair follicle becomes malnourished resulting in further hair loss. Adrenal exhaustion, an underactive thyroid, and certain prescription drugs are also factors in hair loss. Naturopath Steven Langley says "If the tissues are too acid then minerals needed for healthy hair, such as iron, magnesium and zinc, are taken from the hair follicles to buffer this acidity" (see *Acid–Alkaline Balance*).

Hair grows faster in summer and a single hair can live for several years. On average human hair grows between 5 and 6in (12 and 15cm) a year.

Foods to Avoid

- Reduce caffeine from any source. Caffeine increases stress (as it triggers adrenaline to be released) and weakens the adrenal glands.
- Avoid sugar and refined carbohydrates, such as pastries, cakes, desserts, pies and so on, all of which deplete nutrients needed for hair growth.
- Reduce the amount of sodium-based salt in your diet.

Friendly Foods

- Quality protein is the most important food for your hair. Eat organic lean meats, chicken, game, fish and eggs (particularly egg white).
- Whey, milk, yoghurt and cheese are also rich in protein.
- Vegetarian-based proteins are found in seeds, nuts, vegetables, whole grains, such as brown rice, barley, spelt, wholewheat and quinoa, plus legumes, such as peas, lentils, soya beans, tofu, tempeh, lentils, and peanuts.
- Eat more iron-rich foods, such as egg yolks, green leafy vegetables such as spinach, wholegrain breads and cereals, and meat and fish.
- Try adding seaweeds, such as kombu and arame, to meals. You use them as you would a green vegetable and they are a rich source of minerals needed for healthy hair.
- Essential fats are vital for healthy hair and a healthy scalp, therefore eat more oily fish, plus walnuts, pumpkin seeds, sunflower seeds or linseeds (flax seeds) and their unrefined oils, mixed half and half with olive oil. Use for salad dressings and drizzle on cooked foods. Essential fats help you to avoid a dry, scaly scalp and nourish the hair follicles. See *Fats You Need To Eat*.
- Coriander detoxifies heavy metals from the body and is full of nutrients, especially B-vitamins.
- Muesli, cereals and oats are all high in B-vitamins.

Useful Remedies

- Take a good-quality multi-vitamin/mineral, most of the companies on page 13–15 supply specific hair-nutrient formulas.
- Romanda Healthcare makes an excellent formula that contains all the nutrients needed for healthy hair, plus a growth serum and shampoo, which are really excellent (see *Helpful Hints* for contact details).
- Steve Langley has formulated a blood cleanser called Essential Detox Combination that has been shown to help restore hair loss due to stress and mineral depletion. The quality of your scalp depends on the quality of the blood supplying the roots. As we age the quality of our blood is reduced because of the accumulation of toxins. Once the blood is able to carry more oxygen and nutrients, hair can improve. Take 1 tsp in a glass of water 3 times daily, preferably before meals. **NC**
- Zinc, 30mg daily, is essential for hair and nail growth.
- The B-group vitamins are vital if you want to keep your hair, and many people who take a full spectrum of B-vitamins report that their grey hairs disappear. B5, PABA, biotin and folic acid are the anti-greying nutrients and you would need 1000mcg of biotin daily.
- Vitamin B6 x 50mg per day is helpful for women taking the contraceptive pill, which can affect hair loss.
- Find out if you are low in iron, in which case take a liquid, easily absorbable formula such as Spatone. Available from health shops worldwide. Don't take iron unless you need it. If you cook in iron pots, you will absorb some of the iron in your food.
- Red meat contains the amino acid lysine, and people who take lysine as a supplement often experience an increase in hair growth. Take 500mg of lysine twice daily on an empty stomach

before meals. Take this only for a couple of months.

- CT241, plus Colleginase, which contain vitamin C, rutin, hesperidin, cellulose, silica, and vitamins A and D to strengthen hair and nails. **BC**
- The herb ginkgo biloba helps to increase circulation to the scalp. Kudos makes a high-quality, one-a-day (900mg), high-strength capsule. **KVH**
- Herbs that help balance hormones naturally if your hair is thinning because of the menopause, include dong quai, black cohosh, sage, and soya isoflavones. All the companies on pages 13–15 sell these supplements.
- Thinning hair in men caused by excess dihydro-testosterone can be balanced by taking saw palmetto 500mg daily (under supervision – it may need to be higher), and zinc 30mg daily
- Lack of copper is also linked to grey hair. We don't need much of this trace mineral. Try taking a multi-mineral formula for a couple of months.

Helpful Hints

- Take regular exercise, which will stimulate your heart and circulation, thus increasing oxygen-flow, reducing stress, and promoting scalp and hair health.
- There is a myth saying that the more you brush your hair, the thicker and healthier it will grow – it's not true. Too much brushing pulls hair out, breaks it, and scratches the scalp.
- Don't over dry your hair – which makes it more brittle.
- "Women who lose a lot of hair after giving birth should stop panicking" says London and New-York based trichologist Philip Kingsley, "During pregnancy oestrogen levels are higher and this hormone prolongs the natural life span of a hair. The average person loses 70–100 hairs a day, but during pregnancy hair falls out less, because of the oestrogen. Then 4–6 weeks later the woman gives birth and hormones return to normal levels and all the normal shedding that should have happened during the previous months, occurs all at once. As long as these women eat a healthy diet and take the right supplements the hair should soon get back to normal."

- Philip Kingsley has formulated various hormone drops for men and women that nourish the follicle and help prevent hair-loss. They don't make hair re-grow if the hair-loss is permanent, but they help you to keep the hair that you have. For details in the UK call 020 7629 4004. In New York call (212) 753 9600. Website: www.philipkingsley.co.uk. For more help on hair read Philip Kingsley's book *The Hair Bible* (Aurum Press).
- Some doctors have noticed that smokers tend to lose their hair faster than non-smokers.
- Shampoo your hair regularly, this helps to re-moisturise the hair.
- Jojoba oil mixed with a little essential oil of rosemary and massaged into the scalp removes dead skin cells and increases circulation. Be firm, you need the skin on your scalp to move so that blood can circulate more freely. Do this before going to bed and leave the oils on overnight.
- Some yogis say that by doing head- and shoulder-stands they have kept really thick hair because the circulation to their heads is greatly increased. If like me you are not into head stands, simply lie on the floor and put your calves up on a chair or a bed. This not only helps gives your leg veins a rest, it encourages more blood to the head.
- Chlorine from swimming pools damages your hair and is also linked to asthma and heart disease.
- To find your nearest qualified trichologist call 08706 070602, or visit the Institute of Trichologists at www.trichologists.org.uk.
- Try Romanda lotion and shampoos, along with Romanda hair formula powder supplements. Call Jan Adams on the Romanda Advice Line on 0208 346 0784, or write to Romanda Healthcare, Romanda House, Ashley Walk, London NW7 1DU. Website: www. romandahealthcare.co.uk Jan is incredibly helpful and formed the company after suffering hair loss. She also helps people with hair loss after chemotherapy, plus alopecia and patchy hair loss.

- Numerous salons offer hair transplants, which are becoming more sophisticated. Professor Nick Lowe, a dermatologist, offers the latest technique called Micro Grafting, which gives a more natural-looking hairline, rather than hundreds of 'puncture marks'. The surgery is expensive, but the results are amazing. For details in the UK call 020 7499 3223. In the US call (310) 828 8969.
- Philip Kingsley recommends Dr Patrice Cahuzac in Paris. He says her transplant work is the best he has ever seen. Dr Cahuzac often sees patients for their initial consultation in London – but she works in Paris. Rue Clemont-Manot, Paris 75008, France. Tel: 00 33 15 65 20 101
- The Hair Clinic at John Bell and Croydon in London also offers a Micro Grafting service. Address: 50–54 Wigmore Street, London. Tel: 020 7224 4640.

HALITOSIS (Bad breath) (see also *Liver Problems*)

Bad breath is often caused by poor dental hygiene. A build-up of plaque, infected gums, abscesses, and insufficient brushing and flossing are mostly to blame. Make sure you see a qualified dental hygienist at least twice a year. Use fluoride-free floss and mouthwash daily, change your toothbrush regularly, and clean your teeth at least twice a day, preferably after every meal.

Poor digestion, and a sluggish bowel and liver can also cause bad breath. Foods such as meat take a long time to digest and can putrefy in the bowel. One of the simple things you can do is to chew properly as this enhances carbohydrate digestion and makes it easier for the rest of the digestive process. Try not to eat too much food at one sitting, which overloads the stomach and bowel.

Some people find their digestion improves if they avoid eating proteins and carbohydrates together in one meal. For example, if you are eating protein meals such as chicken or fish, eat them with only vegetables and not carbohydrates. Conversely if you eat rice or pasta eat them with only vegetables and not protein. Long-term bad breath can indicate problems with the liver or kidneys, or diabetes, in which case you must consult a doctor. If the bowel is severely congested with impacted matter, the body re-absorbs the toxins into the blood and hence the lungs, and toxins are then breathed out.

Foods to Avoid
- Avoid too much caffeine, sugar and low-fibre, high-fat foods, which all weaken the digestion and cause sluggish bowel movements.
- Smoking not only causes bad breath directly, it can also cause it indirectly as it weakens digestion.
- Cut down on the amount of milk and dairy produce from cows, which is mucus forming and slows bowel function.

Friendly Foods
- Leafy green vegetables such as pak choy, spring greens, kale, cabbage and so on are rich in chlorophyll. Chlorophyll is useful in helping to clear the bowel thus helping to improve the smell of the breath.
- Eat more artichokes, celeriac and chicory – see dietary advice in *Liver Problems*.
- Eat plenty of fresh whole fruits. Pineapple or papaya eaten as a dessert is a good idea as the enzymes in these fruits can help break down the proteins ensuring proper digestion.
- A 'bio' or live yoghurt either for breakfast or as a dessert containing acidophilus and bifidus improves the quality of the bacteria in the bowel, enhancing digestion and making bad breath less likely.

- Add more coriander and fresh mint to foods, and eat fennel or caraway seeds, which help kill the bacteria that cause bad breath.
- Drink fenugreek tea and also green tea, which helps to kill bacteria in the mouth.
- Drink plenty of water.

Useful Remedies

- Betaine hydrochloride (stomach acid), 1 capsule taken with main meals improves protein digestion and ensures that foods are completely digested and don't arrive at the bowel causing fermentation. Not to be taken if you have active stomach ulcers. In which case take a Digestaid, containing enzymes that help break down foods, at the end of a meal to improve digestion. **BC**
- Sprinkle 1–3 dessertspoons of linseeds (flax seeds) or sunflower seeds over salads, breakfast cereals and so on to encourage toxins to move more quickly through the bowel. See my smoothie recipe in *General Supplements*.
- Acidophilus and bifidus capsules with FOS (fructo-oligosaccharides), which increase healthy bacteria. 1–2 capsules taken at the end of the meal can increase healthy bacteria in the bowel and enhance digestion. **BC**
- Take 5–6 drops of chlorophyll daily to help eliminate bad breath. Try the Liquid Nutrient Shot from Dr Gillian McKeith – a liquid blue-green algae, rich in chlorophyll. Available from all good health stores.
- Psyllium husks are great bowel-cleansers. They are a form of fibre that expands with water and they improve bowel movements if you take them daily on an empty stomach one hour before food. Keep going, as their affect can take 3 days to 'kick in'. Make sure that you drink plenty of water with these husks otherwise it can make the problem worse.
- Or try Lepicol capsules or powder (also includes beneficial bacteria) – take daily. Available from health stores and some pharmacies.
- Make a mouthwash of one capful of hydrogen peroxide mixed with four capfuls of water – swill around the mouth, hold for one minute and then spit out. This helps to oxygenate the gums and kill off bacteria.

Helpful Hints

- Make up your own healthy mouthwash using a few drops of essential oils of tea tree, peppermint, thyme and lemon. Mix with warm water and use regularly after meals and before bed. I make up mine with boiled water. I allow it to cool and then I keep the blend in a dark bottle in my bathroom and it lasts for ages.
- Exercise regularly as this ensures healthy bowel function.
- If the bad breath is severe, with your doctor's permission, have a colonic irrigation, which gently washes out the bowel helping to reduce toxicity (see *Useful Information*).
- Contact the Fresh Breath Centre, Conan Doyle House, 2 Devonshire Place, London W1N 1PA; or call 020 7935 1666. Website: www.freshbreath.co.uk
- Ask at your local chemist for a tongue scraper and use regularly to help clear any bacteria off your tongue
- For immediate breath-freshening, use a drop of pure peppermint oil on the tongue. Try Obbekjaers Japanese oil of Peppermint.

HANGOVERS   *(see Alcohol)*

HAYFEVER

(see also *Allergies, Allergic Rhinitis* and *Liver Problems*)

Dr Jean Monro, an allergy specialist at the Breakspear Hospital in Hertfordshire, says "Before the industrial revolution conditions such as hayfever did not exist. But since then we have done a great job of polluting our atmosphere and thus our bodies, hence why hayfever is actually more common in city-dwellers than in people who live in the country. We now know that an accumulation of a variety of pollutants, such as paint sprays or pesticides (there are hundreds of others), act as the *initial* trigger – and these chemicals became the *sensitizers* – and in most cases the membranes within the nose and throat begin to react by becoming inflamed. Then, the next thing that comes along, such as grass pollens, the body treats as a threatening foreign invader which increases any inflammation and induces allergic-type symptoms. But it's important to realise that it's the *chemicals* that sensitise the body in the first place. Chemicals can have a local affect such as on the skin – and then this effect is communicated to the rest of the body by neural (nerve) pathways and a sensitivity is born." This is important news to anyone suffering from hayfever, as Dr Monro and her colleagues have developed vaccines that can help to neutralise any reaction to substances found to trigger a response. For more details see *Allergies*.

Meanwhile, symptoms vary from sore, puffy, itchy, watering eyes, to continual sneezing and a runny or congested nose. Hayfever is sometimes confused with a condition called allergic or perennial rhinitis, as the symptoms are similar to hayfever but occur all year round. Common causes of allergic rhinitis include dust, food allergies and atmospheric pollution. Many people with hayfever and allergic rhinitis are also likely to have a sensitivity to certain foods, the most common being wheat and dairy, but some sufferers have problems with anything from eggs to bananas. As this has been linked to digestive problems for some people, see also *Leaky Gut*.

Foods to Avoid
- Greatly reduce your exposure to any foods with additives and/or preservatives, and that have been sprayed with pesticides and herbicides – eat organic. Keep in mind that non-organic lettuces, for example, can be sprayed up to 11 times before being harvested.
- Any foods to which you have an intolerance; typically these would include wheat, dairy products, eggs, and citrus fruits – especially oranges.
- Dairy foods are mucus-forming and without doubt can exacerbate the problem. While symptoms are acute, avoid milk in any form for at least one week, plus cheeses, chocolate, foods high in saturated fats such as croissants, Danish pastries, meat pies, and white-flour-based cakes and biscuits.
- Many foods high in sugar, such as puddings and sweets, are also high in dairy and fats. Too much sugar will greatly lower immune function.
- Reduce salt, caffeine and alcohol.

Friendly Foods
- Garlic and onions are high in the flavonoid quercetin, which can help reduce the severity of allergic reactions.
- Nettle tea helps to ease the symptoms of allergic rhinitis.
- Dairy-free alternatives to cow's milk are rice, oat and pea milk.
- Have a freshly squeezed vegetable juice, especially beetroot, artichoke, a little garlic, ginger, apple and carrot, which boosts the immune system and helps eliminate toxins.
- Bioflavonoids are important protectors of mucous membranes, therefore eat plenty of blueberries, blackberries, strawberries and kiwi fruit and include plenty of fresh vegetables, brown rice and whole grains in your diet.

Useful Remedies

- Quercetin, 400mg 3 times a day, is a natural antihistamine, which helps reduce puffy eyes and reduces irritation in the nose.
- While symptoms are acute, take up to 2–3 grams of vitamin C daily in an ascorbate form with food, which acts like a mild antihistamine.
- Nettle tablets or tincture 3 times a day has proven to be effective for allergic rhinitis.
- Garlic, ginger and horseradish tincture, as all of these herbs can ease congestion and reduce the symptoms of hayfever; take 1–2ml as needed. **FSC**
- Oralmat is an extract of the rye plant that has proven in medical trials to be hugely successful in reducing allergies of all kinds. It supports healthy respiratory function by strengthening defences against allergens. Dr Princetta, a specialist in the treatment of allergies in Atlanta, Georgia, reports: "The south-eastern United States, and Atlanta, Georgia, in particular, is a well-known allergy area of the world. Even some of my worst allergy patients responded very well to the drops and suffered a minimum of 50 percent less this past spring." Take 3 drops under the tongue (hold 30 seconds or longer) 3 times daily. Children can use one drop. **NC**
- Histazyme contains calcium, vitamin C, the amino acid lysine, zinc, vitamin B6, silica, bromelain, vitamin A and manganese, which all help if you suffer seasonal disorders. Take 1 capsule twice daily. This formula is not to be taken if you are pregnant. **BC**
- If nothing else, take a high-strength multi-vitamin and mineral that contains plenty of the B-group vitamins (see *Kudos 24* in *General Supplements*; p.160).
- Take probiotics daily – healthy bacteria, which help to boost immune function and heal the gut wall thus reducing the toxins that enter the bloodstream. **BC**

Helpful Hints

- It's well worth your while to check for food intolerances – see details of the York Test under the *Helpful Hints* in *Allergies*.
- Begin subscribing to *Allergy* magazine; details under *Allergies*.
- Ask your GP to refer you to the Breakspear. Website: www.breakspearmedical.com. Tel. 01442 261333. The NHS will pay if your GP agrees. Otherwise you can call them direct and pay privately.
- Buy a pot of honey from your local area, preferably with the honeycomb still in it, and take a dessertspoonful daily for about a month before the onset of the hayfever season. The pollen in the honey may protect you from developing full-blown hayfever.
- The plant extract butterbur helps relieve the cold-like symptoms associated with hayfever.
- Alka Life is a green herbal food supplement rich in bee pollen. Sprinkle daily over breakfast cereal for at least one month prior to the hayfever season to help reduce the severity or onset of an attack. Available from health stores, or for your nearest stockists contact Best Care Products on 01342 410303, or log on to www.bestcare-UK.com
- Homeopathy has been successful in treating hayfever with remedies like allium cepa, euphrasia and arundo. Ask for details at your local homeopathic pharmacy or to find a qualified practitioner in your area (see *Useful Information*). The Organic Pharmacy makes a combination mixture in a tablet, which makes this easier. **OP**
- Place a few drops of essential oil of basil and melissa on a handkerchief to help clear the sinuses. Massage these oils into the chest and throat once mixed with a base carrier oil such as almond or jojoba.
- Treat yourself to a good-quality ioniser and place it near your bed to help reduce any allergens in the air around you.

HEAD LICE

(see Scalp Problems)

HEALING AND HEALERS

(see also Electrical Pollution)

Research from the University of Maryland's School of Medicine in 2000 confirmed what healers have known intuitively for more than 2000 years – that hands-on healing and the power of prayer are not figments of our imagination. In fact there have now been so many well-designed, scientific, published experiments showing how hands-on healing can work, the efficacy of healing itself is no longer in doubt. Some hospitals and doctor's surgeries offer healing on the NHS and there are hundreds of Reiki healers working in beauty salons and alternative-treatment centres globally. Some people still believe that healing cannot work unless one has a specific religious belief or strong faith that the healing will work. Yet there are hundreds of documented cases where young babies, plants, children and animals have benefitted from healing. To understand how healing works, it is imperative first to comprehend that we are all electrical beings in a physical shell. If you take a photograph using Kirlian cameras you can clearly see the energy or auric field surrounding a person, animal, plant, vegetable – or in fact any object, even a stone will have an auric field. Roger Coghill, a bioelectromagnetics research scientist based in Wales, says "An individual's energy field or aura is as unique to them as their DNA. When we become ill, our field's characteristics change, this was proven by the American neurologist Albert Abrams in 1916."

After my near-death experience in 1998, which is documented in my book *Divine Intervention* (Cico Books), I truly began to comprehend how healing works. Professor Gary Schwartz at the University of Arizona conducted experiments during 2002 in which a well-known healer, Rosalyn Bruyere, taught 26 doctors and nurses how to give hands-on healing. After the training it was found that the nurses and doctors were able to absorb more gamma cosmic rays (which are the highest frequencies we can measure) – and then their bodies acted like transformers, literally 'turning down' the cosmic ray frequencies into subtle x-ray frequencies, which they then focused and pulsed into patients' energy fields. There are also machines that mimic this process. Biophysicist Harry Oldfield, based in Middlesex in the UK, spent 20 years developing a PIP scanner, which can 'read' the energies being emitted from our bodies. During his early research at some of the UK's leading teaching hospitals, Harry began to notice that, when he compared patients' energy emissions before and after treatments like chemotherapy, the treatments triggered energy distortions, which eventually manifested as negative symptoms. Over the following 20 years he became an expert at correctly interpreting these energy distortions – and eventually concluded that if these distortions could be treated with the correct harmonic frequencies, this could normalize the person's energy field, which would encourage the body to heal itself. Years later he designed electro-crystal healing for this purpose.

When we become sick, cells begin emitting disharmonic frequencies, which can clearly be seen in our energy field on his specialist scanners. Harry has found that every illness shows up in our energy field before appearing in the physical body. To counteract various medical conditions he simply pulses the correct tonal frequency back into the patient to encourage the body to heal itself. This is what healers have been doing intuitively for thousands of years. Harry has trained hundreds of therapists in the UK and globally; for more information on your nearest therapist, Harry Oldfield's PIP scanners and his electro-crystal therapy, visit www.electrocrystal.com

New frequency-based vaccines for allergies work on similar principals – see *Allergies*. This is how dolphins heal. They have been on the planet for 30 million years longer than humans and their brains are highly developed. They can 'scan' someone, much the same as a good healer can, and they then pulse harmonic, healing frequencies back into the patient, which over time can encourage the body to heal itself. And when Harry has scanned healers whilst they are working, he says the transfer of energy can be clearly seen on his equipment. Also he said that sometimes the healing energy emanated from *inside* the healers – usually from within their heart or solar plexus energy centres – whilst at other times they can clearly see energy from outside the healer being absorbed into the healer and then out through their hands.

However, both Harry and Gary make it clear that, in the majority of cases, without a clear *intention* from the healer, little or no energy transfers take place. Also they say that it's vital that the healer should be in a positive frame of mind and not sick themselves when they offer healing to a patient.

Of course some healers are better than others, just as there are better pianists, computer experts, or surgeons.

Recalling that we all emit our own unique range of frequencies, you need to find a healer who is on a compatible range of frequencies to your own, then you generally receive a more beneficial effect. You will soon know after 3 or 4 sessions whether their healing is making any difference, and if you are no better, simply find another healer. It is also possible to facilitate a transfer of healing energies over distances. Remember, energy can neither be created nor destroyed – it can only change into other forms of energy. Your thoughts are energy – they go somewhere – and when the *intention* is done with the whole heart and is for the receiver's greater good, your prayers will reach their destination. And the more people who pray at the same time with the same intention, the more powerful the prayer becomes. According to well-known healers such as Matthew Manning and Uri Geller, it is imperative we transmit only positive thoughts and visualise the person as looking 100% well in our mind's eye or imagination. I have detailed more information on healing and the science of miracles, plus the science behind how spontaneous healing occurs, in my book *The Evidence For The Sixth Sense* (Cico Books).

Helpful Hints

- The human mind is far more powerful than most people can even begin to imagine, therefore if you also truly believe the healing will work this really helps. Remember there is a huge difference between wanting something to work and believing it will.
- I find healing a great additional therapy when used in conjunction with eating the right diet and so on. It literally recharges your internal batteries, which gives your body more energy to heal itself. Most healers find that the great majority of their patients are looking for a single magic bullet to heal their ills. But if they continue eating junk foods, which emit a disharmonic range of frequencies, take no exercise and so on, obviously it's like trying to put a fire out while you remain standing in the flames.
- Then again, I have witnessed many miracles. Cancers have disappeared, crippled people walked again. How can this happen? I firmly believe this a combination of the power of the sick person's mind believing they are well and the ability of the healer to transmit a strong healing signal. Also, spiritual masters can without doubt affect healing miracles without the person's knowledge. See my book *The Evidence for the Sixth Sense* (Cico Books). But I also know that if a person believes 100% with their mind and heart they are truly healed, in that instant they are. Visit www.thetahealing.com for more information on instant healing. This is the website of Vianna Stibal in America who teaches people to go into a theta brainwave state to help

facilitate faster healing.

- You can hypnotise someone and tell them you are putting lighted cigarettes on their skin that will cause blisters. When the therapy is over their skin can be covered in blisters, but no such torture was ever applied. The blisters emanate from the power of the mind. We all have the ability to heal others and ourselves. All we need is an honourable intention, to be in a positive frame of mind and healthy when we offer healing – and to keep an open mind.
- Reiki healing is also becoming very popular. To find out more about Reiki log on to www.reikiassociation.org.uk For non-membership enquiries call 07704 270727.
- Although there are hundreds of really amazing healers in the UK alone, there are three of whom I have interviewed and seen their work and I have interviewed several of their patients. I believe they are exceptional healers. The first is Seka Nikolic, who practices at the Hale Clinic in London, see page 361 for contact details or her website www.sekanikolic.com; the second is Kelvin Heard, who specialises in chronic fatigue or ME. His number is 07710 794627. The third is Susan Anthony, who practices in Wells in Somerset. Her website is at www.psalifemastery.com; or call her on 01749 679900.
- To find your nearest registered, insured healer call the National Federation of Spiritual Healers on 0845 1232777. They have a worldwide network of healers. Visit their website on www.nfsh.org.uk
- Read *Virtual Medicine* by Dr Keith Scott-Mumby (Timpanogos Publishers). Keith offers excellent research details for practically every form of electro-healing, including the Scenar; well worth a read. To order call the Nutri Centre bookshop on 020 7323 2382; they can also help you with any number of books on healing. Dan Benor has written some highly authoritative books on scientific research into healing and meditation.

HEARTBURN　　　　　　　(see *Acid Stomach, Indigestion* and *Low Stomach Acid*)

HEART DISEASE

(see also *Angina, Cholesterol, Circulation* and *High Blood Pressure*)

Heart disease and diseases of the circulatory system account for 1 in every 3 deaths in the UK – 233,000 annually. Around 1 in 5 men and 1 in 6 women die from heart disease. One adult dies from heart disease every three minutes. Yet, the saddest part is that a huge majority of these deaths are preventable if people would just wake up to a healthier diet and lifestyle before it's too late. The majority of younger people who die with heart disease are male. Once women go through the menopause their risk of dying from heart disease increases threefold (see *Menopause*). Your heart is an amazing organ – a simple pump that can beat around 70 times a minute non-stop for 100 or more years, pumping more than 10 million litres of blood around your 100,000km of blood vessels every year. While it works we tend to take it for granted, and yet if more people could think of their heart health from their 30s onwards, then heart and arterial disease would not still be the number-one killer in the Western world.

For some there is a genetic predisposition for developing heart disease, but if you eat healthily and change any negative and unhealthy lifestyle patterns practised by your parents and grandparents, then in most cases you can stack the cards in your favour and add decades to your life. The heart, like any other muscle, needs its own blood supply and receives this via three main vessels called the coronary arteries. Over time, one or more of the arteries can become blocked and if an artery becomes completely blocked, some of the heart muscle may die during a heart attack. Typically symptoms of a heart attack include a severe pressing band of pain across the chest that can spread up the neck and into the jaw or across the shoulders and down into the left arm. This is often termed a 'myocardial infarction', which means death of the heart muscle due to an interrupted blood supply. The muscle may simply stop beating or, more commonly, it goes into an irregular pattern, which no longer works like a pump. Sweating, breathlessness and a feeling of nausea can accompany a heart attack, which needs urgent medical attention.

A heart attack can be fatal, unless someone can apply immediate cardio-pulmonary resuscitation (CPR is something everyone should learn and one day you may save a life with this simple skill). Luckily many people survive their first heart attack. Specialists may recommend drugs and/or by-pass surgery or other operative procedures, but it's important to consider that none of these medical or surgical treatments attempts to solve the cause of the problem, only the result of the problem. While some heart attacks appear to strike out of the blue, there are usually warning signs telling us that something wrong. The most common warning is angina – a constrictive pain in the chest, provoked by exertion. It's the body's signal that the blood supply to the heart is inadequate, owing to narrowed or spasms in the coronary arteries. If you experience angina, it's time to act. You can still turn it around and live another 40 years or more. Some people have gone on to run a marathon after their first heart attack. If you suffer angina or have had a heart attack, then you need to radically change your diet, increase exercise (gently) and reduce stress.

Other known risk factors for heart disease include smoking, excessive alcohol consumption, high blood pressure, high homocysteine levels (see *High Blood Pressure*), high LDL cholesterol levels, being overweight, diabetes, insufficient exercise, eating a high-fat, -salt, and -sugar diet, insufficient intake of fresh fruit and vegetables and excessive stress.

There are also links with heart disease via inflammatory conditions caused by the parasite *chlamydia pneumonia* and the organism *helicobacter pylori*, known to cause stomach ulcers. Poor root canal treatment is also linked to heart disease.

Foods to Avoid
- Cut down on saturated fats found in meats, butter, cheese, cream and hard margarines. Keep in mind that many low-fat foods are high in sugar, which will convert to fat in the body if not burned off during exercise.
- You need to have a balance, but if you have a sweet tooth then greatly reduce the amount of concentrated shop-bought fruit juices, fizzy drinks, desserts, cakes and pastries you eat.
- Reduce dairy foods, especially milk. Jeffrey Segall, from London's North Middlesex Hospital, believes the problem may be the lactose, not the fat. Research published in the Lancet in 1999 showed how changes in a country's milk-consumption pattern, either up or down, accurately predicted changes in coronary deaths 4 to 7 years later.
- Especially avoid any foods containing hydrogenated or trans fats, which are found in most mass-produced biscuits, pies, cakes and so on.
- Don't eat too much fried food; frying damages fats and turns them into dangerous fats that heart surgeons find in your arteries.
- Cut down on sodium-based table salts. Use a low-salt alternative or a little magnesium- or potassium-rich sea salt, available from all good health stores and most supermarkets.
- Greatly reduce your intake of mass-produced burgers, pies, sausages, pastries, cakes and desserts.
- Avoid excessive alcohol consumption; even though a moderate intake – that is, 1 glass a day – is slightly protective, large amounts of alcohol over time is a known risk factor for heart disease.

Aim for no more than 6 units a week on average. See *Alcohol*.

Friendly Foods

- Oily fish is rich in omega-3 essential fats: wild salmon, cod, sardines, mackerel, herring, and fresh tuna are good sources, as are linseeds (flax seeds). Try to eat oily fish twice a week.
- Generally eat more fish of any kind in preference to meats.
- Unrefined, unsalted seeds, such as pumpkin, linseed (flax seed), sesame and sunflower, and their unrefined oils, are also a good source of essential fats. Use unrefined organic linseed oil for salad dressings, as people who consume more linseed oil, which contains omega-3 essential fats, have a lower risk of developing heart disease.
- Eat plenty of fruits and vegetables that are high in carotenes and antioxidants – such as carrots, asparagus, French beans, broccoli, Brussels sprouts, watercress, cabbage, spinach, sweet potatoes, spring greens, apricots, mangoes and tomatoes – which help lower your risk of heart disease.
- Include brown rice and pastas, beans, wholemeal bread and other grains, such as quinoa, amaranth, barley, oats and spelt in your diet.
- Fibre, derived from fruits and vegetables, is very protective and additional fibre from linseeds (flax seeds), oat or rice bran or psyllium husks all help lower the risk.
- Eating pistachios, walnuts, Brazil nuts and macadamia nuts on a regular basis have been shown to help lower LDL cholesterol.
- Wheat germ and soya beans are rich in natural vitamin E, which has been shown to reduce the risk of heart disease. This is particularly true for people with type A or AB blood.

- Use non-hydrogenated spreads such as Biona, Vitaquell or Benecol. There is nothing wrong with a little butter as long as you are eating sufficient omega-3 essential fats. Benecol spread helps to lower cholesterol.
- A vegetarian diet, using a lot of beans, vegetables and grains, dramatically lowers your risk of developing heart disease.
- Sprinkle 1 dessertspoon of soya lecithin granules over breakfast cereals and desserts, which help to break down the 'bad' fats.
- Olive oil raises HDL (the good cholesterol) levels, lowers bad LDL cholesterol, and contains antioxidants that protect the LDL from damage.
- Drink more water – at least 6 glasses daily.

Useful Remedies

- After the age of 50, unless you have a medical condition that requires iron, do not take extra iron supplements as excessive iron in the body is linked to heart disease.
- Complete Heart II is a cardiovascular support formula in a powder form, containing garlic, Co-enzyme Q10, tocotrienols (vitamin E), hawthorn, lipoic acid, bromelain, grape skin extract and amino acids. This blend of herbs and nutrients is available at a fraction of the cost of all these nutrients taken separately. As a dietary supplement, 1 scoop (20g) daily mixed in a jar or shaker with 2–3fl oz (55–85ml) of juice or other beverages, such as organic rice milk. Drink immediately and follow with several ounces of liquid, if desired. For details ask at your health store or call the Nutri Centre. **NC**
- Take a high-strength B-complex, as B6, B12 and folic acid reduce homocysteine levels in the blood.
- Vitamin C and the amino acid lysine can help to reverse arterial blockages. You would need approximately 3 grams of each per day. **HN**
- Homocysteine Metabolite Formula. If you have a high homocysteine level, try this formula which contains vitamin B6 x 30mg, folic acid x 400mcg, vitamin B12 x 400mcg, trimethylglycine x 500mg, l-serine x 100mg. Take 1 capsule per day with a meal. Available from the Nutri Centre

and health stores. **NC**

- Include a good-quality multi-vitamin and mineral that contains at least 400iu of natural-source vitamin E, 150mcg of selenium, 30mg of zinc, 100mcg of chromium and 400mg of magnesium. Almost all the vitamin companies listed on pages 13–15 supply such formulae.
- Try the herbs hawthorn (100–500mg of standardised extract) and ginkgo biloba (60–120mg of standardised extract) daily, either as tea, tincture or capsules. Both are known to improve circulation. The Specialist Herbal Suppliers make a formula containing hawthorn, motherwort, lime blossom and dandelion to help balance the heart and circulation. Start with 5 drops a day and then increase gradually. **SHS**

Helpful Hints

- Stop smoking and avoid places where you will be exposed to second-hand smoke as both increase the risk for heart disease.
- If you are overweight, lose weight (see *Weight Problems*).
- Gentlemen, unless you are very tall, a good rule is to not let your waist exceed 39in (99cm), and ladies 35in (90cm) if you want to avoid heart problems.
- Learn to test your heart health. What's your resting pulse? For 1 minute place your first 2 fingers on the vein crossing the bony protuberance on the thumb side of your inner wrist and check your pulse. While your blood pressure tells you about the health of your arteries, your pulse is a measure of your heart health. If your heart is strong and able to pump blood easily around the body, it will pump slowly and rhythmically, around 60–70 beats per minute. If it's weak, and therefore can't pump as much blood as it should with each beat, it will have to beat more often to keep your cells properly oxygenated, so your pulse will be higher. This is why your pulse goes up when you exercise – your cells need more oxygen so the heart pumps more rapidly. In time, this strengthens the heart and it will be able to pump more blood with each beat, so your resting pulse will slow down. A raised pulse is now considered a 'normal' result of ageing, although there is no reason you can't have a pulse of 70 when you're over 70.
- Try chelation, an intravenous therapy that has saved thousands of people from undergoing major heart surgery. It helps to clear clogged arteries, which reduces the likelihood of strokes and heart disease. For more details contact the Arterial Disease Clinic, who have several clinics in the UK, on 01942 886644. Or call Dr Wendy Denning on 020 7224 2423 or Dr Robert Trossell, at 4 Duke Street, London W1U 3EL, on 020 7486 1095.
- Reduce stress in your life (see *Stress*).
- There is now an easy test to discover your plasma homocysteine levels. Made by York Laboratories and backed by the British Cardiac Patients Association, it's a simple pinprick method that can be done by post. For details call York Labs on 0800 458 2052 or log on to: www.yorktest.com.
- Get some exercise. If you have a heart condition, then with your doctor's permission start walking for 30 minutes every day and gradually build up to an hour a day. Join a gym and go regularly. If you don't have access to a gym, walking, swimming, jogging or cycling along quiet roads or nature trails are a good alternative. A little exercise every day is far more effective than a lot of exercise once a week. Even though exercise raises your heart rate while you're doing it, the overall effect is to strengthen the heart and slow your resting heart rate. Research has shown that even moderate exercise after having a heart attack is one very effective way of preventing a second one. If you have had any heart problems, undertake an exercise programme only under professional supervision.
- Stop smoking. The chemicals in cigarette smoke damage your arteries, oxidise the cholesterol that forms plaque in your arteries, and increase the likelihood of clotting.

h

- Reduce your exposure to toxic metals such as lead, cadmium and mercury. Eat more coriander, which helps to eliminate toxic metals from the body – as does chelation (see above).
- People who are angry and argumentative suffer more heart problems. Millions of people are dying because they don't get things off their chest. Learn to deal with anger and internal emotions – see a counsellor; your life may depend on it.
- Contact the British Heart Foundation, 14 Fitzhardinge Street, London W1H 4DH, or call the Heart Health Line on 0870 600 6566. Website: www.bhf.org.uk.
- Read Patrick Holford's *Say No to Heart Disease* (Piatkus), which is an excellent book explaining the causes of arterial damage and what you can do to prevent or correct high blood pressure and heart disease.
- See *High Blood Pressure* for more on protecting your whole cardiovascular system.

HEPATITIS
(see also *Liver Problems*)

With global air travel hepatitis is on the increase. Hepatitis is a form of liver disease mainly caused by a virus, but can also be due to alcohol and some medication. If present, symptoms may include: a short, mild, flu-like illness, nausea and vomiting, diarrhoea, loss of appetite, weight-loss, jaundice (yellow skin and whites of eyes, darker yellow urine and pale faeces), and itchy skin. Symptoms are not always present when a person is infected, but the virus is still active and can still be passed on. If you suspect that you have hepatitis it is important that you visit your doctor or local sexual health clinic (GUM), where a simple blood test can confirm the presence of hepatitis.

Hepatitis A (Hep A)

The hepatitis A virus (HAV) is extremely common in many parts of the world and is 100 times more infectious than HIV. Usually spread by close personal contact (including sex or sharing a household), it is also spread by eating food or drinking water contaminated with HAV. As the virus is carried in the faeces, poor personal hygiene is the major route of infection. Symptoms can include nausea, loss of appetite, vomiting, fatigue and jaundice, with symptoms usually beginning to clear within a few weeks. If you are run down before the onset of the virus you may feel fatigued for some months afterwards. There is no standard medical treatment for Hep A, but once the virus is cleared from the body you are immune from repeated attacks for life. Hep A immunization offers effective protection against the virus and is worth considering especially if you are going to travel abroad out of Europe, or are living with someone who is infected.

Foods to Avoid
- Avoid water if you are at all unsure of its purity – such as in India and the Far East.
- When you go abroad, avoid eating salads that have been washed in local water. See *Food Poisoning*.
- Avoid raw or partially cooked shellfish, which can harbour Hep A.
- Avoid all alcohol as this adds to liver damage.
- Avoid foods full of saturated animal fats, red meat and dairy (cheese, cream, butter and milk) as these add an additional burden on the liver, as do deep-fried foods, such as crisps, samosas, fried breakfasts and chips. Avoid curries too.
- Simple carbohydrates, such as white rice, pasta, bread, cakes and pastries, give the liver extra

work to do so keep them to a minimum.

- Caffeine, from tea, coffee, cola-type energy drinks, and some painkillers, adds to the overall load of the liver so they are best avoided.
- Try not to consume excess amounts of preserved meats, such as pizza meats, jerky, salami, provolone, sausages, hot dogs or hamburger meats, as these are often high in unfriendly bacteria, which the liver has to clear from the body.
- Toxicity is linked to aspartame so avoid artificial sweeteners; look out for aspartame hidden in hundreds of foods, drinks and chewing gums.
- A high-potassium diet, low in sodium, is known to have a positive effect on the liver. Avoid salt and salty foods, such as chips, sauces, ready-made processed foods, and savoury snacks, to reduce salt intake; and increase intake of fresh fruits and vegetables to increase intake of potassium.

Friendly Foods

- Eat more organic food as non-organic food often contains antibiotic, steroid, hormone and pesticide residues, all of which place a strain on the liver.
- Include salads in your diet – made with fresh raw vegetables, such as tomatoes, shallots, sliced red onion, cucumbers, broccoli, lettuce, endives, radicchio, celery, red radish, avocado, shredded cabbage, carrots and beets and grated horseradish, ginger and so on. You can use a dressing of cold-pressed oil, apple cider vinegar, and/or lemon and lime juice. Try to have a salad 4 to 5 times a week, or ideally every day.
- Drink 8–10 cups of antioxidant-rich green tea daily. Green tea is also rich in polyphenols which have strong anti-viral properties.

- Make yourself raw vegetable and fruit juices regularly. Ideally you should do this every day; however, even if you make raw juices only two to three times a week, you will see tremendous benefits. A basic juice to improve liver function can be made with equal parts of apple, carrot and/or beetroot, and cabbage of different colours – one week use a purple–red cabbage and the next week, a green cabbage.
- Linseed (flaxseed) oil is essential for improving liver function. It is beneficial for damaged liver cells whilst reducing inflammation. Use instead of butter on baked potatoes and for salad dressings.
- Wholegrain foods such as brown rice, millet, brown pasta and rye contain lots of B-vitamins needed for the liver to work effectively.
- Sulphur-rich foods including, onions, garlic and leeks enhance liver function so try to eat a little of one of these daily.

Useful Remedies

- Linseed oil is good for repairing damaged liver cell membranes and reducing inflammation. Use with olive oil in salad dressings or take BioCare's easily absorbable Linseed Oil 1000; 1 capsule, 3 times per day.
- Vitamin E assists in protecting liver cell membranes from free-radical damage and reduces and prevents scarring. Take 400iu daily.
- Liquorice is known for its anti-viral and immune-enhancing action, as well as being beneficial to the liver. Take 1–2 grams once a day of powdered whole root, or 250mg once per day of solid root extract. Available from www.positivenutrtionshop.com. If you are taking liquorice for long periods increase the amount of fresh fruit and vegetables you are eating to address your potassium balance, which can be upset by liquorice.
- Milk thistle extract is very protective for the liver. Kudos makes a one-a-day formula. **KVH**
- Garlic has strong anti-viral properties; take 400mg per day.
- N-acetylcysteine (NAC) effectively enhances liver function. Take 500mg 3 times per day before meals.

- Antioxidants have protective and therapeutic action against hepatitis. Take 250mg of alpha lipoic acid, a potent antioxidant, twice a day
- Vitamin C has strong anti-viral properties, along with being an antioxidant. Take to bowel tolerance levels; 5–10 grams per day. BioCare's magnesium ascorbate powder can be added to a bottle of water and drunk throughout the day.
- Take 800mg of green tea polyphenols daily, which have strong anti-viral action.

Helpful Hints

- Avoid chemical cleaning products in the home as the liver has the job of breaking these down. Instead opt for natural products. Look out for the Ecover range now available in most good supermarkets.
- Hepatitis A occurs more frequently in developing countries, possibly because of over-crowding and poor sanitation. Travellers to areas such as Asia, Africa, India, Eastern Europe and Central and South America are therefore at high risk. While travelling, drink only boiled or bottled water, avoid eating all raw fish and shellfish, and use disinfectant soaps for the hands. (For more help see *Food Poisoning*.)
- Cigarettes weaken your immune system, compromising its ability to fight the virus; do your best to give it up (see *Smoking*).

Hepatitis B (Hep B)

The Hepatitis B virus (HBV) lives on dry surfaces for up to 7 days, making it one of the most communicable diseases and the 9th most common cause of death worldwide. 90% of sufferers recover but 10% are chronically infected meaning they could develop liver damage, which can be fatal. This virus can be spread via blood or other bodily fluids. The most common routes of infection are via unprotected penetrative sex – especially if blood is produced – or by sharing contaminated needles during drug use. Hep B is also contracted by blood transfusions and non-sterile needles, which may be used in hospitals in certain developing countries (all blood used in the UK is tested for Hepatitis B). Non-sterilised equipment used for tattooing, acupuncture or body-piercing is also a risk. As vaccination is 95% effective it's worth considering if you are travelling abroad or living with an infected person.

Foods to Avoid

- See dietary advice for *Hepatitis A*.

Friendly foods

- See dietary advice for *Hepatitis A*.

Useful Remedies
(see also *Useful Remedies* for *Hepatitis A*)

- Selenium reduces Hepatitis B infection by 77%, as well as helping to prevent liver cancer – a secondary complication common in chronic Hepatitis B sufferers. Take 200mcg daily.

Helpful Hints
(see also *Helpful Hints* for *Hepatitis C*)

- If planning to travel outside Europe to developing countries, it is possible to get a small first-aid kit that contains sterile needles to prevent infection. The kit is available from the Hospital for Tropical Diseases in London, or ask at pharmacies.

Hepatitis C (Hep C)

200,000 people in the UK are estimated to have Hepatitis C, with 300 million people infected worldwide. It can take decades for symptoms to appear meaning that 8 out of 10 people are unaware they have it. Unlike Hepatitis A and B there is no vaccine for Hepatitis C. Infection occurs from blood transfusions, needle-sharing (including acupuncture, piercing and tattooing), the sharing of notes used to snort cocaine, working in a medical environment, and sexual contact – especially if a woman is having her period or genital sores are present and bleeding. On rare occasions it can be passed from an infected mother to her baby, mainly during delivery. If you have ever received a blood transfusion in a country where blood is not tested for the Hepatitis C virus (many developing countries), or if you received a transfusion in the UK before 1991 (all blood for transfusion in the UK is now tested), or if you have received medical or dental treatment abroad where equipment may not have been sterilised properly, you may want to have a blood test. As with all types of hepatitis, symptoms may not occur but the virus can still be passed on. Evidence suggests that about 20% of individuals who have Hepatitis C appear to clear the virus from the blood, whilst about 80% will remain infected and can pass on the virus to others. If a person continues to be infected over a number of years they may develop chronic hepatitis, liver cirrhosis or liver cancer. HCV is not spread by sneezing, hugging, coughing, food or water, sharing eating utensils or drinking glasses, or casual contact.

Foods to Avoid
(see *Hepatitis A*)

Friendly Foods
(see also *Hepatitis A*)

- Drink plenty of water, try to drink 8–12 full glasses a day. If you vomit a lot, you should drink more clear liquids.
- Include salads in your diet. Make them with fresh raw vegetables, such as tomatoes, shallots, sliced red onion, cucumbers, broccoli, lettuce, endives, radicchio, celery, red radish, avocado, shredded cabbage, carrots and beets and grated horseradish, ginger and so on. You can use a dressing of cold-pressed oil, apple cider vinegar, and/or lemon and lime juice. Try to have a salad 4 or 5 times a week, or ideally every day.

Useful Remedies
(see also *Hepatitis A*)

- Keep iron levels to a minimum and do not supplement with iron, as the Hepatitis C virus does most of its damage by joining with iron stored in the liver, delivering a massive free-radical attack, which damages liver cells.

Helpful Hints
(see also *Hepatitis A*)

- Blood spills should be wiped up with bleach and all cuts and wounds covered with adhesive dressings. Bloodstained tissues, sanitary napkins and so on must be disposed of safely.
- Tell your healthcare provider and dentist that you have the virus to avoid infecting them.
- Do not share toothbrushes, razors, nail files, clippers or scissors, or any object that may come into contact with your blood.
- Do not share food that has been in your mouth and do not pre-chew food for babies.
- Tell sexual partners you have the virus, advise them to see their doctor and in the meantime use a condom.
- For more help call the NHS Hepatitis C helpline on 0800 451 451, open from 10am–10pm, 7 days a week.
- An informative Hepatitis C website can be found at www.hepatitis-central.com
- To find details about your local STD clinic, go to www.condomessentialwear.co.uk

HERPES

(see also *Cold Sores*)

There are two types of herpes simplex virus: Type 1 causes cold sores, Type 2 is sexually transmitted and is the most common. It can cause extreme pain and swelling of the genital area and is sometimes accompanied by fever. You never eradicate the virus once you have it, but you can keep attacks under control using supplements and by eating a healthier diet.

Foods to Avoid
(see *Cold Sores*)

Friendly Foods
(See *Cold Sores*)

Useful Remedies
- Vitamin C, take 1 gram as a preventative, and between 2 and 3 grams daily during an attack.
- The amino acid lysine inhibits replication of the virus. Take 500mg as a preventative, and up to 3 grams daily spread throughout the day and taken 30 minutes before food, while suffering an attack. Take lysine only when symptoms appear and for about a week afterwards.
- Lemon balm applied topically and taken internally is very useful. Normally available in tincture form. If you use it externally, dilute it in warmish water first or douche in lemon balm tea. If you are unable to find lemon balm, liquorice is a good alternative as it is a strong anti-viral.
- Propolis cream is highly anti-viral. Use daily.
- Olive Leaf Extract acts like a natural antibiotic and boosts immune function. Take 2–3 capsules daily.
- Larreastat, an extract of the larrea bush, has had a 97.5% success rate in treating herpes simplex 1 and 2, and herpes zoster (which causes shingles). Available in capsules or as a lotion. Take 1 capsule up to 3 times a day, and the lotion can be applied up to 5 times daily on to the lesions. **NC SL**
- A multi-vitamin and mineral that contains around 30 mg of zinc.
- Lemon balm (*Melissa officinalis*) helps to stop the spread of the virus and speeds the healing process. Take as a tincture applied to the sores, and take internally. This is a very calming tincture. **OP**

Helpful Hints
- Avoidance of sexual intercourse when you have an attack of Type 2 is very important, as the virus is extremely contagious. If you must have sex then use a condom, but you may well find it is too painful and need to wait until the sores have either healed or completely gone away.
- Avoid oral sex when you have an attack of Type 1 or 2. Remember that oral sex is one way of transferring a cold sore and turning it into genital herpes.
- For further help contact the Herpes Viruses Association on their helpline, on 0845 123 2305. Website: www.herpes.org.uk

HIATUS HERNIA

(see also *Acid–Alkaline Balance* and *Indigestion*)

The gullet or oesophagus takes food from the mouth to the stomach and passes through a sheet of muscle called the diaphragm. A hiatus hernia occurs when the part of the stomach pushes up through the diaphragm and allows acid to escape into the gullet causing heartburn, reflux of food, and indigestion, especially when lying down. It can also cause a fair amount of chest pain, which obviously needs looking at quickly. Most hiatus hernias can easily be seen on an x-ray. Being overweight is a common factor for hiatus hernia. Believe it or not, too much exercise – especially jogging – can trigger this problem.

Foods to Avoid

- Generally avoid large meals, especially ones containing red meat, fried foods such as chips, and creamy-type sauces.
- Alcohol, strong tea, coffee, fizzy drinks, sugar, chocolate, dairy products and all high-fat foods can cause an 'acid' rebound reaction as they are all acid-forming foods within the body.
- Chew food thoroughly and don't drink too much fluid with food.
- If symptoms are acute, avoid eating for a short time, or, at most, eat only lightly cooked small meals regularly.
- Avoid artificial sweeteners, such as aspartame, and artificial additives, which can aggravate symptoms.

Friendly Foods

- Slippery elm and liquorice both soothe the oesophagus, as well as providing a gentle fibre, which can reduce discomfort. Ask at your health shop for de-glycyrrhized liquorice, and chew 20 minutes before each main meal. Liquorice works as well as many drugs, without the negative side-effects.
- Try decaffeinated beverages and drink more herbal teas such as camomile, liquorice and peppermint.
- Food combining has proved very useful to people who have this condition. There are numerous books on food combining, the best being *The Complete Book of Food Combining* by Kathryn Marsden (Piatkus). The basic rule is to avoid eating proteins, such as meat or fish, with potatoes, pasta, rice or bread. And when eating potatoes, pasta, rice or bread, do not eat proteins, but eat vegetables and salads.
- Eat live, low-fat yoghurt after meals to soothe the digestive tract.
- Generally eat a low-fat diet, but see *Fats You Need to Eat* and *General Health Hints* to ensure that you get all the essential nutrients you need.
- Steam, boil, poach, stir-fry, roast or grill your food.
- Eat more wheat germ, soya beans, alfalfa and dark green vegetables (especially cabbage and kale – these are rich in glutamine, which heals the gut), plus a little avocado. These foods are all rich in vitamin E.
- Sprinkle lecithin granules over a low-sugar breakfast cereal daily, which helps to emulsify fats.
- Eat more garlic and fresh root ginger.

Useful Remedies

- Deglycyrrhized liquorice: chew 1–2 tablets 20 minutes before a meal. The liquorice protects the mucous membranes, helps with digestion, and can rapidly ease the discomfort of hiatus hernia. FSC
- Slippery elm: 2 tablets taken at the end of each meal can help reduce any discomfort.
- L-glutamine, found in cabbage, helps to heal any ulceration in the gut. Take 1–2 grams daily before food for 6 weeks.
- Take a good-quality multi-vitamin and mineral.
- Drink half a cup of aloe vera juice daily.
- Calcium fluoride tissue salts: 4 a day to help strengthen the diaphragm.

Helpful Hints

- Eat smaller meals, which are easier on the digestion. Avoid large rich meals at any time.
- Try to relax as much as possible and avoid lying down immediately after eating.
- Do not smoke near meal times.
- Go for a gentle walk after meals, but do not get involved in heavy exercise.
- Many people report relief from symptoms after seeing a chiropractor. See *Useful Information*.

HIGH BLOOD PRESSURE (see also *Circulation, Stress* and *Strokes*)

High blood pressure makes you more susceptible to heart disease, strokes and kidney disease. Blood pressure of 150 over 100 or more is classified as high. A normal reading is 120/80, but 140/90 or less is deemed as raised, but acceptable. There is no reason you shouldn't have a blood pressure of 120/80 when you're 80 if you take good care of your arteries.

While your pulse is a measure of your heart health, your blood pressure tells you about the health of your arteries. High blood pressure, also known as hypertension, is often considered a 'normal' part of ageing, but just because something's common, doesn't mean it's normal. It's important to remember that high blood pressure is a symptom of a problem, not the problem. The problem is that your arteries are too constricted, or 'furred up', to properly relax when your heart pumps the blood through. And narrower arteries make you age faster, as you have a reduced oxygen supply to tissues, so the heart works harder, which raises your blood pressure even more, exposing arterial walls to damage, which triggers further hardening or furring up, and the problem gets worse still.

Think of your arteries as being like a complex system of garden hoses, coming off a single pump – your heart. Every time your heart beats, it's sending oxygen and nutrient-rich blood gushing around your body via your arteries to nourish each of your trillions of cells. These gushes of blood, forced through the arteries with every heartbeat, exert pressure on the walls of your arteries, and this pressure can damage the delicate cells lining your arteries. To reduce the pressure and ensure smooth blood-flow, rather than blood-flow in spurts, the arterial walls are flexible, and are surrounded by smooth muscle that is able to expand and contact in response to the pressure being exerted on the arterial walls by the pumped blood. Over time, many peoples' arteries become gradually harder and narrower, a process called arteriosclerosis; or if the arteries are furred up, the condition is called atherosclerosis. Arteriosclerosis is a major recognized cause of dementia in the elderly (see *Alzheimer's Disease*). The kidneys, liver and other organs suffer reduced blood-flow too, and so cannot perform effectively in detoxifying the body. Lumps of thickened matter (called 'plaques') build up in the artery wall and reduce the diameter of the vessels that the blood-flows through. We now know why this occurs, and it all starts with damage to the arterial wall. This can occur due to abrasion (from high blood pressure), viral or bacterial infection, or high homocysteine levels (a toxic amino acid formed as a byproduct of the metabolism of proteins), or free radical damage. Once the damage is done, the body tries to repair the area, causing scar tissue, and this is made worse by high levels of low-density lipoprotein (LDL – 'bad cholesterol'), that can pass into the walls of the artery where it is oxidised by free radicals into dangerous rancid forms. This in turn is gobbled up by macrophages (part of your immune system), which become engorged 'foam cells'. The whole area attracts more and more oxidised cholesterol, more immune responses, more inflammation, and inevitably the arteries grow stiffer and narrower. So now we can understand why LDL cholesterol is bad for us and why levels of unoxidised cholesterol never was the real problem. Total cholesterol, so often touted as the cause of heart and arterial disease, is less a risk marker than high homocysteine levels. Homocysteine, now thought to be one of the key agents involved in damaging the arterial walls, is a damaging compound produced in the body that's normally recycled or broken down by vitamins B6, B12 and folic acid – nutrients often deficient in overly refined foods. A University of Washington study showed that high homocysteine levels doubled the risk of arterial disease in young women, and that B-vitamins help reduce homocysteine levels (see *Helpful Hints* on page 188 to find out how to get these levels tested).

Another key cause of raised blood pressure is a lack of the mineral magnesium. Remember those muscles around the arteries that enable the walls to contract and relax? Magnesium is needed for muscles to relax after they've contracted (muscle cramps or eye ticks are a symptom of magnesium deficiency), and research has shown that arteries are considerably narrower in those who are deficient in magnesium. In Japan, paramedics inject magnesium directly into the heart of heart-attack victims to relax the muscle and the blocked arteries supplying it. Many heart attacks and strokes are now thought to be due to arterial spasms blocking blood supply to the heart or brain, rather than a clot. Stress and excessive exercise are known to deplete magnesium, which may be deficient in your diet already if you don't eat enough dark green leafy vegetables, whole grains and seeds. This may explain why fit, apparently healthy people sometimes die suddenly of a heart attack or stroke.

A dangerous side effect of arteriosclerosis is an increased tendency toward (and greater dangers from) blood clotting. This is especially true for those with A or AB blood types. Turbulence in the blood caused by rough areas in the normally very smooth arterial walls can increase clotting. Also the plaques can break off and travel along the artery until they get stuck in a narrower blood vessel, commonly known as 'thrombosis'. If these clots reach an area sufficiently narrowed by arterial plaques, they can block the vessel completely and starve the tissues 'down stream' of blood, oxygen and nutrients. If this happens in the vessels supplying the heart or brain, a heart attack or stroke can occur.

Despite all this, there is plenty you can do to help yourself. 85% of all cases of high blood pressure can be treated without drugs, if the person is willing to change their lifestyle and diet. For example in societies where salt is virtually absent, hypertension is equally absent. Too much caffeine, alcohol and smoking, when combined with high blood pressure, greatly increases your chances of suffering heart disease or stroke. Stress is a major factor in high blood pressure, because adrenaline is released into the blood stream, which increases your heart rate, breathing and blood pressure, but also constricts arteries.

Foods to Avoid
- Salt. There is a clear link between the use of sodium-based salt and high blood pressure because sodium causes more water to be retained by your kidneys, so keep the sodium level in your diet low. More water means more blood volume, and therefore higher blood pressure. There are plenty of magnesium- and potassium-based salts, such as Solo Salt, available from health shops. Use sparingly on the food that's on your plate.
- Reduce stimulants. Blood pressure has been shown to drop as much as 20 points when all caffeine is eliminated, because caffeine causes arteries to constrict. Some decaffeinated drinks contain formaldehyde, so look for decaffeinated drinks and coffee that has been decaffeinated using the more natural water method.
- Sugar is also a problem as sugar coverts into fat in the body if not used up during exercise, and be aware that many low-fat foods are high in sugar. Always check the labels.
- Replace refined grains, for example white bread, pasta and rice, with whole grains such as brown rice, breads and pastas, to increase your intake of the B-vitamins B6, B12 and folic acid, which are involved in breaking down homocysteine.
- If you have eliminated all of the above and still have a tendency towards high blood pressure, it might be worth consulting a nutritionist who can check for food intolerances, particularly if you are a migraine sufferer.

Friendly Foods
- Green vegetables, fresh fruit, unprocessed and unsalted nuts, seafood, roast potatoes, butterbeans, currants, dried figs, apricots, almonds, black treacle and sunflower seeds are all rich in minerals such as magnesium and potassium.
- Two bananas or 4 sticks of celery a day (rich in potassium) have been shown to help lower

blood pressure.

- Try Solo instead of table salt, which is potassium and not sodium-based. Potassium can help lower blood pressure because it balances sodium.
- Another useful salt is Organic Herb Seasoning Salt by Bioforce. It is made from organic sea salt, dried celery, leeks, cress, parsley, kelp, garlic and basil and sold globally in health stores and supermarkets. Website: www.bioforce.co.uk.
- If you are not a fan of eating fresh fruit and vegetables, at least drink a couple of glasses of freshly made fruit or vegetable juice. You will miss out on the fibre, but still get much of the nutrient-content.
- Try switching to a more vegetarian-based diet as the more fruit, vegetables, beans and lentils you eat, the greater your potassium intake and, generally speaking, the lower your sodium intake. And vegetarians tend to have much lower blood pressure.
- Eat more garlic, onions, broccoli (which are antioxidant, anti-viral and anti-bacterial) and celery (which is diuretic).
- Use unrefined organic virgin olive, walnut, pumpkin, linseed (flax seed) or sunflower oil for your salad dressings, and eat oily fish 3 times a week (see *Fats You Need To Eat*).
- As high levels of toxic metals, such as lead, can contribute to high blood pressure, buy a good-quality water filter. The fibre in apples (pectin), plus coriander and seaweed (alginates) all help to detoxify metals from the body.
- Natural-source vitamin E helps to thin blood naturally, therefore eat more soya beans, wheat germ, alfalfa sprouts, dark green vegetables, hazelnuts, almonds and avocados. This is especially important for those with type A or AB blood.

- Add more cayenne paper to your food, or take 1 capsule 3 times daily, to help balance your blood pressure. Check with your doctor if you are taking drugs such as warfarin.
- See also *Friendly Foods* in *Constipation*, as constipation can aggravate blood pressure.

Useful Remedies

- If you are taking blood-pressure medication, tell your doctor about any supplements you are taking, as in time your prescription drugs may be able to be reduced, and these supplements help to lower blood pressure naturally and you don't want your blood pressure to go too low.
- Take 500mg of magnesium with 500mg of calcium daily. Both of these minerals have been shown to lower blood pressure.
- Essential fats thin the blood (to protect you from clots) and reduce inflammation (in your arterial walls). Take a 1 gram of fish oil daily or 1 gram of linseed (flax seed) oil, both of which contain omega-3 fats (see *Fats You Need To Eat*).
- Take garlic; 900mg a day. When used long-term garlic can help gently lower blood pressure and thin the blood. Kudos makes a high-strength 1000mg capsule. **KVH**
- Hawthorne, either as tincture or as tablets, is a gentle way of bringing blood pressure back down to normal. 1–3ml of tincture or 1–2 grams of the tablets.
- Begin taking 100iu of natural-source, full-spectrum vitamin E and gradually increase to 500iu a day. Vitamin E thins the blood, protecting you from clotting, and is also a powerful antioxidant that protects fats (such as cholesterol) from free-radical damage.
- Include a high-strength multi-vitamin/mineral in your programme, as the B-vitamins help to support your nerves, controlling muscle contraction and improving your tolerance to stress.
- If your homocysteine level is high, take an extra 10–50mg of vitamin B6, 400–1000mcg of folic acid plus 10mg of B12.

Helpful Hints

- High blood pressure can occur during pregnancy, in which case seek medical attention.
- Cigarettes, plus the chemicals in cigarette smoke, damage your arteries and make the blood

more likely to clot, raising your risk of developing heart disease.

- Reduce stress. Try to find a method of relaxation that you enjoy whether it's meditation, T'ai Chi, yoga, exercising, walking or swimming.
- Have a regular aromatherapy massage using relaxing essential oils, such as rosewood, ylang ylang, clary sage, lavender and marjoram.
- Get a pet. Researchers from the State University of New York have shown how having a pet can protect against the effects of stress better than drugs designed to lower blood pressure.
- Exercise is vital for reducing blood pressure. With your doctor's permission start walking briskly for 30 minutes daily. People who are overweight and don't get much exercise are much more likely to suffer high blood pressure.
- Toxic metals in the body are also linked to high blood pressure. If you have tried all the dietary guidelines without impact, have your metal levels checked.
- Have a nutrition consultant conduct a hair mineral analysis for you. This test costs around £40–£50 and determines your level of calcium, magnesium and other important minerals, identifies any raised heavy metals in your system, plus gives you an indication of your glucose tolerance, and adrenal and thyroid functions. For further information call Sarah Stelling of ARL (UK) on 0131 229 1077, or write to ARL (UK), Edinburgh Centre of Nutrition and Therapy, 11 Home Street, Edinburgh EH3 9JR.
- Have your doctor obtain an ordinary cardiac risk blood profile. This will check your total cholesterol, HDL (good cholesterol), LDL (bad cholesterol), and triglycerides. There is no doubt that raised triglycerides put you in the high-risk category, although this does not mean that triglycerides are necessarily to blame. If you're prescribed cholesterol-lowering drugs, get a second opinion (see *Cholesterol*). Cholesterol is made in the body naturally, and as explained above, oxidised cholesterol is the problem. So increase your intake of antioxidants and eat more fibre to support you body's own method of reducing cholesterol (via the bowels).

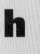

- Additionally, have your homocysteine level checked: it is not tested routinely and you will need to ask for the test. It should be below 8; above 10 is poor; above 12 is definitely dangerous. But the good news is that homocysteine can be brought down by supplementing just 3 vitamins: B6, B12 and folic acid. If yours is high, you need higher levels of these vitamins than you can get in your diet alone (see *Useful Remedies*).
- There is now an easy test to discover your plasma homocysteine levels. Made by York Laboratories and backed by the British Cardiac Patients Association, it's a simple pinprick method that can be done by post. For details call York Labs on 0800 458 2052, or log on to: www.yorktest.com.
- If you need to check for food intolerances, see either a kinesiologist or take a more scientifically accepted blood test from York Laboratories.
- Many men who suffer arteriosclerosis have low levels of testosterone – therefore, gentlemen over 45 should ask their GP to test their hormone levels.
- Patrick Holford's *Say No to Heart Disease* (Piatkus) is an excellent book explaining the causes of arterial damage and what you can do to prevent or correct high blood pressure. He has also written *The H Factor*, which gives all details of homocysteine. Website: www.patrickholford.com

HIRSUTISM

(see Body Hair, Excessive)

HYPERACTIVITY

(see also *Allergies*)

Hyperactivity is also often referred to as Attention Deficit Disorder (ADD), or Attention Deficit Hyperactivity Disorder (ADHD), and they are all closely related. These conditions occur predominantly in children, but sometimes symptoms can continue into adulthood. There is no hard-and-fast definition of this disorder and consequently children who are merely rebellious, find it difficult to pay attention for great lengths of time, or find it difficult to learn generally may tend to be labelled as having ADD. And children that also constantly fidget and are always on the go may well be diagnosed as having ADHD. Typical symptoms include an inability to concentrate or sit still for any length of time, or rapid and severe mood swings, and these children often need very little sleep. Children that are affected often find themselves in trouble and are shunted from school to school. They can become delinquent teenagers and often end up using drugs and alcohol.

All of these conditions are associated with an excessive intake of the sugar, artificial sweeteners, colourings and preservatives that are found in prescription medicines and thousands of foods and drinks. Sensitivities to various foods and substances, such as bubble bath, air fresheners, spray deodorants, perfumes and toothpastes can also trigger these types of behavioural problems. Far too many children still eat huge amounts of junk foods that are devoid of vitamins, minerals and essential fats. Junk foods deplete nutrients from the body, and without any doubt, tests have shown that these children are malnourished, and this lack of proper nutrients can have a devastating effect not only on their bodies, but most importantly on their brains. Also, exposure to neurotoxins, such as lead from water pipes and car fumes, plus cadmium from cigarettes, can make the problem even worse. As can overexposure to these chemicals during pregnancy.

The normal drug therapy is Ritalin, from the amphetamine family. In the US 3% of school-age children take this medication, even though research has shown that it initiates changes in brain structure and function that remain long after any therapeutic effects have dissipated. Ritalin may also increase the incidence of addiction to other substances such as cocaine and smoking in later life. Understandably many parents don't feel comfortable giving this drug to their child; however, others feel it is their only weapon in making the child controllable or teachable.

There is a growing body of negative evidence against this drug, but on the positive side, nutritionists such as Patrick Holford have shown time and time again, that if artificial additives and so on are removed from the diet and proper nutrition is practised, these children improve in leaps and bounds. In prisons in the US and the UK, it has also been shown that when violent prisoners are given a better diet, plus the right vitamins, minerals and essentials fats, they become calmer and 'kinder' people.

Foods to Avoid

- Any foods containing large numbers of additives, particularly the strong colourings like tartrazine. Many sweets are bright and rainbow-coloured. The brighter the sweets the more they should be avoided.
- Greatly reduce or eliminate cola-type drinks, and any foods or drinks containing the artificial sweetener aspartame. Look out for hidden sources such as chewing gum.
- Generally cut out most foods containing sugar, such as cakes, biscuits, chocolates, and snack bars. One specialist once told me that giving sugar to hyperactive children was 'like putting rocket fuel in a Mini'. The odd treat is OK, but try to buy organic, low-sugar snack bars that have been sweetened with apple juice or honey. Most of the mass-produced refined foods

(white bread, pasta and rice; packaged ready-meals and so on) should go. As an occasional treat allow the child to eat a small amount of organic chocolate.

- Citrus fruits and juices are often a problem.
- If your child has a favourite food, be it cheese, eggs, wheat-based foods, milk or orange juice, try cutting these out for 1–2 weeks and see if behaviour improves. It is usually the foods they eat and crave the most that are triggering many of their symptoms
- Buy a book that gives you all E numbers and note which foods have the highest amounts and avoid them like the plague.

Friendly Foods
- As much as possible feed your child organic foods free from pesticides and herbicides.
- Try buying corn-, lentil-, rice- and spinach-based pastas.
- Introduce more whole foods and grains, such as brown rice, millet, oats, quinoa, lentils and vegetables into your child's diet.
- Nature's Path makes a great breakfast cereal range that is sweetened with apple juice. Any health shop sells ranges of wheat-free and/or low-sugar organic source cereals, mueslis and snack bars these days. Chop an apple or banana into the cereal for added fibre and nutrients. Alternatively make up your own muesli – use organic oats as a base, and then add sunflower and pumpkin seeds or linseeds (flax seeds), plus nuts such as Brazils or hazelnuts, to which you can add a few organic raisins or dried apricots. Nuts and seeds are high in essential fats, and in minerals like zinc, which are vital for healthy brain-functioning. This mix can be alternated to suit your preference. One week add more chopped almonds or grated coconut – another week add millet or rice flakes. When serving chop a banana, add fresh blueberries, and use organic rice milk or natural, low-fat yoghurt. Children are now discovering healthier milks such as Tiger White – made from plant extracts, which are non-dairy and high in healthier monounsaturated fats. To find your nearest stockist call 01453 874 000.

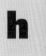

- Try organic rice, oat, or goat's milk or yoghurt, which are less likely to cause a problem. Or try Tiger White 'milk' (see above).
- Use diluted sugar-free pear, apple or even grape juice, which are less likely than the citrus fruits to cause a problem.
- Encourage the child to drink water in preference to fizzy drinks and try to encourage a taste for fresh fruit rather than sugary sweets. If he or she still wants the bubbles add 50:50 fruit juice to plain fizzy water – don't buy flavoured waters, which tend to be high in sugars.
- Add low-sugar fruit yoghurts to colourful fruit for tasty desserts that look attractive. I make jellies with a base of low-sugar cranberry juice, camomile tea, or fresh grapes – I chop fresh fruit into the jelly liquid and allow to set. A wonderful low-sugar treat.
- Sprinkle chopped nuts onto desserts as they are a rich source of minerals, but avoid peanuts. I use organic hazelnuts, Brazil nuts, almonds, coconut, and walnuts. I whiz them all in a blender. Keep the mixture in an air-tight jar in the fridge and sprinkle over breakfast cereals and desserts. The mixture lasts about a week.
- Give your child a serving of quality protein, such as chicken, fresh fish, eggs, tempeh, lentils and beans, nuts and seeds, with each meal of the day. Add pumpkin seeds to a salad – they are delicious.
- Essential fats found in oily fish, seeds and nuts are really important in controlling this type of behaviour. (See *Fats You Need To Eat*.)
- Ensure plenty of iron-rich foods are included in the diet as a lack of iron can decrease attentiveness and narrow attention span. Good choices are cooked tofu, beans and pulses, spinach, eggs (unless your child has an intolerance to eggs), cabbage, prunes, dates and apricots and pumpkin seeds. Eat them along with some strawberries or kiwi fruit, which are rich in vitamin

C, to enhance absorption.

- Use unrefined, cold-pressed, preferably organic olive, sunflower, hemp, walnut or sesame oils for salad dressings, or drizzle over cooked foods. Cook only with the olive oil or use Higher Nature's coconut oil instead. **HN**

Useful Remedies

- Magnesium is known as nature's tranquilliser and many children are low in this vital mineral; 400mg daily. Dr Bernard Rimland, the director of the Autism Research Institute, has found that combining vitamin B6 and magnesium was up to 10 times more effective than Ritalin. 50mg of B6 should be taken in a high-strength B-complex.
- Essential fatty acids are vital. Try Efalex, 1–2 spoons a day over cooked food, or add to salad dressings.
- Give your child a good-quality chewable multi-vitamin and mineral that is free from artificial additives. Solgar's chewable Kanga Vites are flavoured with natural fruit (avoid if citrus is a problem for your child). Nature's Plus also makes a great children's range of nutrients. **NP**

Helpful Hints

- Try to avoid smoking and drinking during pregnancy as both of these have been linked with an increased likelihood of the child becoming hyperactive.
- If the child has allergies or food intolerances, explain to the child how they affect their behaviour and tell everyone in the school or relatives who might be giving the child food or drinks, which they think are perfectly harmless.
- For some children natural compounds found in food, called salicylates, can cause a problem (see *Autism* for more details).
- Homoeopathy has a great track record of dealing with ADD and hyperactivity so, if you can, get your child along to a good homoeopath. Be prepared to be patient as it may not be an overnight success. See *Useful Information*, or call the Organic Pharmacy. **OP**
- Avoid air fresheners of all types, spray deodorants, pot-pourri, and perfumed fabric conditioners, washing powders and liquids. Try Ecover products, which contain far fewer chemicals, available in all major supermarkets and health stores.
- As children with ADHD are 7 times more likely to have food intolerances than other children, get these checked out. Individual Wellbeing Diagnostic Laboratories have an in-depth food intolerance test, and you can also request that they add on food additives to the test. Contact them on 08704 190 435, or check out their website at www.iwdl.net
- Links have been found between hyperactivity and high levels of heavy metals, namely mercury, lead, copper and aluminium. Get these checked out with a simple non-invasive, hair mineral analysis test. To order, call Analytical Research Laboratories on 0131 229 1077.
- Patrick Holford's book *Optimum Nutrition for the Mind* has lots of information including details of the Brain Bio Centre, which he founded and which successfully treats those with ADHD.
- ADD and ADHD are complex conditions, and as it is important that children do not become deficient in any nutrients, enlist the help of a qualified nutritionist. Contact the British Association for Nutritional Therapy by checking out their website at www.bant.org.uk, or calling 08706 061284 to find a nutritionist in your area.
- A great site sharing stories from children affected by ADD and ADHD can be found at www.adders.org
- For more help contact the Hyperactive Children's Support Group via www.hacsg.org.uk, or call 01243 551313.

HYPOGLYCAEMIA   *(see Low Blood Sugar)*

IBS (see *Irritable Bowel Syndrome*)

IMMUNE FUNCTION (see also *MRSA* and *Stress*)

With new strains of bacteria and viruses mutating with alarming speed, the challenge for our immune systems has never been greater. Our immune system is made up of a network of cells, organs and fluids that help defend us against the millions of bacteria, viruses and fungi that bombard us in our daily lives. And one of the most important things you can do to stay healthy, throughout your life, is to keep your immune system in good shape. For example, when I was younger and did not realise how diet and lifestyle affected my ability to fight off illnesses, and when I was under pressure, not getting sufficient sleep, and eating the wrong foods, I was always ill. At times when I felt ghastly, I would turn to a sugary snack to keep me going and I could literally feel my immune system going 'over the edge'. Stress alone can suppress immune function by up to 60% (see also *Stress*). These days I recognise my limits, I know when to stop and get more sleep. I eat a cleaner diet and try as much as possible to keep my stress levels within limits. You need to listen to your body and take notice! Often the first signs of an immune system under threat are a chronic sore throat, regular colds or niggling infections. If this is the case with you, it's time to take action.

Meanwhile, most people don't think of their skin as being part of the immune system, but it forms a physical barrier against attack, and the immune system is in charge of cell regeneration within your skin. The more efficient your immune system, the fresher your skin will look. Then comes your stomach acid, which also helps to destroy harmful organisms, but as we age and under stress, stomach-acid levels fall and more bacteria can get through (see *Low Stomach Acid*). And within a child's bone marrow are 'stem cells' which, as we grow, develop into various types of immune cells some of which mature in the thymus gland, where they become known as known as T cells. The spleen also contains immune cells that manufacture antibodies; and the lymphatic system, often called the master drain, is also a major player in immune function. The lymph system removes toxins and microbes from the body's tissue and along with bone marrow manufactures lymphocytes (a specific kind of white blood cell that comes in 3 types – B cells, T cells and natural killer cells – which keep your immune system in good shape). Lymph nodes are found all over the body, but the ones most people are aware of are situated in the neck, groin and arm pits. During an infection the lymph glands can swell as they produce more white blood cells, this is very common in throat conditions for example. If the lymphatic system becomes congested, the fluid thickens and becomes more gel like, which inhibits proper drainage and detoxification and puts more pressure on the liver and kidneys. This is why a fully functioning lymph system helps you to fight off invading bacteria and viruses. The liver and thymus gland also play a huge role in immune function (see *Liver Problems*).

Unfortunately, as we age our immune system becomes less effective at protecting us and more viruses and bacteria get through our defences. Conversely our immune system can also overreact, which produces chronic inflammation when we eat certain foods, or are exposed to pollen, pollutants and so on. The immune system may even begin attacking the body's own tissue, called an 'autoimmune response', in conditions such as lupus and rheumatoid arthritis.

High cholesterol levels are also linked to a lowered immune response, because cells containing high levels of cholesterol can disrupt our cells' ability to communicate with each other, which is vital for proper immune responses (see *Cholesterol*).

Lowered immune function is also linked to chronic fatigue, allergies, parasite infections, and some forms of heart disease.

Prostaglandins, which are hormone-like substances, become more out of balance as we age. This has the effect of suppressing the immune system and affecting important processes such as body temperature and metabolism. Essential fatty acids, such as EPA (from fish oil) and GLA (from evening primrose, blackcurrant, and borage oils) help to restore the proper prostaglandin ratios, thereby supporting the immune system (see *Fats You Need To Eat*).

Foods to Avoid
- As a person with a sweet tooth, I'm sorry to say that sugar greatly compromises your immune system. If you are run-down and then you eat one, say, sugary breakfast bar, it can literally send your immune system into free-fall – and the next thing you know, you have a cold, or develop cold sores or whatever. So if you know that you are under stress, stay off sugar and allow your immune system time to regroup. Use a little fructose or organic honey if you need sugar, but generally cut down on pies, biscuits, sweets and shop-bought sugary snacks and drinks.
- Reduce your intake of caffeine and alcohol, which place an extra burden on the immune system.
- Avoid any foods containing lots of preservatives, additives and especially the artificial sweetener aspartame, which adds an extra burden on your liver.
- Avoid all smoked foods and cheeses.
- Reduce your intake of saturated fats found in red meat and full-fat dairy produce including milks, cheese, Greek yoghurts, and chocolates, as well as hydrogenated and trans fats (see *Fats You Need To Eat*).

Friendly Foods
- Eat organic as much as possible. Make sure your diet is high in all fresh fruits and vegetables, which are packed with nutrients.
- Eat more fresh fish, chicken, broccoli, cabbage, cauliflower, parsley, green beans, apples, green salads, pumpkin, buckwheat, soya beans and millet.
- Eat sprouts such as alfalfa and brown rice, and algae, such as spirulina and chlorella.
- Eat more purple, red and orange foods: blueberries, bilberries and blackberries are high in immune-boosting nutrients, as are sweet potatoes, apricots, papaya and red peppers.
- Nuts and seeds are packed with essential fats, and minerals such as zinc and selenium (see *Fats You Need To Eat*).
- See also *General Health Hints*.
- Eat more freshly made soups – many supermarkets and take-away shops now sell freshly made organic soups. They are easy on the digestive system and full of nutrients. Add barley, brown rice, lentils and more cabbage to soups.
- When the body is under attack it requires more protein, so eat fresh fish, organic tofu (cooked), fresh chicken, turkey and lean meats.
- If you are desperate for sugar then try Slim Sweet, a low glycemic index sweetener from the Lo-han fruit. Available from all health stores or call the Sloane Health Store. **SL**

Useful Remedies
- Take a good-quality, high-strength multi-vitamin and mineral, and an antioxidant formula daily. See *Kudos 24* in *General Supplements* (see p.160).

- Add organic-source green food powders to your breakfast cereals, smoothies, or vegetable juices, and drink daily. They are packed with nutrition that helps to keep your immune system in good shape. My favourite is Nature's Living, which includes natural soil organisms, wheat grass, whole-leaf barley grass, dandelion leaf, and so on. For details of your nearest stockists call Kiki Ltd on 08450 601060. Website: www.kiki-health.com
- Drink more pau d'arco herbal tea, which can boost immune function.
- Echinacea and astragalus in a combination formula can be taken in capsules or fluid extract to really help boost immune function, if taken daily for 3 months. Astragalus has been shown to increase white blood cell counts. Try Ultimate Echinacea Complex by Holos Health, which is available from the Nutri Centre. **NC**
- Colostrum is the pre-milk fluid produced by all mothers after giving birth. It arrives before breast milk and contains 37 natural immune-boosting factors and 8 growth factors, which support the immune system and regeneration of all types of cells. Recent studies have shown it to be extremely beneficial, not only for the newborn, but for people of all ages. Dose: 2000–4000mg per day. **NC SL**
- Whey protein powder helps to boost immune function, thus inhibiting cancer cell proliferation; protects against free radicals; and boosts cellular antioxidant levels. Dose: 20 grams per day. I use Solgar's Whey to Go.
- Astragalus is a traditional Chinese herb used to strengthen the immune system. At least one clinical trial in the US has shown astragalus to boost T-cell levels close to normal in some cancer patients, suggesting the possibility of a synergistic effect of astragalus with chemotherapy. Dose: 250mg twice a day.

Helpful Hints
- One of the simplest ways to boost immune function is to get more sleep – take a day off to call your own; book a holiday; walk out in the countryside breathing the fresher air – and see how that alone lifts your spirits.
- Laugh a lot: watch films that make you laugh; make friends with people who make you laugh. Laughter and having some fun strengthen immune function.
- Stress alone can suppress immune function by up to 60%. Stress triggers the release of the hormone cortisol, which is thought to shrink the thymus gland (which is where T cells mature and is situated in your upper chest area, just below the hollow in your neck). Therefore, keep your stress levels in check (see also *Stress*).
- Learn to say no and not feel guilty.
- Greatly reduce your exposure to external pollutants, such as cigarette smoke, car fumes, chemical-based sprays and heavy metals.
- If possible take regular holidays in the sunshine, which helps to boost your immune system.
- Think positively – people who are cheerful and who look on the bright side have stronger immune systems.
- Take regular exercise but not to excess. Don't over exercise if you are truly exhausted.
- To help decongest your lymphatic system, apply therapeutic grade essential oils along the spine, under the arm, and in the neck, breast and groin areas – anywhere that is congested. They are amazing. Try a blend of 3 drops of cypress, 1 of orange and 2 of grapefruit. For details call Susie Anthony on 01749 679900.
- See *General Health Hints* for more help.

IMPOTENCE

(see also Libido Problems)

There are many reasons why a man may lose either his desire for sex, or his ability to get and maintain an erection. Both problems are often linked to long-term stress and, by dealing effectively with stress, sexual desire and function can, in many cases, be restored. The related problem of 'brewer's droop' is mainly due to excessive alcohol consumption, which can interfere with the ability to maintain an erection quite severely. Smoking has been linked with reduced ability to maintain an erection; smoking constricts blood-flow that is essential for erectile function. Anyone with erectile problems would do well to consider a cholesterol-lowering diet.

Foods to Avoid
see *Circulation* and *Libido*

Friendly Foods
see *Circulation* and *Libido*

Useful Remedies

- The herb ginkgo biloba when taken regularly improves circulation. Kudos makes a high-strength, one-a-day (900mg) pill. Take daily for one month, then have a month off, then begin again for one month on, one month off. **KVH**
- Take 2 grams of the amino acid L-arginine daily (unless you are suffering an attack of cold sores as arginine will make them worse), as this amino acid has been shown to improve impotence. Or try ArginMax – containing L-arginine, ginseng, gingko, vitamins, antioxidants and minerals to help support sexual function. **NC**
- Stress reduces B-vitamins in the body – therefore, also include a good-quality multi-vitamin and mineral for men that includes a full range of B-vitamins.
- Muira Puama, a South-American herb, is considered nature's most potent viagra. A daily dose of 1 gram of a standardised extract has been shown to be effective as it raises testosterone levels. In one study of 100 men with impotence problems, 66% had increased frequency of inter-course, while 70% reported intensification of libido. The stability of the erection was restored in 55% of the patients, and 66% reported a reduction in fatigue. The herb is suitable for both men and women. **NC**

Helpful Hints

- Measures to alleviate stress are often very effective. Take regular exercise and learn to laugh more. This releases natural endorphins, which lower stress levels and help you feel more positive. Learn to breathe more deeply.
- People who use a large amount of marijuana or take steroids may also find their erectile function diminished.
- By constantly worrying about your lack of sex drive, you often make the situation worse. Studies show that a lack of vitamins C, E, A and B, and the minerals zinc and selenium, can cause a low sperm count and lack of sex drive. Anyone taking regular antidepressants or sleeping pills may be lacking in these nutrients.
- Have your hormone levels checked, as testosterone patches are known to help increase libido in both sexes. Once hormones are balanced sex drive often returns (see *Menopause*).
- Testosterone creams that are applied directly to the genital areas are becoming available. These have been shown to quickly increase libido and erectile function. For more details contact Dr Malcolm Carruthers at the Andropause Centre in Harley Street, London, on 020 7636 8283.
- If the condition continues, or you are worried about infertility as well as impotency, see a doctor who is also a nutritionist (see *Useful Information*).

- Acupuncture can help with impotence by unblocking energy channels within the body to help increase blood-flow.
- To help get you in the mood, try watching a sexy movie – this works for most people!

INCONTINENCE   (see also *Cystitis* and *Prostate Problems*)

Incontinence can lead to urine leaking out when the bladder is put under pressure when you laugh, cough, sneeze or exert yourself. It can also occur when you have eaten to excess and the bloated bowel exerts pressure on the bladder. This type of problem is referred to as stress incontinence and is usually associated with a weakness in the muscle in the pelvic floor.

Exercise can help keep the pelvic floor strong, and childbirth tends to weaken it, hence it is a good idea to do plenty of pelvic exercises after giving birth. I suffered this problem during my twenties after giving birth to my daughter. It became so embarrassing that in my early thirties I found a gynaecologist who specialised in bladder repair and had surgery. It has really made a huge difference and I can now exercise without the embarrassment. Non-chronic but acute urinary incontinence is usually caused by an infection (see also *Candida* and *Cystitis*).

Foods to Avoid
- Any food to which you have an allergy or intolerance can aggravate incontinence. The worst offenders are usually wheat and cow's milk.
- Avoid fluoridated water, toothpastes and mouthwashes. I have received many letters from people who say that when fluoride is eliminated, the problem stops. It also seems to help with children who wet the bed.
- The biggest culprits are usually yeast, wheat, dairy, alcohol and sugar.
- Don't overeat – as when your bowel becomes full, pressure is exerted on the bladder.
- See also *Stress*, as when your adrenals are on limits, you often need to urinate far more often.

Friendly Foods
- Add a little cayenne pepper to your foods. It may initially aggravate the problem, but in the long term usually helps.
- See *General Health Hints*.

Useful Remedies
- A high-strength, multi-vitamin and mineral for women.
- 500mg of calcium with 250mg of magnesium to help muscle control. After 6 weeks you should see benefits.
- The mineral silica – take 75mg daily. The herb horsetail is very useful for strengthening the bladder. You can take 5ml daily.
- Cantharis is a homeopathic remedy for frequent urination associated with any burning. Causticum and *equisetum arvense* (horsetail) help to reduce symptoms when there is a weakness in the bladder.
- Cranberry Plus by BioCare contains cranberry concentrate, vitamin C, and acidophilus, and helps to fight any infection (such as cystitis). **BC**

Helpful Hints
- Check with your doctor who will soon tell you if you have an infection that is causing this problem.
- Try using a set of vaginal cones containing weights to help strengthen the muscles. For information on the Aquaflex system, call the information line on 0161 925 3180. Website: www.neenpelvichealth.com

- Also there is a progressive resistance exerciser called the Pelvic Toner. Website: www.pelvictoner.co.uk. This has proven really useful in improving muscle tone, which can help cure or greatly relieve this problem.
- An osteopath or chiropractor can check the alignment of bones in the pubic area. This can help because if the bones are out of balance, urine-flow in both men and women can be affected.
- Acupuncture has proven helpful to some people. See *Useful Information*.
- Contact the Continence Foundation helpline on 0845 345 0165 (9.30am–1pm weekdays). Website: www.continence-foundation.org.uk

INDIGESTION   (see also *Flatulence, Hiatus Hernia* and *Low Stomach Acid*)

Indigestion covers a variety of symptoms from cramping in the stomach, to heartburn, wind, belching, and even pain in the bowel. It is usually a sign that the digestive system is having difficulty coping with food, and this is frequently due to a lack of stomach acid and digestive enzymes in the small intestine. The problem can be made worse if you eat too quickly and don't chew food thoroughly. Overeating, drinking to excess, eating poor food combinations, or eating when stressed all exacerbate indigestion.

Foods to Avoid

- Red meat and fatty cuts of meat are hard to digest. Cheese, especially melted cheese, is really hard for the body to digest. Keep cheese to a minimum.
- Generally reduce your intake of sugar and sugary foods, such as cakes, biscuits and rich puddings.
- Coffee, tea, chocolates, caffeine in any form, alcohol, peppers, citrus fruits, onions and sometimes garlic can be difficult to digest.
- Salt hinders digestion and assimilation of proteins, so cut down on sodium-based salts.
- Don't drink too much liquid with meals as this dilutes the stomach acid, which you need to digest your meal.
- Avoid fruit immediately after a large meal, unless it's a small chunk of pineapple or papaya.
- Avoid as much as possible rich, creamy foods and heavy desserts such as Christmas pudding.
- Avoid antacids that neutralise stomach acid, the very substance you need to digest your meals.
- Many people with indigestion have problems digesting wheat. Try Ryvita, low-salt crisp breads, rice cakes, or amaranth crackers, available from health shops. Especially avoid warm croissant-type treats, as freshly cooked 'dough' is really hard on your digestion. I know they are delicious, so if you are desperate, just one a week!

Friendly Foods

- Drink some ginger or dandelion root tea with or before meals to stimulate digestion.
- Small meals made from whole foods and small quantities of meat or fish are much easier on the digestion.
- Try eating small amounts of pineapple or papaya before a meal. They contain enzymes that can enhance digestion.
- Add more fresh root ginger to foods, as it is very calming.
- If you like beans and pulses, but they give you wind, cook them with a strip of kombu seaweed, which helps to pre-digest the beans.
- Eat more live, low-fat yoghurts.

Useful Remedies

- Take betaine hydrochloride (HCl; stomach acid); 1 capsule with main meals. If you have active stomach ulcers, or the HCl causes a burning sensation, take a digestive enzyme that is free from HCl.

- Chew 1–2 tablets of deglychyrrized liquorice before a meal. This soothes any symptoms of heartburn or indigestion.
- Acidophilus and bifidus are healthy bacteria, which encourage better digestion and elimination. Take 1–2 capsules at the end of a meal.
- Sip peppermint tea after meals.
- Bitters stimulate stomach-acid production and therefore improve digestion; Dr Theiss Swedish Bitters and Bioforce Centaurium tincture work very well (taken before meals).
- If symptoms are at the bowel level, try a good colon-cleanser, such as psyllium husks. Lepicol powder or capsules contain both psyllium husks and probiotics.
- Aloe vera is a very good digestive-system healer. Taken twice a day between meals, one of the purest and most potent is Aloe Gold from Higher Nature. **HN**

Helpful Hints
- Sit down and eat food in a relaxed setting.
- Go for a walk after eating, which really aids digestion.
- Eat fruit between meals, but avoid fruits you know are a problem such as oranges and grapefruit.
- If symptoms are acute, avoid eating for a short time, or at most eat only lightly cooked, small meals regularly.
- Sometimes when people suffer indigestion, it is because they are unable to digest some information or something going on in their lives. If this is the case it would be worth seeing a homoeopath, who may be able to resolve the underlying issues. See also *Stress*. Meanwhile the homeopathic remedy Nux Vomica 30c helps reduce the incidence of indigestion.
- Consult a nutritionist who will help re-balance your system (see *Useful Information*).

INFERTILITY
(see also *PCOS*)

Sperm counts have dropped dramatically in the last fifty years. A quarter of all couples planning a baby have trouble conceiving. In four out of every ten cases the problems are on the male side, with 30% of men being sub-fertile whilst 2% are totally infertile. If the male sperm count is low this can sometimes be a result of an infection such as mumps. A low sperm count can be due to a poor diet, nutrient deficiencies and/or environmental toxins, such as lead, mercury and cadmium. Food additives, smoking, alcohol, food intolerances, urinary tract infections, plus stress, can all affect fertility. Common organisms such as *Mycoplasma hominis* and *Ureaplasma toxoplasmosis* can infect the urinary tracts of men and women. They don't always cause infertility, but there seems to be a higher number of these organisms in the secretions of couples who have unexplained fertility problems. Smoking and alcohol can also reduce sperm count. Many scientists now openly state that sperm counts in the Western world are dropping because of overuse of herbicides and pesticides, which have an oestrogen-boosting effect within the body that counteracts male testosterone.

Female infertility may be due to blockages in the fallopian tubes, which can be triggered by an infection, such as thrush or cystitis, or by chlamydia and other sexually transmitted diseases. Whatever the cause diagnosis requires a medical examination. Sometimes there is a problem with ovulation, usually due to a hormone imbalance. Other conditions, such as endometriosis, low thyroid function, a diet deficient in nutrients especially zinc and magnesium, and/or environmental toxins are also common causes of infertility in women. Candida, a yeast fungal overgrowth, is also linked to infertility. When women are under a lot of stress the body releases adrenaline, eventually exhausting the endocrine system and affecting hormone levels, which can prevent conception.

Foods to Avoid

- Coffee, chocolate and cola, which all contain caffeine, have been shown to affect impotence and reduce the chance of conception.
- Sugary snacks, puddings and confectionary provide empty calories and in turn upset hormone balance. Keep to an absolute minimum; see below for healthy fertility-boosting snacks.
- Alcohol alone can reduce your chances of fertility. It affects zinc levels, reduces sperm count, causes malformation of sperm, and impairs sperm motility in men; whilst preventing implantation in women. The effect is worse when combined with caffeine.
- Avoid foods high in saturated fats, junk foods, pre-packaged meals, sugar and salt which deplete the body of the nutrients needed for conception.
- Avoid dairy produce, which can lead to malabsorption of essential nutrients if you have an intolerance; see *Allergies*.
- Wheat is high in phytates, chemicals which block absorption of some minerals. Avoid foods containing wheat as much as possible. This includes, bread, cakes, biscuits, pasta and pizza bases.
- Recent research showed that soya may well have a negative effect on fertility so is best avoided.
- Avoid food additives, preservatives and artificial flavourings and sweeteners. Individually tartrazine is known to lower zinc levels and other additives lower magnesium. The London Food Commission found that of 426 chemicals listed, 35 were found to individually cause reproductive problems ranging from impotency to birth defects. No one knows the real effect on fertility or the foetus of a chemical cocktail.
- Non-organic food is high in pesticides and other hazardous substances, which have a hormone-disrupting effect. Offspring in cattle exposed to high levels of pesticides are known to be born with higher levels of malformation.
- For a woman when the tissues are more alkaline, this helps with conception – as the body functions more efficiently when the pH is alkaline. For full information see *Acid–Alkaline Balance*.

Friendly Foods

- Good-quality protein is needed for hormone health and sperm synthesis. Choose from lean organic poultry and meat, eggs, fish and vegetable sources, such as seeds, nuts and beans.
- Fibre found in whole grains – brown rice, millet, quinoa, barley and oats – help to reduce excess oestrogen levels and clear out old hormone residues.
- Make sperm stronger by eating more brown rice, lentils, beans, organic nuts and seeds – all rich in fertility-boosting zinc. Enzymes on the sperms heads need zinc in order to push through the egg to fertilize it. Zinc has a huge impact on women's fertility too.
- Eat oily fish, such as mackerel, salmon, sardines or herrings, at least once a week as they are rich in omega-3 essential fats needed for hormone health.
- Add some sunflower seeds, pumpkin seeds and linseeds (flax seeds) to any low-sugar breakfast cereal, as they are high in minerals and essential fats.
- A lack of selenium in the diet has been shown to reduce egg production in females and leads to reduced testicular growth and problems with sperm maturation in men. Eat more brown rice, seafood, oats, barley and garlic.
- Nuts, barley, rye, oats and brown rice are also rich in the mineral manganese, a lack of which leads to defective ovulation and testicular degeneration, as well affecting libido in men.
- Fresh fruit and vegetables are rich in vitamin C, which helps sperm motility. Choose from kiwi

fruit, strawberries, broccoli, cabbage, red and yellow peppers, frozen peas, blackcurrants and oranges.

- Carry a small bag of mixed seeds around for fertility-boosting snacks. These are full of the minerals zinc, manganese, chromium and essential fats.
- Use organic olive, sunflower, walnut and linseed (flax seed) oils for your salad dressings.
- If you have any iron deficiency, eat more lean meats especially calves' liver, turkey and chicken, plus eggs and dried apricots.
- Leafy green vegetables, cereals, honey, beans and nuts are all good sources of magnesium, which may also be deficient. See *Acid–Alkaline Balance*.
- Try caffeine-free alternatives like dandelion tea or dandelion root coffee as these can have beneficial effects on the liver and consequently enhance hormone production.

Useful Remedies

- Nourish has researched and developed a natural treatment plan for couples to help them take control of their reproductive health. The recommended 4-month course comes in convenient monthly packs and contains nutrients and other ingredients that are vital for conception and your baby's healthy development. Tel. 01534 857197
- A multi-vitamin and mineral – many companies now make special formulas for women who are trying to conceive. The Pregnancy Pack is available from Health Plus on 01323 872277. Website: www.healthplus.co.uk
- In order to produce testosterone at optimal levels any multi for men needs to contain at least 30mg of zinc, 200mcg of selenium and 250mg of magnesium
- Both partners should take a B-complex plus 5000iu of vitamin A, which are needed for egg and sperm production. Once pregnant the vitamin A can be reduced to 3000iu daily if required.
- Full-spectrum, natural-source vitamin E, 200iu a day has been shown to help reduce both male and female infertility by helping to balance hormone levels and enabling egg and sperm to fuse.
- For women take 40 drops of agnus castus in the morning, or 1000mg in tablet form. This herb helps regulate the hormonal cycle.
- Both partners should take 1 gram of vitamin C daily.
- The celloid mineral complex potassium chloride; 150mg can help clear the fallopian tubes. **BLK**
- L-arginine and -carnitine are two amino acids that are needed for sperm production and to prevent sperm becoming too 'sticky', which can interfere with conception. You could take 1.5–3 grams of each daily. Do not take the arginine if you have herpes (cold sores) or shingles.

Helpful Hints

- Anthony Porter, a reflexologist since 1972, who went to China and other parts of the Far East to teach reflexology during the 1980s, found that their methods combined with his own gave even better results. He has taught his advanced techniques to thousands of reflexologists internationally and says "With ART we can not only balance various parts of the body (which is what happens with normal reflexology), but we can also feel more subtle changes within the 7,000 nerve-endings or reflex areas of the feet, and after working on them, this has a profound therapeutic affect." Medical research with a leading gynaecologist has shown huge success using ART to help women conceive. To find an ART therapist in your area log on to www.artreflex.com
- Eat organic and get more nutrients, as hormone and antibiotic residues are known to affect fertility in both men and women.
- Your weight can affect your fertility, check out your Body Mass Index – a measure of your weight in relation to your height. A BMI of 20–25 is ideal. Below 20 is underweight and above 25 is overweight.
- Hypnotherapy has been proven to be an effective aid when dealing with infertility. Studies show

that it can also increase conception rates for couples undergoing IVF treatment. See *Useful Information*.

- Regular acupuncture has proven very successful for many couples – see *Useful Information*.
- For more help read *Natural Solutions to Infertility* by Dr Marilyn Glenville (Piatkus). For more information on Dr Glenville's work log on to www.marilynglenville.com
- Cigarette smoke is high in the toxin cadmium. This toxin competes against zinc, which is vital for fertility. This is one of the reasons why smokers are less likely to conceive. Stop smoking – and avoid alcohol.
- Ask to be screened for any urinary infections and sexually transmitted diseases, many of which lay dormant and are often symptom-free. 69% of couples screened have an infection.
- Much of the water in the UK is contaminated with high levels of fluoride, aluminium, copper and cadmium, which compete with essential minerals in the body. Pesticide residue and traces of the contraceptive pill (which can have hormone-disrupting qualities) are excreted via urine, which eventually finds its way into the water system, and can also affect fertility. The Fresh Water Filter Company Ltd offers a broad range of water filters. Call them on 0870 442 3633, or visit their website at www.freshwaterfilter.com
- Limit the amount of chemicals in your home and garden, such as wood preservatives, perfumes, insect sprays and so on. Use eco-friendly products.
- Avoid too much exposure to mobile phones, computers, and electrical equipment.
- If either partner is taking prescription drugs or regular over-the-counter remedies, check for their known side-effects.

- Remember to try not to get too stressed, as stress in either partner can lower the chances of conception. I have received letters from many couples who, when they gave up trying so hard to conceive, bought a pet or adopted a child, the next thing they knew a baby was on its way!
- Sitting for long periods raises the temperature in the testicles, which may reduce male fertility. If you are deskbound, for example, or a long-distance driver, wear loose-fitting underwear and trousers, and get plenty of exercise.
- Contact Foresight, who specialise in giving couples information about how to plan for a healthy pregnancy and increase fertility naturally. The service includes nutritional status analysis, although this is usually done in consultation with a recognised Foresight practitioner. Foresight can be contacted by writing to 78 Hawthorn Road, West Bognor, West Sussex PO21 2UY. Tel: 01243 868001. Website: www.foresight-preconception.org.uk

INSECT BITES (and Repellents)

Apart from the obvious discomfort that they cause, insect bites can occasionally transmit serious disease and cause severe allergic reactions, such as anaphylactic shock. If you know that you or a family member has a particular sensitivity to stings and bites, it is important to discuss this with your GP to make sure you take the appropriate medication away with you. You may also find the *Allergy* section very useful. For people who suffer anaphylactic shock, you need to carry adrenaline injections with you at all times. For anyone travelling to tropical countries, where malarial mosquitoes exist, take precautions seriously. In Africa a child dies every 30 seconds from malaria. In the Caribbean both my husband and myself have suffered Dengue fever from mosquito bites, and I would never want to feel that ill again. The key, as always, lies in prevention. If you are unfortunate enough to be attacked by a swarm of bees, immediately close your eyes and mouth and wait for help. If you happen to be near water and can swim, then jump in.

Foods to Avoid

- Sugar makes your blood taste sweeter, especially to mosquitoes. If you are visiting the tropics, stop eating sugar at least a week before you travel.

Friendly Foods

- Garlic eaten on a regular basis may well make you smell less appetizing to stinging insects. Or take a one-a-day garlic tablet, such as Allimax.
- Malaria-carrying mosquitoes are attracted to the smell of human feet. Limburger cheese or other strong cheeses smell just like your feet, so by putting a bit of the cheese in your room at least 5ft (2.5m) away from you the mosquitoes are distracted.

Useful Remedies

- Thiamine (B1), 300mg and 50mg of zinc per day. When these are excreted in our sweat they give off an odour that repels insects. As all the B-vitamins work together, also take a B-complex.
- Brewer's yeast, either as tablets or powder, is a rich source of vitamin B1, which changes the smell of your sweat, making you less attractive to insects.
- Some people have found that taking feverfew, the herb that contains pyrethin (an effective insecticide), really helps. Also, the herb catnip repels mosquitoes.
- Use Bug Ban by Herbcraft – spray liberally over the body as often as is needed.
- Quantum Buzz Away is deet-free and made from a combination of essential oils, such as cedarwood, eucalyptus, lemongrass and peppermint.
- Try a calendula, pyrethin, arnica and echinacea spray for the bites – to reduce the inflammation and itching. OP

Helpful Hints

- Use lemongrass or citronella candles at dusk to repel insects.
- 'Colibri' products (from Maroma) are made with botanical extracts and 15 natural essential oils (including lavender, lemon grass, citronella, peppermint, geranium, margosa and eucalyptus). These provide a natural alternative to chemical repellents. The range includes incense sticks and cones, candles, body lotion, body spray, and rollers. SL
- Try an essential oil preparation for repelling insects. Mix 10 drops of lavender oil, 10 drops of orange oil, 5 drops of eucalyptus, 5 drops of citronella and 10 drops of neem oil into a base of 50ml apricot or almond oil. Apply sparingly on exposed areas of skin, especially ankles and wrists. Most good health food stores will carry these oils. If you do not have the time to do all this, the Organic Pharmacy make an insect repellent spray containing most of these oils. OP
- Try Alfresco body lotion, containing melissa, geranium, lavender and other essential oils, which has been proven to help repel insects. For details call 020 8348 6704. Website: www.alfresco.uk.com
- Avoid wearing any perfumed toiletries at night, and use cotton night clothes that cover the arms and wrists.
- Use a mosquito net. In Africa, trials on children showed incidence of malaria was cut by 80% when nets were used at night. These are easy to buy at travel shops.
- Ainsworth Homeopathic Pharmacy can supply a general travel kit, which includes items for bites, traveller's tummy, sunstroke and so on. They can also provide individual homeopathic remedies for tropical diseases such as homeopathic Malaria, and Caladium, which change the smell of your sweat making you less attractive to insects. Tel: 020 7935 5330. Website: www.ainsworths.com

INSOMNIA

(see also *Melatonin* and *Sleeping Pills*)

If there is truly one subject I could fill a book on it's this one. I have suffered chronic insomnia for almost 30 years and I really do know what it's like not to be able to get to sleep because your mind is racing, and then when you do drop off to be wide awake again at 3 or 4 am. Thanks to our modern way of life – open-all-hours, stress and anxiety – 1 in every 4 people now says they experience regular sleep problems. In order to go to sleep, you need to switch your brain from its normal busy or beta-brainwave state to a more relaxed alpha state. The best way to achieve this is by meditation (see *Meditation*), self-hypnosis, or relaxation tapes.

No-one functions well when they are short of sleep, as it not only compromises your immune system but can severely affect your day-to-day performance. Studies have shown that, when it comes to driving, lack of sleep can have almost as drastic an effect as drinking alcohol. Lack of sleep has also been shown to increase inflammation in the body.

Many people, including myself, when absolutely desperate, resort to prescription sleeping pills. The problem can then become chronic and addictive. Hence it's best to use sleeping pills only on the odd or occasional night – as a preventative to stop the body and brain becoming overtired, which often makes it even harder to get to sleep. In the long-term prescription sleeping pills can affect your memory and upset delicate brain chemistry. It's worth noting that if you tend to wake regularly between 3 and 5am you are likely to be suffering adrenal exhaustion from stress, or if you wake between 1 and 3am then it's likely that your liver is struggling. In which case you need to cut down on fats, coffee and alcohol, and eat lightly for a few days. (See also *Liver Problems*.)

People who suffer muscle-twitching or restless legs also tend to suffer sleep deprivation. See *Restless Legs*. There can be many explanations for not getting enough sleep, and if you can get to the root cause, this often helps to let go of the fear of not sleeping.

Foods to Avoid

- Caffeine is one of the most important substances to avoid after around 5pm in the afternoon. Having said that, I have friends who can drink espresso and sleep like a log. I'm not one of them; if I drink filter coffee after early evening I can be awake until the early hours. Remember that caffeine is not just found in tea and coffee, it's also in cola, chocolate, cocoa and some over-the-counter cold remedies.
- If you drink a fair amount of alcohol you tend to feel sleepy, but unfortunately because of the way it is metabolised in the body, you might sleep for 2–3 hours and then wake up again and find it very difficult to get back to sleep.
- Food intolerances can make the problem worse. In one study cow's milk appeared to be the problem but it can be any food to which you have a sensitivity. Keep a food diary. See *Allergies*.
- Don't eat big meals late at night.
- Avoid red meat and too much protein, which tend to wake up the brain. Eat protein for breakfast or lunch.
- Avoid cheese at night – it contains amino acids that can keep you awake.

Friendly Foods

- Try to make the last meal of the day a carbohydrate-based one, such as pasta, potatoes or brown rice. These starchy foods can have a slight soporific effect. Eating carbohydrate-rich foods before sleep also encourages the body to produce a brain chemical called serotonin, which can help reduce anxiety and improve the quality of sleep.
- Serotonin is made from a constituent of protein called tryptophan, so include more foods such as fish, turkey, chicken, cottage cheese, beans, avocados, bananas and wheat germ in your diet.

- Sprinkle wheat germ over breakfast cereal; my favourite is Nature's Path who make great cereals from amaranth, quinoa and kamut that are sweetened with a little apple juice.
- Some people find that a banana an hour before they go to sleep helps them sleep longer as bananas are a good source of tryptophan, which is calming.
- Many people have porridge for breakfast, but often having it as a supper or late-night snack made with organic rice milk and a chopped banana encourages sound sleep. If I wake at night, or cannot get off to sleep I often have a small bowl of sugar-free kashi cereal, with a chopped banana, a few sunflower seeds and raisins, with a little organic rice milk, and it helps me to get to sleep almost immediately.
- If you are a regular tea- or coffee-drinker, gradually switch over to the decaffeinated varieties. Don't do this too quickly as caffeine withdrawal headaches can be quite unpleasant.
- Drink camomile tea (or any night-time formulas) before going to bed.
- If you suffer low blood sugar problems, eat a banana with a Ryvita or oat-based biscuit, or a cracker with a little honey just before going to bed.
- Eat more lettuce at night – it contains the natural sedative lactucarium, which encourages deeper sleep. You can also heat crisp lettuce in stir-fries and so on; it's delicious.

Useful Remedies

- I use a homepathic mix of oats, passiflora, valerian and coffee (Coffea) – one pill under the tongue just before bed and again if you wake in the night. It works well for me. **OP** (or ask their pharmacist to make up a remedy that matches your constitution and symptoms).
- Valerian and passiflora are two herbs that help enhance sleep patterns, and have been compared successfully with the prescription drugs benzodiazepines. These help people to get to sleep faster, enhance the quality of their sleep, and leave them less cloudy headed when they wake up. Try Valerian Formula. **FSC**

- Calcium and magnesium are nature's tranquillisers, take a two-in-one formula with your evening meal that includes 600mg of calcium and 300–400mg of magnesium.
- Hops are a good alternative for people who don't get on with valerian. They are available generally in tincture form: take 1–2ml about an hour before you want to go to sleep. People suffering depression should avoid hops.
- Take 100mg of a plant extract 5-hydroxytryptphan (5-HTP), derived from the plant griffonia, twice daily, to help boost serotonin levels naturally. The second pill should be taken at bedtime. **HN**
- The amino acid theanine is found in green tea, and it produces calming effects within the brain. I have taken this for several months, and I am definitely able to switch off more easily than I used to. It does not make you drowsy or groggy. It helps you to relax by increasing alpha-brainwave activity. It also increases levels of dopamine, a brain chemical that improves mood. Try 100mg twice daily. Take them 30 minutes before food and the second one before going to bed. **NC SL** (**NB:** Drinking green tea during the day is a great boost to your health, but it also contains caffeine, so avoid drinking the tea at night. Otherwise buy a decaffeinated version.)
- Take a B-complex every morning to support your nerves and keep you calmer.
- Melatonin is a hormone secreted by the pineal gland, which regulates our sleep–wake cycle. It is produced at night and is nature's way of preparing the body for sleep. Several studies have shown that melatonin deficiency can affect sleep patterns after the age of 35. Dosages to begin with can be rather hit and miss. I suggest you start with 0.5mg a night, and see how you go. Then gradually increase to say no more than 3mg (melatonin can induce more vivid dreams), and see which dose gives you the better sleep. It has been used successfully for years for jet lag and is freely available in health shops outside the UK, but within the UK you would need a prescription. It can be ordered for your own use by calling Pharm West on Freephone 00 353 46

943 7317. Website: www.pharmwest.com (See also *Melatonin*.)

- The Life Extension Foundation in the US make a Natural Sleep Formula, which also contains co-factors such as calcium and B-vitamins. Find them on www.lef.org

Helpful Hints

- One of the most important factors in sleep management is to get up at the same or a similar time every morning, regardless of when you go to bed.
- Try reading a novel before switching out the lights – this takes your mind away from the day's activities and helps you to wind down. If you can't get off to sleep, don't panic. Get up and do something relaxing, like reading a few more pages of a novel, until you start to relax and let go; then go back to bed. Don't **try** to go to sleep, allow yourself to fall asleep naturally. Eat the breakfast cereal I suggest on the previous page – it works every time for me.
- Exercising on a regular basis can often improve sleep patterns, but don't exercise too late in the day as the endorphins released by the brain can be quite stimulating.
- Find a way to reduce stress levels, as stressed individuals definitely have poorer sleep patterns.
- Meditation is particularly useful as it helps you to clear the mind and get rid of all those extraneous thoughts. People who meditate on a regular basis enjoy better-quality sleep. (See *Meditation*.)
- To help your body make more melatonin naturally, get out in the sunshine during the day, and then at night sleep in a fully darkened room – the darker the better.
- Smoking can also be a factor in insomnia so if you want another reason for giving up, poor sleep patterns might be the last push you need.
- Massage your chest with a mixture of essential oils of lavender, clary sage, marjoram and basil, or add them to a relaxing bath. Or, buy a burner and let the aroma fill your room.
- Potter's Nodoff Mixture is a traditional herbal remedy to promote natural sleep. It tastes dreadful but helps a lot of people. Available from all good health stores. For your nearest stockist contact Potter's (Herbal Supplies) Ltd. Tel: 01942 405100. Website: www.pottersherbal.co.uk
- Don't read any work papers close to bedtime – it stimulates your mind.
- Turn the bedside clock to the wall, so you will not panic about the time.
- Advanced reflexology, homeopathy, acupuncture, and hypnotherapy have all proved useful in restoring natural sleep patterns (see *Useful Information*).
- Paul McKenna, the world-renowned hypnotherapist, has made some great sleep CDs and tapes. Tel: 0845 230 2022. Website: www.paulmckenna.com
- Inner Talk also make some very good tapes – for details call 01628 898366. Website: www.innertalk.co.uk
- Persistent insomnia can also be exacerbated by food intolerances, in which case it would be wise to consult a doctor who is also a qualified nutritionist (see *Useful Information*).
- Many people have found a herbal remedy called Valerian Hops Complex containing hops, oats and valerian very helpful. Take 20–30 drops in a little juice half an hour before bed. Contact BioForce. Tel: 01294 277344. Website: www.avogel.co.uk
- Invest in a really comfortable mattress – simply being cosy, and not too warm and not too cold really helps. In winter buy a sheepskin mattress cover and in summer use cotton sheets.
- Read *Alternative Medicine – A Definitive Guide to Sleep Disorders* by Herbert Ross.

INSULIN RESISTANCE   (see also *Diabetes* and *Low Blood Sugar*)

If any blood sugar imbalance (see *Diabetes*) is not addressed, over time it can develop further into insulin resistance or Syndrome X, and finally into full-blown diabetes. Doctors are increasingly concerned about the problem of insulin resistance as a causative factor in degenerative diseases. Insulin is a hormone secreted by cells in the pancreas. Its major function is to lower blood sugar levels and promote the storage of sugars as fats. Its release is stimulated by the consumption of any type of carbohydrates from fruits and grains to starchy vegetables and cakes. It also slows the breakdown of any stored fats. Of all the hormones associated with ageing, insulin is the king player when it comes to ageing. High insulin levels cause ageing, disease, hormone imbalance and deterioration of virtually every body system. According to US diabetes expert, Dr Ron Rosedale MD, almost everyone eating a typical Western diet is overproducing insulin.

The staple of this Western diet is carbohydrates. Bread, rice, pasta and so on are digested into simple sugars, such as glucose, when they enter the gut. Eating large amounts of carbohydrates, such as cakes and biscuits, can result in a 'sugar rush'. Basically, insulin makes cells more receptive to glucose, so they can either metabolize it, or store it for future use as glycogen or fat. This takes glucose out of your blood and into your cells, lowering your blood sugar levels. "However," says nutritional physician Dr Keith Scott-Mumby, "when this process has been abused for many decades, it's liable to break down. Eventually the body ceases to respond to glucose as it should and despite ever-increasing levels of insulin, glucose in the blood begins to rise. The cells can no longer utilise it properly. Insulin receptors on the surface of cells seem to have switched off and stopped listening to the signal from insulin, hence the term for this condition. Insulin resistance is dangerous. Apart from the obvious risk of progression into Syndrome X and eventually diabetes, high insulin levels result in excess sympathetic nervous system activity, which keeps the individual tense and prone to fatigue. What's more, because insulin is usually only released when there's an excess of blood sugar, conversion of fat back to sugar for use as fuel is blocked by the hormone, so weight loss becomes increasingly difficult."

SYNDROME X

In 1988 our understanding of disordered blood sugar control was advanced considerably by Dr Gerald Reaven of Stanford University, who published a paper describing what he called 'Syndrome X'. A 'syndrome' simply means a group of symptoms that appear together in a characteristic pattern. In this case, the syndrome consists of 5 common features: obesity, insulin resistance, high blood pressure, high LDL (the bad) cholesterol and low HDL (good cholesterol). Because Dr Reaven had no idea what caused this group of symptoms to occur together, he named it Syndrome X. Doesn't sound so frightening now does it? As we age, all the manifestations of Syndrome X are more frequently seen, but even elderly people without these problems tend to have increasing insulin resistance. Patients with Syndrome X do not have the dangerously raised glucose levels of diabetes. But they do have insulin resistance and higher-than-normal levels of circulating glucose. The high level of insulin stimulates the kidneys to re-absorb sodium, which in turn results in a tendency to high blood pressure. Dr Reaven believes that half of all people with high blood pressure have insulin resistance (see *High Blood Pressure*). Unfortunately, high levels of insulin also reduce blood enzymes that prevent or dissolve blood clots. Thus, along with the undesirable changes in blood fats, comes a possible increase in the likelihood of blood clotting, making the risk of heart attack or stroke far greater than for healthy individuals. Abnormal glucose and insulin metabolism are also associated with increased free-radical formation. And the more free radicals you have in your body, the more likely you are to become ill.

Foods to Avoid

- White flour, white sugar, corn syrup, white potato and other starch-rich foods will increase blood sugar problems. Yet these are the ingredients commonly used in most mass-produced, refined foods. Bread, cakes, biscuits, pasta, pastries and other confectionary items, French fries, food-thickeners, coffee whiteners, white rice, and skimmed milk (milk with the fat reduced has proportionately more sugar).
- Avoid sugar and foods containing sugar, such as fizzy drinks, chocolate, sweets and many processed foods (check labels), plus reduce your intake of honey, dried fruit and juices as they are all rich in fast-releasing sugars. Try diluting fruit juices. If you are desperate for sugar use a little fructose, which is many times sweeter than ordinary sugar, so you use less, and fructose has a lower Glycemic Index and therefore less of an effect on your blood sugar. Keep in mind that sugar ages your skin and your cells.
- Artificial sweeteners may seem like a good solution, although they do nothing to reduce your sweet tooth and because they place a strain on the liver, can add to weight gain and other health problems.
- Caffeine found in coffee, tea and cola drinks is a powerful stimulant. A cup of coffee contains around 100mg of caffeine, cola 50mg, tea 60mg, green tea 25mg, a slice of chocolate cake 25mg, and 1oz (25g) dark chocolate 30mg. Stimulants encourage sugar to be released into the blood stream.
- Replace chocolate with fresh fruit. Replace coffee and tea with coffee alternatives available in all health shops. Try green, peppermint or fruit teas.
- Alcohol is such a refined carbohydrate that much of it is converted to fat in the body. We are not suggesting you eliminate it altogether, but just be aware that it is fattening.
- Note that many foods advertised as being low in fat are often high in sugar, which if not used up during exercise will turn to fat in the body and reside on your hips!

Friendly Foods

- Eat more lentils and beans. Dr Jeffrey Bland and fellow researchers at the Functional Medicine Research Centre in Gig Harbour, Washington, have found that legumes create a very low insulin response and that increased intake of lentils, chickpeas, beans and peas is desirable in the management of Syndrome X.
- In general, vegetables have a beneficial effect on blood sugar and insulin, but certain vegetables appear to be even better at maintaining blood sugar and insulin levels, including members of the brassica family (cabbage, cauliflower, broccoli), and other green leafy vegetables.
- Soya products – especially fermented soya products, such as tempeh – are also desirable as they help balance blood sugar levels. Soya helps improve glucose transport as well as containing soluble fibre that slows the absorption of glucose from the gut, thereby reducing insulin response.
- See also the dietary guidelines in *Diabetes*.
- Make time for breakfast, this 'kick starts' your metabolism for the rest of the day and is crucial for better energy balance. "In 6 years of advising people on how to improve their energy levels," says nutritionist Shane Heaton, "I've never met anyone who skips breakfast and has good energy levels for the rest of the day. I don't think it's possible." He recommends a piece of fruit followed (15–30 minutes later) by muesli or porridge. Oats, rich in B-vitamins and fibre, are ideal, providing good, slow-burn energy, although the most important thing is to choose breakfast foods you enjoy.
- By eating breakfast your energy will improve (not to mention your concentration, mood and motivation) throughout the day. Any cravings for stimulants will decline, you'll sleep better, and you'll wake feeling more refreshed in the morning.

- Eat more foods in their natural state. Include complex carbohydrates and whole foods contain higher levels of nutrients and fibre, such as brown rice or even better brown Basmati rice, wholewheat/rye bread, porridge oats, fruits and vegetables. These foods also tend to have a low Glycemic Index.
- Eat proteins and carbohydrates together. This flies in the face of the Hay Diet and Food Combining, which does make sense (and works for people with gastric problems such as hiatus hernia), as it's true these foods are digested at different rates, however **if** you have trouble balancing your blood sugar levels, eating carbohydrates alone all the time can constantly disrupt your efforts to stabilise your energy levels. Balancing carbohydrates and proteins (in a ratio of 2 to 1, so twice as much carbohydrate as protein) at each meal or snack can help slow the release of sugars from the carbohydrates. For example, eat some nuts or seeds with fresh fruit, fish with rice, or lentil pâté/houmous with rice cakes.
- Choose more foods with a low Glycemic Index. This is a guide as to how much and how quickly sugar is released from certain foods, compared with straight glucose, which is set at 100. Some foods are fast, others are slow. For example, white bread scores 70, while rye bread is just 41. Bananas are 62, while apples are 39. You don't have to choose only low Glycemic Index foods all the time, but where possible, choose alternatives with lower scores, and when you do eat high Glycemic Index foods, mix them with protein or low Glycemic Index foods to slow the sugar release. For a complete list of low Glycemic Index foods read *The 30 Day Fatburner Diet* by Patrick Holford (Piatkus). Website: www.patrickholford.com
- Drink more water, aim for 6 glasses per day. Dehydration is a key cause of fatigue and can make you crave fast-energy foods that contribute to blood sugar imbalance.
- If you are desperate for sugar then try Slim Sweet, a low Glycemic Index sweetener from the lo-han fruit. From all health stores.

Useful Remedies

- A high-strength, multi-vitamin and mineral complex that provides a good range of antioxidants, chromium, and plenty of B-vitamins. See *Kudos 24* in *General Supplements*; p.160.
- The mineral chromium is the main constituent of 'glucose tolerance factor', a substance that helps with the delivery of sugar to cells. It's used widely by nutritional therapists to help balance blood sugar and reduce cravings. Take 100–200mcg twice daily with meals. American research has shown that when people who tend to eat a high-carbohydrate diet are given 200mcg of chromium daily, this one step helps reduce incidence of diabetes by 50%. Most multis contain around 150mcg.
- Fish oil supplementation has been found to not only improve insulin sensitivity in diabetic animals, but also prevent diabetes-induced nerve damage.
- Antioxidant nutrients have also been found to improve insulin sensitivity. Take a good-quality antioxidant formula containing 100–400mg of vitamin E and 20–50mg of alpha-lipoic acid, both known to improve insulin response. **HN**
- UltraGlycemX is a specially fortified, vegetarian, powdered beverage mix, designed for the nutritional support of glucose metabolism and insulin regulation. **NC**
- Vitamin C is involved with energy production, so if your energy levels are low and your stress levels are high, take 1000mg of vitamin C twice daily with food.
- If stress is a real problem in your life consider trying the herbs rhodiola or Siberian ginseng. They're both adaptogenic herbs, so help you adapt to stress and can really help improve your tolerance to stress of all kinds. Take 200–300mg of a standardised extract of either herb daily with meals.

Helpful Hints

- Apart from dietary changes, one of the best ways to improve glucose control and insulin sensitivity is through regular aerobic activity. This doesn't have to be intense exercise and can be as moderate as a regular walking programme. Twenty minutes per day of walking on level ground has been shown to improve insulin sensitivity and glucose management.
- Moderate alcohol consumption is OK. A recent study by Dr Reaven and colleagues indicated that light-to-moderate alcohol intake was associated with improved insulin sensitivity, while more than 2 drinks per day worsened it.
- Reduce stress. Stress is a major hindrance to stabilising blood sugar levels because the fight-or-flight mechanism (designed to help you run or fight when a lion jumps out of the bushes at you!) floods your blood with sugar ready for action. If we constantly suffer from low blood sugar, we can sometimes learn subconsciously to use stress as a way to keep us going. We might stay in a stressful job, make situations more stressful than they need to be, seek out stressful situations (often subconsciously), take too much on, do things at the last minute, be late everywhere we go, and so on. Blood sugar imbalance itself is a major stress on the body and at the same time lowers your stress tolerance, so by improving your blood sugar balance your tolerance of other stresses in your life should improve. In addition to the other guidelines here, manage your stress levels with exercise, yoga, T'ai Chi, meditation, massage, having 'down time' every week, and learning to relax (for more help see *Stress*).
- Stop smoking – cigarettes are a stimulant, which many people use to keep themselves going, having one after meals to avoid the energy slump and at regular intervals throughout the day. If you find smoking relaxing, you're addicted. The feeling of relaxation is very likely the alleviation of withdrawal symptoms (commonly anxiety, stress, tension, nervousness, and so on). Those who stop smoking and gain weight do so because they usually replace the cigarettes with other stimulants, such as sugar, or sugar-containing foods or drinks. More sugar means more weight.
- The worst thing you can do if your energy levels are poor is go long hours without eating. So eat small, frequent meals throughout the day – every 2–3 hours or so – and avoid skipping meals. This isn't as hard as it sounds. For example, have breakfast, morning tea, lunch, afternoon tea, dinner, and a late snack. People who miss meals often experience hypoglycaemic (low blood sugar) symptoms. Obviously I'm not talking about junk-food snacks. Healthy snacks throughout the day may include fruit, nuts, seeds, rice or oat cakes with houmous or other spreads, raw vegetables (such as, carrots), rye crackers with lentil pâté, alfalfa, and so on.
- Read *The X Factor Diet*, by Leslie Kenton (Vermillion).

INTERMITTENT CLAUDICATION

(see also Angina, Circulation and Heart Disease)

This condition is characterised by a pain in the legs, usually in the calves when walking. It is caused by blockages in the arteries supplying blood to the legs and is due to the hardening of the arteries in the lower body. To deal successfully with intermittent claudication you need to resolve the hardening of the arteries. Diets and therapies that help lower cholesterol levels and reduce the build-up of deposits on the arteries are the most important treatment. See also *Cholesterol*.

Foods to Avoid

- Greatly reduce your intake of animal fats and saturated fats, including margarines and highly refined mass-produced cooking oils. Avoid red meat, chicken skin, too much butter, full-fat milk and most mass-produced pies, sausages, cakes and so on.

- All fried foods should be avoided.
- Cut down alcohol to only 2 units a day.
- Percolated coffee or microwaved coffee elevates cholesterol, which in turn can lead to intermittent claudication. Avoid them.

Friendly Foods

- Oily fish is rich in the omega-3 fats that help to thin the blood naturally.
- Garlic and onion should be used liberally in food as they help to lower LDL cholesterol levels.
- A diet rich in soluble and insoluble fibres from fruits and vegetables, nuts and seeds, linseeds, oat or rice bran and psyllium husks.
- Eggs are fine as long as they are boiled, poached or scrambled and not fried.
- Look for non-hydrogenated spreads in the supermarket such as Biona, Vitaquell and Benecol. Use olive oil instead of butter.
- Drink at least 6 glasses of water daily.
- See *Friendly Foods* in *Cholesterol*.

Useful Remedies

- Take natural-source, full-spectrum vitamin E, 400–600iu a day, which has been shown to improve walking distance and decrease the discomfort of intermittent claudication. It probably needs to be taken for a minimum of six months to be effective. Check with your GP if you are on blood-thinning drugs as vitamin E will thin your blood naturally and reduce the risk of heart disease.
- Vitamin B3 in the form of Inositol Hexaniacinate, 2 grams a day for at least three months. This form of B3 can help lower cholesterol and studies have shown it to be very effective for intermittent claudication. As this form of vitamin B can trigger an intense flushing of the skin as it increases circulation, **be sure to ask for no-flush B3.**
- Ginkgo biloba daily, has been shown to decrease pain and increase walking distance in sufferers. Kudos makes a high strength (900mg), one-a-day. **KVH**
- Taken together the amino Lysine, 1500mg daily, and 2 grams of vitamin C help to clear the arteries. **HN**
- The amino acid L-carnitine also helps to reduce the pain so that people can walk further. It is expensive, but worth a try. Take 2 grams twice daily.

Helpful Hints

- Try chelation therapy – this involves an intravenous drip being administered by a private doctor, which over time helps to clear the arteries. I give full details of this treatment in my book *500 of the Most Important Ways to Stay Younger Longer* (Cico Books). Meanwhile there are several clinics in the UK – for details call 01942 886644 or log on to www.chelation.com. Dr Robert Trossell also gives this treatment at 4 Duke Street, London W1U 3EL. Tel: 020 7486 1095. Or call Dr Wendy Denning in London on 020 7224 2423.
- Don't smoke as there is a strong link between smoking and the development of intermittent claudication.
- Gentle exercise is definitely beneficial even though it may be uncomfortable. Do see your GP before starting on an exercise programme. People who exercise regularly are much less likely to develop intermittent claudication.
- Acupuncture and reflexology (especially Advanced Reflexology) are great for improving circulation and reducing pain. See *Useful Information*.

IRRITABLE BOWEL SYNDROME (IBS)

(see also *Constipation* and *Diverticular Disease*)

One in every 12 visits to the doctor is because of a digestive complaint – with irritable bowel syndrome accounting for half of these visits. In fact 20 to 25% of people in the western world are believed to suffer from IBS – to varying degrees – and this condition is three times more common in women than in men. Sadly in most cases your GP is fairly ill-equipped to deal with this particular problem, as IBS is an umbrella term used to describe a set of symptoms that are often contradictory and can differ hugely from person to person.

They do, however, fit into two categories: spastic colon-type IBS, where gripping pain is common, as well as alternating constipation and diarrhoea. Painless diarrhoea-type IBS causes urgent diarrhoea, usually upon rising and often after a meal. Common symptoms of both types are: abdominal pain (which may be continuous or may come in frequent bouts, and can be a dull ache or, in extreme cases, excruciating), and constipation or diarrhoea – or both alternating from day to day or week to week. Bloating, wind, headaches, nausea, anxiety, cramps and depression are also often associated with IBS.

There are many contributory factors in IBS, which all need to be fully investigated. According to the British Allergy Foundation, around 45% of people who contact them suffer from food intolerance at some time in their lives, and many of these people have IBS-type symptoms. The most commonly offending foods are wheat, dairy, coffee, tea and citrus foods – although an intolerance can be present to the most innocuous of foods that you would never suspect. Stress can also play an important part as your digestion shuts down during stressful times meaning that digestive juices don't get to do their job properly, which leaves incompletely digested particles of food to irritate the gut. A lack of digestive enzymes and stomach acid (see *Acid Stomach* and *Low Stomach Acid*) can also lead to incompletely digested food irritating the gut.

Parasites are a growing and often overlooked factor: 20% of all people tested have parasites, and 49% of people with IBS are known to have the parasite *Blastocystis hominis*, and 20% of people with IBS have the parasite *Dientamoeba fragilis*. If you have ever travelled abroad or had a bout of food poisoning either while on holiday or in the UK, or if you allow pets to walk on food-preparation surfaces, eat raw fish (sushi) or lightly cooked meats, or store meat above vegetables in your fridge, then parasites could be a factor.

You and your doctor should also consider dysbiosis – an imbalance of good to bad bacteria in the gut. Any yeasts, such as candida (see *Candida*), parasites and bad bacteria present in the bowel upset this delicate balance and can cause symptoms of IBS. This imbalance of bacteria can also be triggered by a poor diet that has insufficient fibre, and is high in alcohol, fatty foods and/or sugar. Antibiotics will also upset this balance.

Occasionally the symptoms of IBS can reflect a more serious underlying condition, so it is very important to see your doctor in case you have Crohn's Disease, ulcerative colitis, or diverticulitis, which are often mistaken for IBS. People with IBS need to support their liver by watching their intake of fats, caffeine and alcohol. See also *Liver Problems*.

Foods to Avoid

- Refined wheat is high in gluten, which can be irritating to the gut and is usually the biggest factor in IBS. Cow's milk comes next. Cut these two foods from your diet for two weeks and see if there is any improvement.
- Flour from any source gunks up the bowel in sensitive individuals; for the first seven days around an attack it's a good idea to avoid any foods containing flour. When I was tested for

food intolerances, wheat was fine, and yet wheat-and-flour based products cause me to suffer IBS-type symptoms. I'm OK if I eat flour and wheat now and again – but are you going for a cure or simply a coping strategy? With IBS it's a case of really listening to your body and knowing when enough is enough. Unless, of course, you have a severe intolerance to specific foods, in which case complete avoidance may be necessary.

- Other problem foods are often eggs and citrus fruits, especially oranges; and foods with a high tyramine content, such as cheese, port, red wine and sherry, beef, liver, herring, sauerkraut, and yeast extracts.
- If you suspect Candida see *Foods to Avoid* under *Candida*.
- Melted cheese is very hard for the body to digest – avoid at all costs.
- Refined foods – white rice and pasta, as well as cakes and pastries, alcohol, fried foods, high-sugar foods, and those foods high in saturated animal fat (found in meat and dairy) all deplete good bacteria in the gut and help feed the bad guys.
- Avoid heavy, rich meals, and especially avoid fried foods.

Friendly Foods

- There are plenty of alternatives to wheat. Ask at your health shop for wheat-free breads and use amaranth, spelt, millet, buckwheat, quinoa, oat and rye crisp breads, and rice and corn cakes, which are delicious. But if symptoms are severe, then eliminating all products containing flour for a few days usually helps.
- If symptoms are severe, you might also need to drop oats, barley and rye – other gluten-containing grains – try a small amount and see what happens.
- You can now buy lentil-, corn-, rice- and potato-based pastas.
- Try organic rice, almond or oat milk, or try goat's or sheep's milk, which are easier to digest.
- Eat more brown rice as this is cleansing and healing to the digestive tract, as well as potatoes, fish, lean poultry, fruits and vegetables.
- Peppermint, fresh mint, fennel, camomile and rosemary teas can all enhance digestion and ease discomfort.
- Try to eat more foods that you wouldn't normally eat. Exotic grains like quinoa and amaranth are good protein sources and rarely cause problems.
- Instead of orange juice, try low-sugar diluted apple, pear or pineapple juice.
- Add more ginger to your food, which soothes your gut and has anti-parasitic properties. This is why Japanese sushi – raw fish, which can contain parasites – is often served with ginger. (See also *Leaky Gut*.)
- Pumpkin seeds have anti-parasitic action so munch on some daily
- Many sufferers report that eating a banana often helps to ease symptoms.
- Eating pineapple, which contains bromelain, helps to digest protein. Having some pineapple at the end of a meal that contains protein will aid digestion.
- In order to make stomach acid for efficient digestion, you need vitamin B6 and the mineral zinc. These are found in sunflower seeds, soya beans, walnuts, lentils and lima beans, buckwheat flour (this is a grass and is not related to wheat), bananas, avocados and chestnuts, brown rice, lentils, pumpkin and sesame seeds, almonds and cooked tofu.
- Eat lighter meals: soup and fish-based meals are easier on the digestion than a pizza with melted cheese! Avoid rich sauces.

Useful Remedies

- As absorption of nutrients is often a problem in IBS and you may be low in stomach acid (see *Low Stomach Acid*) dilute 1 tsp of apple cider vinegar in water and drink with each meal. You can increase to 6 tsp if needed. If symptoms persist, instead try taking one Nutri's Nutrigest available from www.positivenutrition.co.uk along with meals. This contains some stomach acid mixed with digestive enzymes. *Take it after the first few mouthfuls*, do not chew it, and never take it on an empty stomach. Avoid all of these remedies if you have active stomach ulcers, or if they create a feeling of warmth in your stomach. Instead take a pancreatic digestive enzyme formula that is free from HCl, which can irritate the gut.

- Try a combination of cayenne capsules (which help stop any bleeding), pure slippery elm tea (which soothes and heals the gut), and Colit capsules, containing wild yam (an anti-spasmodic), plus bayberry and agrimony, which tighten and heal the tissues. Take 3–9 capsules daily depending on severity of symptoms. **SHS**

- Take 1 acidophilus or bifidus capsule twice a day to replace healthy bacteria in the gut and improve digestion. BioCare's Bio Acidophillus is shown to survive stomach acid and make it to the gut where it needs to do its job. **BC**

- Take a high-strength B-complex to make sure you have all the nutrients necessary to digest carbohydrates, proteins and fats. Look for 50mg of most of the B-vitamins.

- Aloe vera juice, 20ml taken before meals, has helped a lot of people, as it helps increase stool bulk, enhances digestion, and eases the discomfort of IBS.

- Take 1–3 dessertspoons of organic linseeds (flax seeds) daily (build up slowly, a teaspoon at a time), providing 10–20 grams of linseeds. The mixture of soluble and insoluble fibres in linseeds helps to stimulate the bowel gently, while providing stool bulk, thus enabling the bowel to function normally and comfortably. Linseeds have also been successful both in alleviating constipation and diarrhoea, but they must be taken with plenty of water.

- See remedies under *Constipation* and *Diarrhoea* if either is your main problem.

- Gamma Oranzyl – rice bran oil – works on the brain to reduce spasms in the gut and has been used to great effect for sufferers of IBS. BioCare combine it in a formula called Permatrol with NAG (N-acetylglutamine), which feeds the good bacteria, and L-glutamine, which helps to repair an inflamed and irritated gut wall. Take 1 capsule of Permatrol before meals, 3 times a day.

Helpful Hints

- Chew, chew, chew and chew again, As you chew you send signals to the digestive system to produce its digestive enzymes, and thoroughly chewed food also gives the enzymes less to do, making them more effective.

- Avoid fruit that ferments easily, such as bananas, apples, pears and melon. Instead eat more berries and tropical fruits, which do not ferment as easily.

- Oil of peppermint has anti-spasmodic properties – massage it on your abdomen and drink peppermint tea after meals. Fennel tea is another herb that aids digestion.

- Gentle exercise on a regular basis enhances bowel function. Yoga, Pilates, swimming and walking are all good forms of exercise that do not overtax the system and enhance relaxation.

- Remember to eat in a relaxed fashion; being stressed while you eat makes it very difficult for normal digestive function to work at its best. Sitting down for 10 minutes either side of a meal is advised. Try to avoid eating food on the run.

- Remember, if you have an intolerance to one food, you are actually likely to be intolerant to more than one. Very few of us react to just one food, and in most cases we react to four or five. IWDL do a thorough food-intolerance test and can be contacted on 08704 190 435. Website: www.iwdl.net

- Call Smart Nutrition who offer help to IBS sufferers and can test for levels of good and bad bacteria, candida and parasites. Tel: 01273 737000, or check out their website at www.smartnutrition.co.uk

- Check out www.ibsnetwork.org.uk for more information.

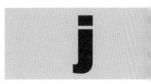

JET LAG

Jet lag is a disturbance of the sleep–wake cycle triggered by air travel across time zones. Jet lag has become a part of modern living. It's obvious that if you travel for many hours across varying time zones, your whole system is going to be affected. Usually, the more time zones you cross, the worse the symptoms. These symptoms include difficulty falling asleep at the new bedtime, and sleepiness and fatigue during the day. In addition, your circulation can become sluggish triggering problems such as leg-, ankle- and foot-swelling, or in extreme cases DVT. Also, as you are breathing recycled air, along with myriad bacteria and viruses, you are at risk of contracting a whole host of diseases from a simple cold to something more serious such as tuberculosis, which is making a comeback. You are exposed to considerable amounts of radiation, which can lower immune function; your pineal gland can become confused, thus affecting melatonin-production, which plays havoc with your internal body clock.

Also you are moving between local magnetic fields, and while your body adjusts you can feel very tired indeed. See *Helpful Hints* for more on magnetic fields.

Children under the age of 3 seem to suffer little jet lag as they are not set in their ways, and so more adaptable. Also the less rigid you are in your everyday life, the less likely you are to suffer jet lag.

A deep-vein thrombosis (DVT) is a blood clot that develops in deep veins, most commonly in the leg, and can happen during a flight or several days after it (or after any period of inactivity or restriction in circulation). DVT can cause considerable pain and sometimes acute swelling. If the clot travels to the lungs, then a pulmonary embolism may result. Symptoms of DVT are extreme pain, usually in the lower limbs and/or pelvic area, although in rarer cases it can also occur in the arm or pelvis.

If you suspect DVT then you need immediate medical help. If you are at home in the UK, this would be a good time to dial 999, or ask someone to take you to the emergency department at your local hospital. DVT is more common in people aged over 40, especially those who are overweight, and in people with circulation or heart problems, and in people who are A or AB blood-types. For more details on DVT, you can find lots of information on www.bupa.co.uk, or have a look at vascular surgeon John Scurr's site at www.jscurr.com

Foods to Avoid
- On long flights eat smaller meals and reduce your intake of tea, coffee, alcohol and cola-type fizzy drinks, which all dehydrate the body. Caffeine can contribute to poor sleep patterns, so ask for decaffeinated varieties.
- Sugar depletes minerals and lowers immune function, which can be a real problem in the airless cabins where bacteria and viruses spread so quickly.
- Alcohol is 2–3 times more potent when you drink it in the air.
- See also *Circulation*.

Friendly Foods
- Try to eat light and healthy foods the day prior to travel, and drink plenty of water. I realise that

airline food can leave a lot to be desired, but eat at regular intervals on the flight to help balance blood sugar levels.

- Foods that help to calm you down and aid restful sleep are turkey, cottage cheese, avocados, pasta, bananas and skimmed milk.
- Camomile, lemon balm or passiflora teas are great for relaxation. Take a few tea bags with you.
- Ask the cabin crew to give you a few bottles of mineral water and drink it throughout the flight. Or take it on with you.
- Eat more garlic during the week or so before flying – it's anti-bacterial and anti-viral, and thins blood naturally.

Useful Remedies

- Take one gram of vitamin C with bioflavonoids every 2–3 hours with a full glass of water.
- Take a high-strength multi-vitamin and mineral.
- Try Emergen C, a powdered vitamin C and electrolyte formula that helps replenish depleted minerals. Sold at all good health stores and pharmacies.
- The amino acid L-glutamine helps improve concentration on long flights – take 1–3 grams during the flight 30 minutes before meals.
- The amino acid L-theanine (extracted from green tea) helps the brain to produce more alpha waves and helps you relax without making you groggy (see *Insomnia*).
- Melatonin produced in the pineal gland has proven highly effective for reducing jet lag. Take 1–3 mg one hour before sleep, preferably at the local bedtime. In the UK this is available only on prescription, but can be bought at virtually any American airport or health store. And you can order from Pharm West for your own use by post in the UK. **PW**

- If you cannot get hold of melatonin, try 5-HTP. This supplement is available in the UK from Higher Nature (Serotone 5-HTP + co-factors). It increases tryptophan levels in the brain, which stimulates sleep (take 100mg about an hour before sleep time). Do not take it with antidepressants. **HN**
- If you are worried about being cramped and contracting DVT, take some high-strength ginkgo biloba and gotu kola (500mg daily), a few days before and during your flight. These natural remedies increase circulation. The gotu kola helps increase circulation in the lower limbs, and a positive side-effect is sometimes a slight loosening of the bowels! **KVH**
- Natural-source, full-spectrum vitamin E thins the blood and reduces the risk of clotting on long flights. Take 400iu at least two weeks prior to travel and during the journey. If you are taking blood-thinning drugs, check with your GP.
- With your GP's permission start taking one baby aspirin daily for a week before the flight, as well as during it, and for a couple of days after you arrive. This can reduce the likelihood of suffering DVT.
- There is also a supplement called Zinopin, which contains pine bark extract (pycnogenol) and ginger. It contains the anti-clotting activity of aspirin – without the negative side-effects. Ginger is also useful against travel sickness. Available from all good pharmacies.
- A homeopathic mixture containing arnica and cocculus helps to reduce symptoms of jet lag by helping the body to readjust to local time. **OP**

Helpful Hints

- Get a good night's sleep before your flight, which will help reduce jet lag. When you arrive, if practical, take some exercise, such as a walk or a swim.
- Try to stay up until the local time to go to bed. When I travel west to the US, I usually manage to stay up until the local bedtime (around 8pm), but if I'm going east I find this harder, and often take a nap. Basically, the sooner you get on to local time the better. Get as much sunlight as you can as soon as you arrive by going for walk, which helps to re-set your body clock.

- To help reset your body clock, attach a Super Magnet to the top of your head for 15 minutes before landing. One of the reasons you get jet lag is because your body clock is trying to adjust to the new magnetic field. By using the magnet you can reset your body clock to the local magnetic field. To order a Super Magnet call Coghill Research on 01495 752122.
- If you have a long wait for connections, try to have a shower, which will help relax your muscles and get your circulation moving again.
- Have a small meal when you arrive to help you to sleep. Otherwise low blood sugar can cause you to wake in the middle of the night.
- There is a great nose spray called Air Defence by Natural Care, which really helps to reduce sneezing on planes and helps protect you against invading bacteria and viruses. SL
- Buy some good support stockings or socks, such as those made by Medi-travel (www.mediuk.co.uk). These are now sold at all major airports. A neck pillow can also be useful as then you can try to relax and sleep more comfortably.
- Keep walking around the plane as much as you can. Use the aisles to do a few squats and raise your arms up and down; stretch out as much as you can.
- Keep in mind that DVT can also occur after long car journeys and in people who sit too long at their desk. To keep blood flowing, and when safe to do so, press both feet firmly into the ground and flex your leg muscles. Or flex your feet up and down and round and round to get your circulation moving.
- Massage your lower legs from the feet upwards every hour or so – go quite deep to 'rev' up your circulation.

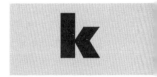

KIDNEY STONES

(see also *Acid–Alkaline Balance*)

Your kidneys filter the plasma of your blood and extract all the waste and unwanted toxins, which are then excreted in the urine (a sterile liquid). Also, the residues of antibiotics, prescription drugs and hormones, and vitamins and minerals are excreted in the urine. The kidneys maintain the acid–alkaline balance of your blood within very narrow limits; and if the blood becomes too acid or too alkaline, life is not possible. Without functioning kidneys you would not survive for very long.

These remarkable organs weigh just a few ounces each and yet, if they cease to function (known as kidney failure), they must be replaced with a huge dialysis machine. Two of the main threats to our kidneys are blood pressure and toxins. If you tend to have a poor diet, or take little or no exercise, it's likely that you may develop hypertension, which, sooner or later, plays havoc with the kidneys (see also *High Blood Pressure*). Other toxins that affect the kidneys are found in our air, water and food. Mercury, arsenic, pesticides and a huge amount of chemical pollutants all pose potential problems to the kidneys. Cadmium, from cigarette smoke, is a major kidney poison, and the accumulation of this metal in the kidneys is one of the reasons why smokers often succumb to illness sooner than average – they simply cannot clear their bloodstream of the harmful waste products as efficiently as non-smokers. If the kidneys have to work harder, they may weaken under the strain.

If over time we eat a poor diet, kidney stones can start to form as miniscule crystals that look like gravel, which can damage the delicate tubules in the kidneys and impede proper urine flow. Kidney-stone episodes are more common in the summer when urine becomes more concentrated, when we tend to sweat more. The stones are generally made from minerals, such as calcium, and deposits of uric acid, the most common component of which is calcium oxalate. Kidney stones can cause excruciating pain as they try to move out of the kidneys and into the bladder. Passing a kidney stone is one of the worst pains in all of medicine. So, try to make sure this never happens to you.

Vegetarians have a 40–60% lower chance of developing stones than meat-eaters; and voracious meat-eaters tend to suffer more stones. Having kidney stones in the body also makes bladder infections much more likely. If you ever pass blood in your urine or have persistent back pain, then it's very important that you see your GP. People with high homocysteine levels also tend to suffer more kidney problems (see *Cholesterol* and *Heart Disease*). You can lower homocysteine levels through your diet and by taking B-vitamins.

Foods to Avoid

- If you tend to eat a lot of foods high in oxalic acid, such as chocolate, cocoa, tea, spinach, rhubarb and chard, don't eat these foods too regularly.
- Beetroot, instant coffee, grapefruit, oranges, gooseberries, peanuts and strawberries also contain oxalic acid – reduce your intake of these if you suffer from kidney stones.
- Reduce or avoid high acid-forming foods, such as red meat, full-fat dairy products, sugar and sweet foods.
- Sugar is the worst food for your kidneys, as it stimulates the release of insulin from the pancreas, which in turn stimulates calcium excretion through the urine. Over time this can increase the risk of kidney stones.
- Cut down on all fizzy canned drinks and reduce alcohol and caffeinated drinks.
- Antacids, excess milk and bicarbonated drinks, such as soda water and fizzy water can all add to the problem.
- Avoid sodium-based salts. Ask at your health shop for magnesium- and potassium-based sea salts instead, and use them sparingly.
- See also *Gout*, as you also need to avoid high purine foods.

Friendly Foods

- Add cranberry juice, parsley tea, dandelion leaf tea, mullein tea and barley water, which all help to break down any stone formation.
- Drink plenty of plain, pure water, and increase to 8 glasses daily in summer.
- Eat black cherries, which help to remove uric acid crystals out of the body.
- Drink carrot, celery and parsley juice, or make "smoothies" with these ingredients. Celery does contain a little oxalic acid, but makes a great kidney cleanser as it is rich in potassium, which helps to flush the kidneys.
- Eat plenty of garlic, horseradish, asparagus, parsley, watermelon, apples, cucumber, kale, parsnips, turnip greens and mango, which are all great kidney foods.
- All magnesium- and calcium-rich foods help you to avoid kidney stones and encourage healthier kidneys. Try green leafy vegetables, apricots, blackstrap molasses, honey, curried vegetables, watercress, soya flour, yoghurt, muesli and sesame seeds. Raw wheat germ is high in magnesium and vitamin E.
- Try rice or oat milk as non-dairy alternatives to cow's milk. Or try low-fat goat's or sheep's milk now and again.
- Use organic, unrefined olive, walnut or linseed (flax seed) oils in salad dressings.

- Sprinkle lecithin granules over your food. These help to emulsify saturated fats that can contribute to stone-formation. Lecithin also contains choline and helps to protect the kidneys from the damage of arteriosclerosis and hypertension. Take 2 tbsp a day.
- Kelp and all seaweeds are a great source of calcium, magnesium and trace minerals.
- Eat more fresh fish, especially pilchards, wild salmon, cod, sea bass and so on.
- Try spelt, amaranth or millet breads and crackers, as spelt, millet and amaranth are alkaline foods.
- Eat more barley- and lentil-based dishes.

Useful Remedies
- A great remedy for kidney stones is hydrangea root, made into a herbal drink with water, and consumed over the course of one day. Often one treatment can make a big difference. **SHS**
- Take a good B-complex – especially if you are under stress (these are usually in any good multi-vitamin/mineral formula, which you also need).
- Vitamin C – 2 grams daily with food – is a good detoxifier.
- Take vitamin D3 via a cod-liver-oil capsule.
- Choline protects the kidneys from inflammation. It is available as the amino acids methionine and s-adenosyl methionine (SAMe), which is super-strength methionine. Take 500mg a day of methionine, or 50g of SAMe. **NC SL**
- Drink more organic green tea, which helps to re-alkalise the system.
- New Era tissue salts, silica, and calcium fluoride help to break down kidney stones. Take 4 of each daily.
- The herb horsetail acts as a diuretic, which promotes kidney function. It can be taken either as capsules or a tincture to help reduce stones, but do not use it if your kidneys are already damaged.
- Take 1 cup of nettle tea 3 times a day. It is best made with the dried herbs available in tea bags or as loose tea from good health stores.
- Include either a liquid multi-mineral, such as Concentrace, available from Higher Nature, or a multi-mineral tablet in your regimen. **HN**
- Take calcium citrate, 500mg, with each meal as the calcium binds to the oxalate and reduces the likelihood of kidney stones forming. However, calcium taken on an empty stomach can increase the risk of kidney stones so it is very important to take it with a meal.
- The amino acid lysine helps decrease urinary calcium. Take 1000mg daily. **HN**

Helpful Hints
- Taking 1 tsp of neat lemon juice every half an hour during the day for two days may help to smooth the kidney stones.
- Reflexology, massage, manual lymph drainage, and other therapies that encourage toxins to move out of the tissues can temporarily overload the kidneys. Warn your therapist to be gentle if you have a kidney problem. Drink plenty of water afterwards.
- Skin-brushing and lymphatic drainage massage also help remove toxins.
- If you need painkillers, avoid paracetamol, which has a negative effect on the kidneys. If you are taking a diuretic medicine, then you need to make sure that you get enough potassium. We need potassium to shed the more toxic sodium. Excess sodium leads *directly* to hypertension (high blood pressure) and kidney damage. You can take a potassium supplement – around 100mg daily; or use a potassium chloride table salt, which is available from most pharmacies and health stores.
- Some homeopathic remedies are excellent for strengthening kidney function. Populus and Solidago are well-known kidney remedies. HEEL also do *Mucosa compositum*, which helps the healing process. Available from all good homeopathic pharmacies.

- Avoid excess sweating, which may mean moderating your exercise routine and staying out of the midday sun. Do not consume strong (concentrated) drinks, which means no sodas, carbonated pops or alco-pops. If you do take alcohol, make sure that you swallow plenty of water with it. Remember that salty food is also proportionately deficient in water; take less salt. Avoid dehydration at all costs.
- Exercise on a regular basis. Inactivity is more likely to lead to a calcium build up, leaving you more prone to developing kidney stones.
- If you are at all concerned about the amounts of supplements you need for your unique symptoms, call and speak to a qualified nutritionist at any of the companies mentioned on pages 13–15.

LEAKY GUT

(see also *Allergies, Candida, Irritable Bowel Syndrome* and *Low Stomach Acid*)

At any age the small villi (small finger-like protrusions) in the small intestine can become irritated or eroded, which allows larger, undigested food molecules and toxins to pass through our gut wall into the blood stream, which affects both the liver and the lymphatic system and places a greater strain on our immune system. These undigested food molecules are treated as foreign invaders and provoke an immune reaction. Our bodies then begin reacting to food as though it were an infection entering our system and sends out antibodies to fight it. This is one of the possible mechanisms that trigger rheumatoid arthritis, and is now recognised as a major trigger for most food intolerances and allergies and, in some people, migraines.

Various toxins accumulate in our body, especially in the small intestine (gut) and large bowel. The accumulation tends to be a combination of undigested food, impacted faeces, bacteria, fungi, parasites and dead cells. As the toxins build up, the gut wall can become irritated and damaged, which enables partly digested food molecules to cross it and make their way into the blood stream.

If you have a leaky gut you are unlikely to absorb or utilise the beneficial nutrients from your food as effectively as non-sufferers.

Leaky Gut Syndrome has now reached epidemic proportions, thanks mostly to stress, eating too many of the wrong foods, eating in a hurry, and so on. People with irritable bowel syndrome tend to have a leaky gut. Generally, if you suffer bloating, constipation and/or diarrhoea, crave sugary, refined foods, feel tired all the time, and/or notice that your food comes out the other end looking fairly much the same as it went in, you may well have a leaky gut. Candida, a yeast fungal overgrowth, is also a common cause of, or results from, a leaky gut. Most people with a leaky gut also tend to have low stomach acid (see *Low Stomach Acid*).

Foods to Avoid
- Grains from wheat, rye, oats and barley, if not properly assimilated, will continue on into the bowel and feed the bad bacteria, which can cause bloating. Eliminating grains for even a week will help to reduce a leaky gut.
- Sugar encourages fermentation and growth of unfriendly bacteria in the bowel, so keep sugary

foods and drinks to a minimum.

- If you tend to bloat a lot after meals, don't eat large amounts of fruit directly after a large protein meal, as fruit likes a quick passage through the gut. If it gets stuck behind proteins, such as meat, the fruit will ferment, which adds to the problem. Alcohol, vinegar and most pickled foods contribute to fermentation.
- Any foods to which you have an intolerance will only aggravate the problem, the most common being wheat, citrus fruits and sometimes cow's milk.
- Melon is particularly bad for a leaky gut – this should only ever be eaten on its own.
- Avoid heavy, fatty, large meals, which place a strain on the digestive system and the liver.
- Cut down on low-fibre foods, such as jellies, ice cream, burgers, biscuits, cakes, pies, pastries and so on.

Friendly Foods

- If you are desperate for sugar, use a little organic honey or zylosweet (HN).
- Include in your diet more natural low-fat, live yoghurt containing the friendly bacteria acidophilus and bifidus.
- Pineapple and papaya are rich in enzymes, which improve protein digestion, making it less likely that undigested proteins end up in the bowel.
- Beetroots, artichokes, radishes, celeriac and dandelion are all good liver-cleansers, which also improve digestion. They contain inulin, which helps encourage the growth of bifidus within the large bowel. This helps to reduce the load on the liver in the long term (see *Liver Problems*).
- Unsalted sunflower, pumpkin and sesame seeds, linseeds (flax seeds), and nuts are all rich sources of fibre. A great way to get more nuts and seeds into your diet is to place 1 tbsp each of sunflower, pumpkin, sesame seeds and walnuts, hazel or Brazil nuts in a coffee grinder or food mixer and pulse for a few seconds. Keep them in a screw-top jar in the fridge and sprinkle over cereals, salads, desserts, fruit, yoghurts and so on. The mixture will stay fresh for about a week.
- Drink plenty of water – at least 6 glasses a day.
- Garlic and onions help fight infections and encourage growth of friendly bacteria in the bowel.
- Organic-source chlorella is a great way to detoxify the system. Stir into smoothies or juices, or sprinkle over cereals and fruit salads.
- Use fresh root ginger in your cooking, which soothes and heals the gut.
- Green cabbage is rich in the amino acid L-glutamine, which helps heal a leaky gut. Eat more raw or steamed cabbage, and use the liquid from the cooking to make gravy and sauces.
- Eat plenty of fresh vegetables; and if you eat fruit, eat it between meals.
- Figs, apricots, apples and bananas all help to reduce constipation.
- Try quinoa, buckwheat or millet and plenty of brown rice.
- Most health shops sell pastas made from soya, millet or rice flour.
- Sprinkle rice bran over cereals.
- Drink more green tea.

Useful Remedies

- Take 2 capsules of acidophilus and bifidus bacteria after main meals to replenish healthy bacteria. This aids digestion and elimination. **BC**
- Take a digestive enzyme capsule with meals, such as Polyzyme Forte. **BC**
- L-glutamine, the amino acid, helps to heal a leaky gut. Take between 1 and 4 grams a day, on an empty stomach, for the first month and then reduce to 1 gram daily. Children can take Colostrum – a quarter teaspoon twice daily on an empty stomach. **NC**
- Take a high-strength, easily absorbable multi-vitamin and mineral supplement daily. (See *Kudos 24* in *General Supplements*; p.160)

- Sprinkle Alkalife Green Food, which is rich in wheat germ and green foods that re-alkalise your system, over cereals and desserts. To order contact Best Care Products on www.bestcare-uk.com
- Add 1–3 dessertspoons of raw, ready cracked linseeds (flax seeds) to your cereals or yoghurts every day. Keep the seeds in the fridge.
- After taking these supplements for 3 months, your gut should be in better shape and you could then reduce this regimen to a good multi-vitamin and mineral, plus a digestive enzyme daily.

Helpful Hints
- It is vital that you chew food thoroughly and more slowly, which helps break down the food more effectively. Many people with a leaky gut swallow large food particles in a hurry, which places a great strain on an already labouring digestive tract.
- Smoking increases the toxic load on the body and can make the situation worse.
- Make sure you get plenty of regular exercise and always walk for at least 15 minutes after a meal to aid digestion.
- Lower your stress levels (see *Stress*). Eat only light meals when stressed.
- Remember not to eat on the move – as much as possible eat in a relaxed, comfortable situation. At the very least sit down to eat.
- Read *Good Gut Healing: the No-nonsense Guide to Bowel and Digestive Disorders* by Kathryn Marsden (Cygnus Books).

LEG ULCERS
(see also *Circulation* and *Cholesterol*)

This is a very common problem in the over-60s, which is caused by restricted circulation, and a lack of oxygen and nutrients reaching the skin. Leg and foot ulcers are more common in diabetics because of changes in circulation and the nerve-endings near the skin.

Foods to Avoid
- Avoid foods that impede circulation including animal fats, especially red meats, sausages, meat pies, burgers, full-fat cheeses and dairy produce, as well as hard margarines made from refined vegetable oils.
- Avoid all fried foods and don't use mass-produced vegetable oils.
- Cut down on alcohol, and on low-fibre foods, such as jelly and ice cream, white breads, mass-produced pies and cakes.
- See dietary advice in *Circulation* and *Cholesterol*.

Friendly Foods
- Eat more leafy green vegetables, especially cabbage, kale, celery, pak choy, spinach and broccoli, which contain high levels of carotenes and minerals.
- Eat more salads and sprinkle sunflower, pumpkin and sesame seeds over them, as these seeds are high in essential fatty acids, minerals and fibre.
- Oily fish are rich in omega-3 fats, which thin the blood naturally and aid healing.
- Sprinkle wheat germ and lecithin granules over breakfast cereals to lower 'bad' cholesterol.
- Add almonds, Brazil nuts, hazelnuts and walnuts to fruit dips as they are all high in zinc, which aids skin-healing.
- High-protein foods, such as whey protein, are a very rich source of glutamine, which speeds the healing process. You can buy powdered whey at all health shops.
- Eat more garlic and onions which are anti-bacterial.
- Drink more organic green tea to help boost your immune system. It is delicious with a small amount of honey.

Useful Remedies

- Take zinc, 30mg, 1–2 times a day with meals. This is absolutely essential if you are suffering from slow wound-healing.
- Take gotu kola, 500mg, 3 times a day with meals. This herb has been used historically for wound-healing and when combined with zinc can be very successful. It helps increase circulation in lower limbs and can have a slight laxative effect – for many people this is a bonus!
- Vitamin C, 1 gram daily with food, is essential for healing connective tissue.
- If the ulcers are superficial and not too deep, aloe vera gel applied topically can speed healing, ease the discomfort, and protect from infection.
- Many elderly people cannot be bothered to cook proper meals, so if this is the case make sure you take an easily absorbed, high-quality multi-vitamin and mineral. (See *Kudos 24* in *General Supplements*; p.160)
- Ginkgo biloba helps to increase circulation. Take 120mg of standardised extract daily until symptoms ease.
- Try Kudos's "Circuplex", which contains butcher's broom (which improves the strength and tone of the veins), rutin, ginkgo biloba, hawthorn and grape seed extract. **KVH**
- Try Solgar's horse chestnut seed extract, which contains the active ingredient aescin. This ingredient has been shown to be very effective in supporting venous problems, and has the ability to strengthen capillaries and enhance circulation. **SVHC**

Helpful Hints

- Try Bach Rescue Remedy cream once the skin starts to heal – available from good health stores.
- V-Nal Cream (from Bional) contains a combination that includes horse chestnut, butcher's broom (an anti-inflammatory), elderflower, and soothing aloe and witch hazel. It is recommended for circulation in the legs and feet.
- Place raw Manuka honey on the site of the ulcer, which will speed the healing process. You can also buy Manuka Honey Dressings (made by Comvita), which are easier to use.
- Raise your legs above hip level when resting, and move your feet backwards and forwards slowly to increase the circulation in your lower legs. Try to walk for at least 15 minutes twice a day.
- Regular acupuncture and reflexology will greatly help to improve your circulation (see *Useful Information*).
- Wearing magnets in your shoes greatly aids circulation as magnets bring more blood to the affected areas and thus oxygenated blood, which helps to speed the healing process. These are now sold at good health stores and large pharmacies. Magnopulse in the UK also make magnet-filled dressings to place directly over wounds, which have been shown to heal faster with the magnet therapy. For details call Magnopulse on 0117 971 0710. Website: www.magnopulse.com

LIBIDO PROBLEMS   (see also *Impotence*)

It is important to remember that everyone has different appetites and you should not assume you have a "libido problem" just because you do not want sex as often as your friends or people in the media. Moreover, it is quite normal to experience a decline in desire as the years go by. Other pleasures, equally fulfilling, shared with your partner may take the place of sex, which then occasionally surfaces at moments of great tenderness, romance or nostalgia.

Libido is only a problem, as such, when an otherwise harmonious couple have sexual needs that are wildly different. As always, a compromise is a good solution – one partner trying harder to get in the mood and the other trying to reduce high demands.

Impotence in men and frigidity in women are extreme cases of lowered libido, where one or other partner cannot or does not wish to perform. This section gives advice covering all aspects of altered or diminished sexual function.

Dr Keith Scott-Mumby, a British doctor now living in Los Angeles, says, "Without doubt the single biggest factor that impairs sexual performance is poor general health. Conditions as varied as obesity, hypertension, stress, digestive disorders, depression and alcoholism will all result in lessened interest in sex. The number one turn-off for everyone is stress. Living a life full of worry, with an uncertain or threatening future, is bound to result in lowered libido."

He also points to the natural age-related decline in sexual function: "Hormone levels fall off slowly at first but by the fifth decade this natural slow-down process accelerates. Women experience a dramatic shift at the menopause. Men suffer a more gradual process that is widely overlooked, known as the andropause.

"Beyond the menopause, lowered oestrogen levels for women may result in vaginal dryness and soreness. This obviously interferes with sexual desire and performance. The onset of andropause for men is an indicator of diminishing testosterone levels and this leads to loss of libido – interestingly, healthy women also need low levels of natural testosterone, which drives their libido." If you would like to contact Dr Mumby, log on to www.alternative-doctor.com

Foods to Avoid

- Make a real effort to lose weight if you have piled on those pounds. You'll feel sexier, look better and experience the energies you lost years ago.
- Avoid refined carbohydrates, sugar, high sodium salt foods, and the saturated fats found in red meat, full-fat dairy produce, sausages, chocolates, meat pies and other manufactured foods.
- Eliminate caffeine and drink only de-caff or better-still herbal tea, and low-sugar or diluted fruit juices.
- Reduce your alcohol intake to 20 units a week or less. Remember Shakespeare's words "Alcohol promotes the desire but takes away the performance."

Friendly Foods

- Pumpkin and sunflower seeds, linseeds and oysters are rich in zinc – vital for a healthy sex life.
- Plenty of garlic and onions in your diet improves circulation and helps lower LDL, the 'bad' cholesterol.
- Sprinkle cayenne pepper and turmeric over your food to add spice to your life; you can also take them in tincture or capsule form.
- Eat more fresh fruits and vegetables and replace red meat with fresh fish and chicken.
- See *General Health Hints*.

Useful Remedies

- The herbal remedy ginkgo biloba, when taken regularly, improves circulation. Kudos makes a high strength one-a-day (900mg). Then break for a month and begin again, making a cycle of 3 months on, 1 month off. **KVH**
- Korean ginseng, taken 500–1000mg a day, helps to reduce the underlying stress that is often linked to this problem. This is shown to be more effective when taken for a month, then stopped for a month and so on.
- Suma, the South American root, can help restore libido. Take 500–1000mg daily for up to 3 months.
- Damiana, a herb from Mexico and India, is a natural aphrodisiac for men and women. Take 125–500mg a day until libido is restored. **NC**
- Stress reduces B-vitamins in the body – therefore also include a good-quality multi-vitamin and

mineral for men that includes a full range of B-vitamins.

- Muira puama, a South American herb, is considered nature's most potent viagra. A daily dose of 1 gram of a standardised extract has been shown to be effective as it raises testosterone levels. In one study of 100 men with impotence problems, 66% had increased frequency of intercourse, while 70% reported intensification of libido. The stability of the erection was restored in 55% of the patients and 66% reported a reduction in fatigue. The herb is suitable for both men and women. **NC**
- The herb maca has been found to improve libido in men and women as it helps to balance hormones, so if the problem is hormonal try 1 capsule 3 times daily (500mg). **KVH**

Helpful Hints

- Measures to alleviate stress are often very effective. Take regular exercise and learn to laugh more. This releases natural endorphins, which lower stress levels and help you to feel more positive. Learn to breathe more deeply.
- If there is a problem, you must discuss matters openly with your significant other. If one partner's needs are not being met it can lead to frustration and even hostility. It is unfair to put your partner in a position where they have no ethical means of satisfying their physical desires.
- Quit smoking. You'll be glad you did. Smoking has been linked with reduced ability to maintain an erection, because it constricts the blood-flow that is essential for erectile function.
- Ylang ylang, rose and jasmine therapeutic oils applied to the lower abdomen area can help revive a flagging sex drive in men and women. Look at the resources page on www.psalifemastery.com for details of Young Livings Oils.
- People who use a large amount of marijuana or take steroids may also find their erectile function diminished.
- By constantly worrying about your lack of sex drive, you often make the situation worse. Studies show that a lack of vitamins C, E, A, B and the minerals zinc and selenium can cause a low sperm count and lack of sex drive. Anyone taking regular antidepressants or sleeping pills may be lacking in these nutrients.
- Have your hormone levels checked – testosterone patches are known to help increase libido in both sexes. Once hormones are restored often sex drive returns (see also *Menopause*).
- If the condition continues, or you are worried about infertility as well as impotency, see a doctor who is also a nutritionist (see *Useful Information*).
- Acupuncture can help with poor libido by unblocking energy channels within the body, which helps increase blood-flow (see *Useful Information*).
- Discuss whatever turns you on with your partner. If you find that difficult, discuss sex in general until you are more comfortable with this topic. To help get you in the mood, try watching a sexy movie, which works for many people!
- Try reading *His Needs Her Needs – Building an Affair-proof Marriage* by Willard F. Harley, Jr.; or take a look at the website at www.marriagebuilders.com
- Try reading *What Your Doctor May Not Tell You About the Menopause* by John R. Lee, MD; or take a look at the website at www.johnleemd.com
- Try reading *Maximize Your Vitality and Potency: For Men Over 40* by Jonathan V. Wright, MD; or visit the website at www.tahoma-clinic.com)
- All these books can be ordered from the Nutri Centre Bookshop on 020 7323 2382.

LICHEN PLANUS

Lichen planus is a chronic condition of the skin and mucous membranes, typically the lining of the mouth. This is thought to be caused by a virus and has some features in common with other skin problems, such as eczema and psoriasis. Sores on the skin are often localized on the wrist and ankles, but they can be widespread.

Foods to Avoid
- Anything that weakens the immune system, such as concentrated sugars, refined carbohydrates, even concentrated fruit juices, and any food to which you have an intolerance.
- Foods that are a problem for many sufferers are tomatoes, pineapples, mushrooms, coffee, red meat, chocolate and ice cream. Keep a food diary and note when symptoms are worse, so you can identify and remove those foods from your diet.
- Alcohol, vinegars and oily, spicy foods can make the problem worse – avoid them.
- Avoid dairy produce from cows as much as possible.

Friendly Foods
- Eat more fresh fish of any kind, but try to make it oily fish, such as wild salmon, cod, sardines or mackerel. Oily fish are rich in omega-3 essential fats and vitamin A. Aim for twice a week.
- Beta carotene converts to vitamin A in the body and aids the healing process. Therefore, eat plenty of carrots, green vegetables, French beans, cress, spinach, cantaloupe melons, spring greens, watercress, sweet potatoes, apricots (fresh and dried), pumpkin, butternut squash, parsley and mangoes. A little butter is also fine as it is rich in vitamin A. Organic is best.

- Organic unrefined and unsalted nuts and seeds, such as sunflower, pumpkin, sesame, linseeds (flax seeds), and Brazil nuts and walnuts, are high in zinc, which can speed up healing.

Useful Remedies
- Take vitamin A, 20,000iu a day for up to 2 months, as there is speculation that lichen planus is due to a vitamin-A deficiency. If you are pregnant or planning a pregnancy only take 3000iu daily.
- Take a good-quality multi-vitamin and mineral.
- Take 30mg of zinc in addition to the multi once a day. Zinc and vitamin A are complementary in their action. Zinc is essential for wound-healing and a healthy immune system.
- Organic aloe vera juice – 20ml taken before every meal – speeds healing, and reduces discomfort as well as boosting the immune system.
- Anti-viral herbs are echinacea, liquorice and St John's wort. They can all be used internally and applied topically to the skin.

Helpful Hints
- Try to rest as much as possible. Don't overwork and don't over-stress your system as it is much harder for the body to heal.
- Use washing powders and detergents suitable for sensitive skin.
- Ultraviolet light often brings relief, but try this only under proper supervision.
- Moderate amounts of sunshine can help too, but avoid sunbathing between 11am and 3pm.
- Chickweed ointment has been useful to some people.
- Homeopathy has helped many sufferers (see *Useful Information*).

LIVER PROBLEMS

Your liver is the most overworked organ in the body, having to break down all the increasing toxins found in our environment (including our air and water) and our food. It is, in essence, the chemical factory of your body that builds or recycles substances you need for good health and breaks down those you don't. If your liver isn't functioning properly, toxins that would normally be filtered by the liver accumulate in the body. Most people's livers today work only at around 35–40% of their potential capacity because of the large amount of toxins we ingest. When it's working properly the liver can clean up to 99% of bacteria and toxins from the blood. Around 4 pints (2.25 litres) of blood pass through the liver every minute for detoxification, and every day the liver manufactures about 2 pints (1 litre) of bile, which helps carry away toxins via the bowel.

Typical symptoms of a sluggish liver are, feeling constantly tired even though you have slept, nausea (especially after a fatty meal or alcohol), skin disorders such as acne, eczema and psoriasis, muscle and joint pain, age spots on the skin, and regular infections. Also, most people don't associate being constipated with poor liver function, but blood from the bowel goes first to the liver, via the portal venous system, hence a bowel loaded with rubbish is going to overwork the liver.

Other symptoms of poor liver function can include yellowing whites of the eyes, yellow-looking skin, fever, nausea, difficulty digesting fatty foods, and an increased sensitivity to cigarette smoke, strong perfume, petrol and other chemicals.

Because the brain is unable to disarm a wide range of toxins it relies on the liver to clean the blood before it gets there. So, over the long term, an under-performing liver can have dire consequences for the brain and nervous system, including memory loss, Parkinson's Disease and Alzheimer's Disease.

While detoxification is the key function of the liver, it also produces bile to aid fat digestion (as well as eliminate toxins); manufactures and balances hormones; stores various vitamins and minerals; assembles amino acids; makes cholesterol; controls glucose and fat supplies; and plays a key role in immunity.

Your digestive system is closely involved in the health of your liver, as the blood from your digestive system, where nutrients are absorbed from your food, goes directly to the liver for filtering before it goes anywhere else in the body. If your diet is good and your digestion and absorption are working well, then the nutrients needed for good health will make it to the liver and then on into the body. However if your digestive system is generally toxic, thanks to a poor, low-nutrient, high-fat diet, constipation, poor gut flora, and so on, these toxins, and any others you ingest, will similarly be delivered directly to your liver which adds to the liver's workload.

The good news is that the liver is capable of regenerating itself, so with a good diet and lifestyle and the right supplements there's no reason you can't maintain liver function at an optimal level at any age. And if you look after your liver, your skin literally glows with health.

Begin by eliminating as many unnatural chemicals as possible from your home and environment. Keep in mind that many manmade chemicals (especially in plastics and pesticides) have a hormone-like effect within the body – therefore the incidence of hormone-related cancers (including breast, ovarian, testicular and prostate cancer) are all increasing. These chemicals are commonly found in plastic food-packaging, non-organic food, plastics and laminates, synthetic fabrics (clothes, carpets, furniture), dry-cleaning chemicals, air-'fresheners' (a misnomer, most of them poison the air), cosmetics, paints, glues, food additives, medicines, household cleaning products and wallpaper… but the list is virtually endless, and they are all around us.

You could drive yourself crazy trying to avoid all these things, but you would be surprised at how many healthier, safer alternatives to all the above are available if you are willing to seek them out.

Foods to Avoid

- Avoid excess alcohol, which is a liver toxin. 1–2 units per day is generally considered not harmful, although the best gauge is how you feel afterwards or the next day. If you feel worse than you should, your liver is probably struggling to detoxify the alcohol.
- Reduce your consumption of non-organic food as much as possible, as certain foods such as lettuces are often sprayed up to 11 times with pesticides and/or fungicides before they are harvested.
- When you can't avoid non-organic fruits and vegetables, wash them thoroughly, or use a weak vinegar/water solution to remove the majority of the pesticide residues, which are designed to resist being washed off easily by water (in other words, rain). Until recently even the UK government advised peeling fruit for young children to reduce the risk.
- If you're trying to detox or suspect your liver is under-functioning, avoid eating or drinking grapefruit. It contains narningenin, a compound known to slow liver detoxification. A glass of grapefruit juice can significantly affect the action of some medications, which explains why some very expensive medications are prescribed with grapefruit juice, it slows down the body's ability to remove the drug, thus increasing it's efficacy.

- Avoid eating excessive protein, as protein metabolism gives the liver a lot of work to do. Generally reduce your animal-protein (meat, chicken, dairy) intake, and increase the amount of vegetable protein in your diet from beans, lentils, nuts, seeds, fermented soya products, such as tempeh or miso, plus whole grains, such as brown rice.
- Reduce your intake of saturated fats, especially hydrogenated or trans-fats, fried and highly processed foods. Don't avoid all fat, essential fats from oily fish and seeds are vital for proper liver function (see *Fats You Need To Eat*).
- Caffeine, paracetamol, aspirin and most other medications place a strain on the liver. A good alternative to coffee is dandelion coffee, available in health food stores.
- Melted cheese is very difficult for the liver to process – avoid as much as possible.
- Eggs are an excellent source of nutrients – but for anyone with liver problems, they are hard to digest. Keep it down to two a week.

Friendly Foods

- Increase your intake of all fruit and vegetables, especially those rich in antioxidants, such as organic carrots, tomatoes, alfalfa sprouts, peppers and watercress.
- Eat more berries, grapes, cabbage, broccoli, Brussels sprouts, and kale. Aim for 40% of your diet to be raw in summer. This is not nearly as hard as it sounds if you eat plenty of fresh fruit and salads.
- Eat artichokes, black cherries, pears and celeriac, all of which help support the liver.
- Eat more beetroot, raw or cooked – it's one of the best vegetables for the liver because it aids digestion, improves liver function, and reduces constipation.
- Sprinkle a dessertspoon of lecithin granules over breakfast cereals, fruits and yoghurts, as lecithin helps the body to digest fats, which eases the burden on the liver.
- If you know that your liver is a problem, eat lighter meals regularly and avoid heavy, rich meals. If you eat too much in one sitting, especially fatty or fried foods and alcohol, then you place an enormous burden on the digestion and liver, which could make you feel nauseous.
- Foods that naturally raise glutathione levels (see below) in the body are fresh asparagus, avocado and walnuts. Spinach and tomatoes are also great foods for raising glutathione – but

they need to be eaten raw.

- Curcumin, the pigment that gives the spice turmeric its yellow colour, has shown a great ability to increase gluathione production. Found in curries and mustards, curcumin also has fantastic anti-inflammatory properties. People who suffer MS, Parkinson's Disease and Alzheimer's Disease tend to not eat too many curries. For the best effect, toast the curcumin seeds and then lightly grind them before adding them to foods. You can now buy pure curcumin capsules. **SHS**
- Eat organically produced food as much as possible, the Food Standards Agency in the UK acknowledges that pesticide residues are likely to be considerably lower in organic food than in conventional produce. You are also likely to encounter far fewer food additives and no unnecessary artificial colourings or flavourings.

Useful Remedies

- As always, start with a good-quality multi-vitamin, which provides a baseline of nutrients you can then add to. Make sure it contains 15–30mg of zinc. Many multi-vitamins now also contain most of the nutrients below. Try Kudos 24 (see *General Supplements*; p.160).
- Take 1 gram of vitamin C daily.
- Take a 1 gram of fish oil or 1 linseed (flax seed) oil capsule daily. Make sure the fish oil you buy is free of toxins such as PCBs and dioxins.
- Magnesium is required by literally hundreds of enzymes throughout the body, many of which have a detoxifying function. Take at least 350mg daily; twice that if you have backache, twitching and/or can't sleep.
- The best-known remedy for the liver is the herb milk thistle, which contains the bioflavonoid silymarin, which promotes cell regeneration in the liver, increases levels of glutathione in the liver (see below), and has been shown to repair liver damage from alcohol. For optimum effects you need 600mg of standardised extract daily. Kudos makes a high-strength one-a-day (900mg) milk thistle. **KVH**

- The most powerful antioxidant and detoxifying compound in the liver is glutathione, a naturally occurring amino acid combination. Unfortunately it is not particularly well-absorbed via capsules; however alpha lipoic acid (50–100mg a day) and N-acetyl cysteine (NAC; 500–600mg a day taken in-between meals) and vitamin C increase production of glutathione in the liver, as well as protecting the liver and being first-rate antioxidants in their own right. Within the body you also need B-vitamins and selenium to make more glutathione.
- Another key nutrient needed by the liver is sulphur. It can be supplemented as MSM or the amino acids cysteine and methionine. Take 500mg of all three daily. Also include sulphur-rich foods in your diet, including garlic, asparagus, cabbage and broccoli.
- The nutrients choline, inositol and l-methionine, prevent the accumulation of fat in the liver, thereby enhancing general liver function (take 300–400mg of each, 1–3 times per day). Methionine also aids liver de-toxification.

Helpful Hints

- Standard tests for liver function involve measuring levels of key enzymes. If they're raised, it means that your liver is struggling. This indicates a chronic problem and while it's useful in indicating a problem exists, it doesn't tell you the best way to help recovery. A better, non-invasive test, that is available through nutritionists, is a comprehensive Liver Detoxification Profile. This urine test tells you exactly which detox phases and pathways in the liver are under-performing and you can then be advised which nutrients are needed to restore normal function (to find a qualified nutritionist see under *Useful Information* at the back of the book).
- Stop smoking and reduce the amount of time you spend in traffic, there can be more pollution inside your car than outside! If you are walking or cycling, avoid busy roads where possible.
- The intravenous therapy called chelation is marvellous for delivering large amounts of nutrients,

especially glutiathione into the body. Full details about chelation are in my book *500 of the Most Important Ways to Stay Younger Longer* (Cico Books); or call Dr Robert Trossell on 020 7486 1095, or Dr Wendy Denning on 020 7224 2423.

- Indoor air pollution is now recognised as a real problem, and the availability of more natural household cleaning products, paints and fibres has improved dramatically in recent years. Visit your local health food store for natural cleaning products, such as Ecover and see health, environmental, and/or organic magazines like *The Ecologist* for details of more natural products.

- Use a water filter to remove unwanted chemicals from your drinking supply. Reverse osmosis (RO) filters remove 99.999% of all known chemicals, but they also remove minerals. So, if you drink only RO water you will need to take a multi-mineral daily. RO water will even filter anthrax spores. For details of RO water contact the Pure H2O Company on 01784 221188. Website: www.purewater.co.uk. Or the Fresh Water Filter Company on 0208 597 3223. Website: www.freshwaterfilter.com

- Another good option is to drink bottled still, natural mineral water – Volvic and Fiji or Belgian Spa Water are the preferred choice of many nutritionists. A filter jug containing a simple carbon filter is the bare minimum, but don't forget to change the cartridges regularly.

- Because the liver is responsible for balancing hormones, if it's not working efficiently, hormones can accumulate inappropriately or become unbalanced, triggering problems like facial hair. Also many women who take the pill and orthodox HRT have put on weight – this could be because these hormones place a greater strain on the liver.

- According to Traditional Chinese Medicine, the liver does most work between 1 and 3am in the morning. Liver dysfunction will often wake a person up at these times.

- The liver detoxes more efficiently when we are lying down and relaxed, so make sure you are getting sufficient sleep.

- Don't eat large meals late at night or drink alcohol after 11pm if you know your liver is in trouble.

- Repressed anger and resentments affect liver function, so deal with any stress-type issues.

- Coffee enemas have long been known to stimulate liver function as they increase bile flow from the liver and gall bladder and aid detoxification. A great book to read is *Tired or Toxic?* by Sherry Rogers (Prestige Publishing).

LOW BLOOD PRESSURE (HYPOTENSION)

(see also *Low Blood Sugar*)

The most classic symptom of low blood pressure is a feeling of light-headedness on standing, especially from the ground up. It is more common in women. Orthodox doctors in the UK do not think of low blood pressure as a problem, however, in certain European countries the condition is often treated. Because the blood is responsible for carrying oxygen and nutrients to the body's tissues and organs, low blood pressure can often trigger problems with energy levels and mental function. The condition is frequently a sign of weakness in the adrenal glands (see *Stress*). These glands sit on top of your kidneys and have an important role to play in your hormonal system. Adrenal weakness is often a result of overworking and excessive stresses, compounded by dietary deficiencies. Far too many of us have a lifestyle that overstresses our adrenal glands. We work too many hours, don't get sufficient sleep and tend to rely on coffee and sugar to get us through the day or to pick us up when our energy levels drop. In the long term all these factors weaken adrenal function.

One of the most common complaints received by staff in health food shops these days is that of feeling tired all the time. The first question you need to ask yourself is, do you start the day with a good breakfast or find that you can't face breakfast and the only thing that gets you going is two or three cups of tea or coffee. What you are doing is putting a stimulant into your body that puts even more stress on your adrenal glands.

Foods to Avoid

- Caffeine and sugar in any form will particularly deplete the adrenal glands. Remember that tea, coffee, chocolate and cola all contain caffeine. You might remember not to put sugar in your tea or coffee, but are you having several biscuits with it? Everything in moderation.
- Refined foods such as bread, biscuits, cakes, pizza, burgers and pies all deplete the body of the B-vitamins necessary to keep the adrenal glands in good shape.

Friendly Foods

- Liquorice is one of the quickest and simplest ways of restoring adrenal glands to normal function. Look for pure liquorice sweetened with molasses sold in most health stores.
- Eat more quality protein, such as fresh fish, chicken, lentils, beans pulses and tempeh. Protein helps to normalise blood pressure.
- Whole grains, which include brown rice, quinoa, millet and amaranth, are highly nutritious. Eat more of them.
- Eat plenty of fresh fruit and vegetables, particularly fresh juices – if you are feeling low in energy, rather than reaching for a coffee, try a glass of carrot, beetroot, apple and ginger juice.
- Green tea has a small amount of caffeine, which will give you a boost – and contains many health benefits. Or try ginseng or liquorice teas, which will support your adrenal glands.
- Eat more avocados and wheat germ, which are rich in vitamin E.
- Use potassium- and magnesium-based salt, such as Solo Salt, in your diet. BioForce also make excellent herbal salts.

Useful Remedies

- Liquorice Formula, taken 1–3ml a day for up to three months, is a blend of herbs to nourish the adrenal glands. Over time it will help increase energy and can also help to normalise blood pressure. **FSC**
- Take high-potency B-complex – 1 twice daily with meals. Take B-vitamins with breakfast and lunch, but not with supper, as they keep you more alert.
- As the mineral magnesium is often lacking in people with hypotension, take 250–500mg daily with food.
- Ginseng taken 1–3 grams a day for 60 days helps to balance the body. If the blood pressure is low it can help to bring it back up and ginseng has the added benefit of being an excellent adrenal restorative.
- Try Dr Christopher's Blood Circulation capsules, which contain ginger, cayenne and hawthorn. These help to normalize blood pressure (high or low); 1 or 2 capsules three times daily with meals. **SHS**

Helpful Hints

- Take sensible amounts of exercise but also make sure you are getting sufficient rest.
- See *General Health Hints*.
- See *Stress*.

LOW BLOOD SUGAR (HYPOGLYCAEMIA)

Low blood sugar, also known as hypoglycaemia, is something that 95% of us experience at some time if we go without food for too long – the most common cause is skipping breakfast. I have met a number of young women who suffer regular blackouts, fainting spells, and dizziness that their doctor cannot explain. But when they relate their diet of missed meals and sugary drinks and snacks I know almost immediately what the problem is.

The level of sugar in the blood is critical to how you feel. If it is too low, you may well feel very tired, find concentration difficult, become shaky, feel very hungry and drowsy, possibly have headaches, and feel anxious. These myriad symptoms can simply result from skipping breakfast.

If you are one of those people who won't eat breakfast for the sake of an extra 15 to 20 minutes in bed, or simply can't face it in the mornings and then rush off to work, by mid-morning you are going to feel even hungrier than you did when you left the house. Most people then reach for coffee and a doughnut, tea and biscuits, something that will quickly raise blood-sugar levels. Unfortunately, not long after consuming this type of food, our blood sugar drops even lower than it was before. This is a result of the body producing an excess of insulin to compensate for the sugar load. One of the problems with skipping breakfast is that even if your first meal of the day (lunch) is a good wholesome one, your blood-sugar levels are still likely to be very erratic, bouncing up and down all day long. This can lead you to becoming irritable with your colleagues or extremely emotional in response to even small problems.

Other people with low blood sugar will find it crucial to have their meals at regular times. If their lunch hour is normally midday and someone asks them to leave it until 2pm, they may feel weak, suffer memory problems or simply find it hard to concentrate. If they are dealing with the public, they are much more likely to be short-tempered and less approachable. If they are trying to complete a task, the work is likely to be of lower quality than it would have been if they had eaten at the regular time.

The brain's only food source is pure glucose and, if you have not eaten for a while, the hypothalamus area within the brain will just demand more sugar. Basically, if your hypothalamus is not happy, no amount of willpower will stop you craving something sweet. Nutritionists have known for years that the easiest way to control blood sugar is to eat small, healthy meals more regularly, but most people don't do this. The average person in the West eats 35lbs of snacks a year, which cause weight gain and a very unstable blood sugar. The result is a huge increase in diabetes. As symptoms of low blood sugar are similar to those of high-blood-sugar diabetes, have a check-up with your doctor. However, a single blood test is unlikely to show any problem with low blood sugar, because unless you are actually suffering a dip in blood sugar at the time of the test, results could be normal. See also *Insulin Resistance*.

Foods to Avoid
- Most people with low blood sugar rush from one sugar fix to the next. In extreme cases they might eat 6–8 chocolate-type snacks daily. Cravings for caffeine, sugar, refined carbohydrates, such as croissants, biscuits, pastries and pizzas, are all common. Not only do all these foods have a negative effect on blood sugar, they are also low in fibre, vitamins and minerals.

Friendly Foods
- Fibre helps to slow down the release of sugars, and if absent, the sugars in any foods get into the bloodstream too quickly. Great fibres are linseeds (flax seeds), oat or rice bran, sunflower seeds, and psyllium husks.
- Begin the day with a good breakfast, such as low-sugar muesli or cereal, porridge, eggs, or beans on toast.

- If you have time for only a small meal, try to make sure it is high in protein rather than carbohydrate, which will keep you more satisfied in the long term.
- At the very least eat a banana and a low-fat fruit yoghurt.
- Eat more brown rice, barley, oats, lentils, amaranth, spelt, and wholemeal bread and pastas; also try corn, spinach and rice pastas.
- Make sure you eat a portion of good-quality protein with each meal – such as fish, lean meats, chicken, turkey, cooked tofu, eggs or whey protein powder.
- Eat smaller meals more regularly or eat three sensible meals a day.
- Snack on fresh fruit and low-sugar snack bars available from health shops. Or use low-fat hummus on an amaranth cracker or rye crispbread.
- Drink freshly made or organic fruit and vegetable juices.
- Snack on low-fat yoghurts with added sunflower seeds and raisins to reduce sugar cravings.
- Have a piece of wholemeal toast or an amaranth cracker with a little low-fat spread and low-sugar jam or honey.
- Drink more herbal teas and pure dandelion coffee. (NB: some brands contain 50% lactose, which is a form of sugar.)
- Drink more water.
- Make salad dressings with a combination of any unrefined organic oils, such as sesame, walnut, olive or sunflower.
- Essential fats help sustain energy levels and help balance blood sugar. See *Fats You Need To Eat*.

Useful Remedies

- In the US studies have shown that when people who eat a refined Western diet, are given 200mcg of the mineral chromium twice daily, the incidence of late-onset diabetes was halved. Chromium is greatly depleted in the body by sugar and junk foods. Once you cut down on sugar and white carbohydrates, you may crave sweet foods. Therefore, begin taking 400 mcg of chromium daily. It takes a few days to kick in but really does help reduce cravings. After 2 weeks reduce to 200mcg.
- Take 200–500mg magnesium once a day with food. Magnesium helps regulate blood-sugar levels.
- Take a strong B-complex with 30mg of niacinamide B3. **(Make sure it's a no-flush type niacin, as niacin can cause skin-flushing.)** B3 is essential for the control of blood-sugar levels.
- Take vitamin E, 500–600 units, a day as vitamin E has been shown to help improve insulin response in the body.
- BioCare make Sucro Guard, developed by Dr John Briffa. Taken between meals it contains all the above nutrients in one capsule. **BC**

Helpful Hints

- If you suffer acute symptoms, such as fainting fits, blackouts, extreme weakness and trembling, it is important to restore blood sugar levels as quickly as possible. In an emergency you need to get glucose into your body. While I would generally not recommend high-sugar foods and drinks, this is one occasion when you can use them. Drink Lucozade or similar, or eat a sugary biscuit. This is not a long-term solution!
- Your own GP can refer you to the nearest doctor who is also a qualified nutritionist (see *Useful Information*).

LOW STOMACH ACID   (see also *Acid Stomach* and *Indigestion*)

When we eat food, particularly protein-based foods, our stomachs should produce a lot of gastric juice in response. This juice is a mixture of mucus, which protects the stomach lining, and a very strong acid, hydrochloric acid. High levels of hydrochloric acid are needed for proper digestion before the food goes on to the small intestine and the nutrients start to be absorbed. Due to various aspects of our diet, lifestyle and age, the amount of acid we produce over time tends to decline. Low levels of stomach acid are associated with poor digestion and, more importantly, the poor absorption of nutrients we need for good health.

Conditions strongly linked with low-stomach-acid levels are asthma, allergies, leaky gut and gall stones, and the problem can be a factor in stomach ulcers. Many people feel they make too much stomach acid, whereas in reality they often produce too little. A lot of people will take an antacid, which neutralises what little acid was available, making digestion even harder. Undigested foods can end up leaking into the bloodstream causing food allergies. Undigested food can rot in the bowel causing wind, bloating, and overgrowth of unhealthy organisms such as candida (see *Candida*).

Foods to Avoid
- Cut down on alcohol, sugar, caffeinated foods and drinks and cow's dairy products, which can all cause an acid reflux.
- Don't eat in a rush and keep heavy, rich meals containing red meat and creamy sauces to a minimum.
- Avoid all fried foods, which are hard to digest.
- Avoid eating proteins, like fish or meat, with potatoes or pasta.
- Avoid drinking too much liquid with meals.
- Stop chewing gum – this makes the stomach think that food is about to arrive, which triggers stomach-acid production.
- Avoid eating large amounts of fruit directly after a large meal.

Friendly Foods
- Chew your food thoroughly and take your time eating.
- Eat fruit generally between meals or include a little papaya and pineapple with meals, which are packed with digestive enzymes.
- Bitter-tasting vegetables are great for stimulating digestion – eat more rocket, radicchio and celeriac, as well as ginger. These foods encourage gastric-juice production.

Useful Remedies
- As levels of stomach acid tend to drop as we age or when we are under stress, take 1 betaine hydrochloride (stomach acid) capsule with a glass of water just before your main meals. If you have active stomach ulcers, use a good-quality digestive enzyme that is free from HCl instead.
- Try Peppermint Formula, 10–20 drops before a meal. If you suffer with symptoms of overeating, and/or feeling bloated and uncomfortable take 10–20 drops after a meal. **FSC**
- Acidophilus and bifidus are the healthy bacteria that help to regulate digestion. Take 1–2 capsules at the end of the meal.

Helpful Hints
- Chewing food thoroughly really helps to improve the digestive process.
- Some people have found separating proteins and carbohydrates at one meal has improved their digestion no end. Buy a book on food combining – Kathryn Marsden's are still the best.
- Eat small meals regularly, try 4 snack-type meals daily. Avoid eating when stressed.
- Dr John Briffa suggests this home test for low stomach acid. Take a level teaspoon of bicarbonate of soda and dissolve in some water. Drink this mixture on an empty stomach. If sufficient quantities of acid are present in the stomach, the bicarb mixture is converted into gas, producing significant bloating and belching within 5–10 minutes of drinking the mix. Little or no belching denotes low stomach acid.
- If you have pronounced longitudinal ridges in your nails, this is a common sign of low stomach acid.
- Drink mint or peppermint, fennel or fresh mint herbal teas to aid digestion.
- Walking for 30 minutes each day aids digestion.

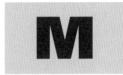

MACULAR DEGENERATION (see also *Eye Problems*)

Macular degeneration (also known as AMD – aged-related macular degeneration) is the slow deterioration of cells in the macula, a tiny yellowish area in the central part of the retina, which is responsible for visual sharpness. This deterioration affects your ability to read, write, drive and so on. Macular degeneration is now the leading cause of blindness in people over the age of 55, and 25% of people in the West over the age of 65 have symptoms of AMD – symptoms that increase over time.

There are 2 types of macular degeneration: wet and dry. 90% of people with macular degeneration have the dry type, in which small, yellow spots, called drusens, form underneath the macular. Drusens are waste products that accumulate because of lack of antioxidants to clear them from the eyes. The drusens slowly break down the cells in the macular, causing distorted vision. In the wet type, abnormal blood vessels begin to grow toward the macular, causing rapid and severe vision loss.

Scientists now believe that AMD is triggered by oxidative stress, caused by free-radical reactions in the body, especially in the retina because of its high consumption of oxygen. Free-radical reactions occur as the normal by-products of living, eating and breathing, but also from over-exposure to ultra-violet radiation, and from smoking, a poor diet and a compromised immune system. The condition is also linked to the hardening of the arteries and poor circulation (see under *High Blood Pressure* and *Circulation*).

Some people believe that macular degeneration is inherited, but diet is a far more important factor. However, women with light-coloured irises are more at risk of AMD.

Foods to Avoid
- Full-fat dairy foods, plus meats, hamburgers, mass-produced pies, sausages, cheeses, chocolates and sugary, fatty foods – all the usual suspects.
- Definitely avoid too many fried foods and hydrogenated or trans fats, which are found in most margarines and mass-produced vegetable oils (see *Fats You Need To Eat*).
- Cut down or eliminate sodium-based salt; instead use a natural mineral-based salt, which is available from all good health stores.
- Avoid monosodium glutamate (MSG), which is a potential retinal toxin.
- Avoid excessive alcohol, but the occasional glass of wine is fine. Too much alcohol interferes with liver function, and reduces protective glutathione levels in the eyes. (As glutathione is so important, see *Liver Problems* for more details.)
- At all costs avoid foods and drinks containing the artificial sweetener aspartame.

Friendly Foods
- The most important foods for reducing and preventing AMD are carotenes (especially lutein and zeaxanthin).
  * *Lutein* is found in all dark green leafy vegetables, such as spinach (raw is best), kale, broccoli, spring greens, cabbage and so on.
  * *Zeaxanthin* is found in yellow and orange fruits and vegetables, such as carrots, yams, peaches, persimmons, pumpkins, sweet potatoes, mangoes, apricots and cantaloupe melons.

- Other great eye foods are onions, apples, green tea, cherries, pears, grapes, cranberries, red onions, garlic, mustard greens, alfalfa sprouts, asparagus and butternut squash.
- Generally, eat more whole foods, such as brown bread, rice and pastas.
- Eat oily fish and other fish in preference to meats.
- Eat more blueberries, bilberries and blackcurrants.
- In addition, green drinks made from organic grasses, blue-green and sea algae, herbs and other nutrients are very helpful. Most health shops sell excellent organic green-food-based powders.
- Vitamin-E-rich foods help to reduce the risk of developing AMD. These include hazelnuts, almonds, cod liver oil, raw wheat germ, avocado, and tomato purée.

Useful Remedies

- Take a high-strength, multi-vitamin and mineral daily as a base. Make sure your multi contains 200mcg of selenium and 50mg of zinc. See *Kudos 24* in *General Supplements*; see p.160.
- Bilberry has been called the vision herb for its powerful effect on all types of visual disorders. British Royal Air Force pilots during World War II reported improved nighttime vision after consuming bilberry. The fruit supports the structural integrity of the tiny capillaries that deliver oxygen and nutrients to the eyes. Take 200–300mg daily.
- Bioflavonoids, such as quercetin and rutin, are neither vitamins nor minerals but plant pigments, rich in antioxidants that protect the eyes from sunlight damage. Take 1000mg daily of a mixed bioflavonoid supplement.

- Glutathione is essential for vision. This is an antioxidant found in large concentrations in the eye. Diminished levels of glutathione occur during ageing, which makes the lens nucleus susceptible to oxidative stress-induced clouding. Take 500mg daily. See *Liver Problems*.
- Cysteine is important for a healthy retina. Taken as N-acetylcysteine (NAC) it increases production of glutathione, one of the most important antioxidants in the eye. Take 500mg daily
- Taurine is another potent antioxidant that is highly concentrated within the eye, normally found in high concentrations in the retina. A deficiency of this amino acid alters the structure and function of the retina. Taurine also helps to prevent cataracts. Take 500mg daily.
- If you don't eat plenty of carotene-rich foods, you definitely need to take a high-strength, natural-source carotene complex.
- Vitamin C helps to make collagen, which strengthens the capillaries that nourish the retina, and protects against UV light. The eye contains the second-highest concentration of vitamin C in the body next to the adrenal glands. Take 1 gram daily in an ascorbate form.
- Most of the companies listed on pages 13–15 make all-in-one eye formulae that contain most of the above.

Helpful Hints

- Make sure you get sufficient exercise, which helps increase circulation.
- Acupuncture can help increase circulation to the eye area, as can Advanced Reflexology. For a therapist near you log on to www.artreflex.com

ME (MYALGIA ENCEPHALOMYELITIS) OR CHRONIC FATIGUE

Around 250,000 people in Britain are recognised as having chronic fatigue or ME, but I believe that hundreds of thousands more go undiagnosed. Many people feel tired all the time and just struggle on, but only when the crushing exhaustion becomes incapacitating do people seek medical help. Orthodox medicine basically offers antidepressants, which will not help in the long term and certainly do not address the root cause of the problem.

Symptoms range from chronic, debilitating tiredness to depression, muscle pain, headaches and decreased concentration to name but a few.

This condition appears multi-factorial in origin. If you are stressed, have suffered a viral illness, such as flu or glandular fever, are exposed to a lot of electrical equipment, or have running water under your home, any, or all these factors can play a part. ME is also linked to the polio vaccine, low blood sugar, heavy metal toxicity, liver congestion, food intolerances, candida, adrenal exhaustion and deficiencies in minerals such as magnesium; there are also possible parasite links. If you have long-term low blood pressure this denotes your adrenal glands are struggling.

It is possible that some individuals could have all of these conditions, which eventually result in chronic fatigue; and while it is true to say that there is no single answer for ME, there are a number of things that seem to help the majority. Even so, as we are all unique, what helps one person may not work for another, but without doubt eating the right diet and taking the right supplements will make a difference. If you contract a viral infection – you must give your body a chance to rest and recover, which gives you more chance of avoiding long-term illness.

Foods to Avoid
- Avoid any foods and drinks containing caffeine, sugar and alcohol – all of which lower immune function, weaken the adrenal system and play havoc with blood sugar levels. Also most pre-packaged foods high in sugar are also high in saturated fats, salt, additives and preservatives.
- Most mass-produced, tinned foods and takeaways (unless they are freshly made) are lacking in magnesium. 40% of ME patients have low levels of this vital mineral.

- Some people mistakenly use guarana (or drinks like Red Bull) as an energy source when they are very low in energy. Unfortunately, the primary reason they give you energy is the caffeine content, which will only serve to weaken you in the long term. Never mix Red Bull with alcohol.
- If you find yourself constantly craving foods such as wheat, sugar and snacks, are bloated, have an urgency to urinate, suffer mood swings and are always tired, you may well have candida (see *Foods to Avoid* under *Candida*).
- Almost everyone with chronic fatigue will have multiple food intolerances. The most common being wheat and dairy from cow's milk. See *Allergies*.

Friendly Foods
- See also *Insulin Resistance*.
- Essential fats are vital for people with ME – they support the endocrine system, boost immunity, and help balance blood sugar. Therefore eat more organic sunflower and pumpkin seeds and linseeds (flax seeds). See *Fats You Need To Eat*.
- It is vital that you eat good-quality protein, such as organic meat, chicken, fresh fish, or beans at least twice a day. Protein helps to balance blood sugar for longer periods.
- Include plenty of vegetables and fruits in the diet, but don't eat too much fruit if you have candida.
- Replace wheat with amaranth, oat and rice crackers, and ask for wheat and yeast-free breads at your health shops.
- Try experimenting with other grains, such as millet, quinoa, kamut, spelt and so on. Nature's Path makes a great range of cereals from these grains, which you can enjoy with organic rice or milk.
- Remember to include plenty of cereals, leafy greens, such as cabbage, kale, spring greens, pak choy, broccoli, celery, wheat germ, soya-based biscuits and pastas, Brazil nuts, walnuts, almonds, curries, black strap molasses, honey and beans, as they are rich in magnesium.

- If you find you are intolerant to dairy there are now plenty of alternatives. Oat, almond or rice milks are all nutritious and can be used instead of cow's milk. There is also a non-dairy milk called Tiger White made from chufas, which is rich in monounsaturated fats. It has a lovely mild, nutty taste.
- Drink plenty of water, even if you are not thirsty, to help detoxify your system.
- Eat sunflower, pumpkin and sesame seeds, which are packed with essential fats and fibre, and use extra-virgin unrefined olive or sunflower oils for salad dressings.
- Add coriander to your foods, which really helps to detoxify heavy metals from the body.

Useful Remedies
- L-carnitine – an amino acid – has been shown to help reduce symptoms of chronic fatigue. You would need to take 3 grams daily before food. This is expensive, but, if you can afford it, worth a try.
- Take Siberian ginseng, 1–3 grams a day, which helps the body adapt to stressful circumstances. Take it for 60 days and then stop for 30 days before starting again. Don't take ginseng if you are pregnant.
- Liquorice Formula is a blend of herbs for the adrenal system, it is anti-viral, helps to alleviate pain and strengthens the adrenal glands. If your blood pressure is low, take it for 3–6 months until the blood pressure is normal then take a rest. **FSC**

- Enada is a stabilised form of vitamin B3, which was originally formulated at the Parkinson's Institute in Vienna to help alleviate the terrible fatigue that accompanies Parkinson's Disease. In independent medical trials globally, for 70% of ME patients, it has been found to raise energy levels and greatly reduce or eliminate the 'brain fog' often associated with ME. Initially take 10mg every morning, 1 hour before food and then after 2 months reduce to 5mg daily. Springfield Enada is available from health stores worldwide.
- Take magnesium malate, 500–1000mg per day, which helps to reduce muscle soreness.
- Milk thistle and dandelion are two herbs that support and detoxify the liver, which is often overloaded. Take 1ml 3 times daily.
- Take a high-strength multi-vitamin and mineral twice daily – see details of *Kudos 24* in *General Supplements*; see p.160.
- Take echinacea, as a tincture or a tablet, either every week from Monday through Friday, breaking only at the weekends; or every day for three weeks on, one week off. This will boost the immune system and help fight off any other infections.

Helpful Hints
- Take some gentle exercise. One study found that people were able to walk for 3 minutes, then rest for 3 minutes, until they had done a total of 30 minutes walking, without any negative effect on chronic fatigue.
- Try a gentle stretching programme to gradually tone the muscles and help drain the lymph system, which is often overloaded.
- Learn to relax. Meditation is a great way to give the body and brain a complete rest (see *Meditation*).
- Homeopathic Sarco Lactic Acid 6x taken twice daily for 7–10 days helps reduce symptoms.
- If you want more information on being checked for parasites, which are often linked to ME, then see all details under IBS (*Irritable Bowel Syndrome*).
- Have a friend massage your aching muscles with a mix of the essential oils of thyme and lemongrass. To help lift depression, try a mix of neroli and rose in a good base oil.
- Oxygen therapies are well worth looking into. Mark Lester in London uses an ozone cabinet and ozone therapies to treat patients. He also uses oxygen supplements to great effect. Tel: 020 8349 4730; or log on to www.thefinchleyclinic.com

- For a free information pack, or for more help, contact Action for ME, PO Box 1302, Wells BA5 1YE; or telephone 01749 670799. Website: www.afme.org.uk Email: info@afme.org.uk
- Many readers have been cured of ME by energy healers. Although there are hundreds of really amazing healers in the UK alone, there are three I have interviewed and seen for myself who are exceptional:
  * The first is Seka Nikolic, who specialises in ME. She practices at The Hale Clinic in London. See page 361 for contact details or visit www.sekanikolic.com.
  * The second is Kelvin Heard who also specializes in ME. His number is 07710 794627.
  * The third is Susan Anthony, who practises in Wells in Somerset. Her website is at www.psalifemastery.com; or you can call her on 01749 679900. (For more information on healing which is helpful for ME patients see under *Healing*.)
- If your symptoms persist, try having your house dowsed for electrical or geopathic stress. To find a dowser, call The British Dowsing Society. Tel: 01684 576969. Website: www.britishdowsers.org
- Cranial osteopathy has helped many people with ME, as it frees up nerve endings, which releases energy in the body. See *Useful Information*.
- With ME it is best to consult a doctor who is also a qualified nutritionist, as you may need injections of magnesium and B12 (see *Useful Information*).

MEDITATION

I realise that meditation is not a health condition that needs healing – but science has discovered that meditation offers so many health benefits to help us in today's stressed world that I have decided to include it. In the past meditation was associated with the hippy or New Age culture. But these days science has validated its numerous benefits. People who meditate regularly look younger, enjoy better mental clarity and more peace of mind, feel more contented with their lives, have a reduced heart rate and lower blood pressure, breathe more easily, and if they become ill, recover more quickly. Under pressure people who meditate remain calm and are generally less anxious.

During everyday life your brain emits beta waves. I call them busy waves – you are reading this page in beta. But if you sit quietly for around 20–30 minutes daily, your brain starts to produce more alpha waves, which are associated with relaxation. This gradual increase in alpha-wave activity results in the left and right frontal areas of the brain, known as the 'pre-frontal cortex', becoming more harmonious as brain waves start to rise and fall together. Eventually this changes the *quality* of the brain's functioning, including levels of intelligence and creativity. The more you meditate the brainier you could become! The calming alpha waves are automatically transmitted to every cell in the body, which helps to balance your whole system.

Parapsychologist Dr Serena Roney-Dougal, based at a research centre in Glastonbury, Somerset, has spent five years researching meditation. She says "Most people think of meditation as a great way to relax – but relaxation is simply one of the many positive side-effects of regular meditation. Over time meditation increases one's sense of wellbeing and heightens spiritual awareness. There are hundreds of verified medical studies showing that regular meditation helps to lower high blood pressure and decrease stress-hormone production, and encourages deeper sleep. If more people could meditate every day, we would not only be happier, but also our health service would not be stretched to breaking point." I could not have said it better myself.

Regular meditation also slows the ageing process, because it decreases the amount of thyroxin produced by the thyroid gland, which acts as the metabolic regulator – or 'body clock'. High levels of thyroxin mean that all body processes speed up (see *Thyroid*), whereas lower levels of thyroxin allow the body to slow down to an optimal level. Regular meditation helps to keep the thyroid balanced.

Meditation also stimulates the pineal gland situated in the centre of the brain, in Indian tradition this place is known as the 'third eye' or the Ajna Chakra, which acts as the 'off' switch for many of the hormones that contribute to a host of health problems. It also reduces the release of the stress hormones adrenaline and cortisol, which are major contributing factors in heart disease, strokes and ulcers, and it helps you to better tolerate stressful situations. Researchers have also found that people who meditate regularly sleep more easily, as they produce more of the hormone melatonin. Naturopath Steve Langley, who studied meditation in a Zen monastery in Kyoto, Japan, says, "Being in the alpha state has been proven to increase our immune system, and even deeper states can help raise levels of the anti-ageing hormone DHEA."

Meditation costs nothing, you can practise it daily on your own or with friends and it has proven health benefits. The single biggest reason people don't meditate is because they say they do not have the time. Well, it seems if we could make time, the benefits would far outweigh any negative effect of losing 15–20 minutes per day. In some areas learning meditation is available on the NHS.

When to Meditate

- Meditation is best practised in the morning before you begin the rush of the day; or at dusk. Even if you just sit quietly for 10 minutes daily, this will help.
- If you like to meditate before going to bed, make sure you eat a light meal early. Then have a walk, and then settle for your meditation.

How to Meditate

- Turn off the phone; find a space and time when you will not be disturbed. Sit in a straight-backed comfortable chair and sit with your back straight and your feet firmly on the ground. Take a few deep breaths. Then, breathe in and close your eyes and RELAX, say the word to yourself and, as you see the word in your mind's eye, allow the feeling of calm to flood from the top of your head right down to your toes. Then simply invite a golden or white light to come from the Heavens and imagine it flowing, like a liquid, through the top of your head, down to your toes and into the ground. At this point I visualise my mind as a bowl of clear white light that is totally empty and I enjoy the peace I find there. Many people have a mantra such as *Om* or 'I am', which they repeat silently over and over to help reduce their 'brain chatter'. You could also simply try the word 'space' – as what you are trying to do is to access the space between your thoughts. It takes a while to learn to meditate, but with practice you will get better. There are thousands of meditations; it is just a question of finding which one really suits you.

Useful Remedies

- The herb sceletium, from South Africa, has been used for centuries to reduce anxiety, improve mood and increase one's sense of connection and perception. Take 100–200mg 1 hour before meditating. Nutritionist Patrick Holford has formulated a Connect Formula containing this herb and others that aid meditation. **HN**
- Bach Flower Remedies – white chestnut and walnut taken in water will help still the mind.
- Drink more green tea, which contains an amino acid called L-theanine. This helps the brain to produce more alpha waves. You can also buy L-theanine in health shops to generally help keen you calmer during the day and to sleep better. For more information, see *Insomnia*.

Helpful Hints

- Cats purr in alpha waves, so get a cat and stroke him or her when you want to relax!
- There are now hundreds of books teaching you how to practise this age-old art. One of my favourites *is The Meditation Plan* by Dr Richard Lawrence (Piatkus). His book *Realise Your Inner Potential* (which is also available on DVD) is also wonderful as it contains some magical meditations. For more details call 020 7736 4187; or log on to www.richardlawrence.co.uk
- For more information on the science of meditation, read Herbert Benson *The Relaxation Response* (Avon Books).
- Frankincense oil placed in a burner helps the mind to relax, or use incense sticks, or dab a small amount of the oil on the third-eye area, as this powerful plant resin helps induce a calmer state.
- Light a candle, or even better, several to create the right atmosphere.
- Chanting induces similar results to meditation. Again, find a chant that suits you best.

MELATONIN

(see also *Insomnia*)

Melatonin is a hormone secreted by the pineal gland, which is located in the brain, behind our eyes.

Melatonin is crucial for controlling our biological rhythms and is secreted mainly at night, see-sawing with serotonin, its counterpart, which is secreted during the day. Melatonin helps you to sleep; whilst serotonin raises mood and makes you feel positive. Serotonin, called the 'happy neurotransmitter', is converted to melatonin by the pineal gland.

Professor Richard Wurtmann, of the Massachusetts Institute, proved to the scientific world that ageing is caused by healthy cells being attacked by free radicals when the pineal gland no longer secretes sufficient amounts of melatonin to protect them. Secretion of this natural anti-ageing agent starts at the age of 3 months and then drops before puberty. It continues to decline and falls dramatically around age 45. The other systems in the body seem to take this as a signal to slow down – and the ageing process begins in earnest.

In thousands of published studies, melatonin has been shown to protect against almost every disease associated with ageing, including cardiovascular disease. Melatonin helps to lower LDL (the 'bad' cholesterol) and lower blood pressure; it also reduces the effects of osteoporosis, Alzheimer's, and Parkinson's Disease.

Furthermore, melatonin boosts immunity, by increasing our 'Natural Killer' (NK) cells (the ones that attack and destroy wandering microbes and cancer cells), and is one of the most effective antioxidants studied so far. One study found that as little as 2mg of melatonin led to a 240% increase in NK cells.

The strong relaxant effects of melatonin means that it can be helpful in schizophrenia, depression, anxiety, panic attacks and sleep disorders. The list goes on and on. Melatonin also acts effectively against wrinkles, as it enhances the elasticity of the skin, the suppleness of the joints, sexual activity, and bone and muscular strength.

Melatonin also promotes the release of Human Growth Hormone, which is the master anti-ageing hormone. It seems no coincidence that both these hormones appear in our blood stream only at night.

Some drugs also interfere with melatonin-production, chiefly the NSAIDs, such as aspirin, ibuprofen and indomethacin. Their action is caused by the intentional suppression of semi-hormone messengers called prostaglandins, some of which are inflammatory, but some of which we need to manufacture melatonin. Paradoxically, lack of sunshine during the daytime also reduces melatonin secretion at night. This is because during the daytime we are supposed to be making serotonin, a precursor of melatonin. Serotonin fights depression (Prozac and St John's wort both work by inhibiting the breakdown of serotonin), but too little attention is given to the fact that we need it to make melatonin, which also fights depression.

Foods to Avoid

■ Too much caffeine and alcohol inhibit the release of melatonin. Avoid them as much as possible after 6pm if you are a poor sleeper.

Friendly Foods

■ Tryptophan, which increases production of melatonin, is found in such foods as turkey, bananas, sunflowers seeds, and milk. You can now buy organic Slumber Milk from most supermarkets, which helps increase melatonin levels.

■ If you are taking NSAIDs, you need to eat more essential fats, especially the omega-3s, eicosopentanoic acid (EPA) and dicosohexanoinc acid (DHA), which counter the inflammatory prostaglandins, and are good for the brain. EPA and DHA are found in fish, egg yolks, animal organs and marine algae (for more information on essential fats see *Fats You Need To Eat*).

Useful Remedies

■ Melatonin is not available over the counter in health stores in the UK as it is in the USA. You can purchase it for your own use from Pharm West on 00 353 46 943 7317, or ask a friend travelling to America to bring some home for you.

■ The most common side-effect of taking too much melatonin is feeling drowsy when you wake up. This can be prevented by taking less melatonin the following night. Begin by taking 1mg and see how you go, you can increase to 3mg and up to a maximum of 5mg. See what suits you best.

■ Tryptophan increases the production of melatonin and serotonin. Take 100mg at night before bed in the form of 5-HTP (for more details see *Insomnia*).

■ For good melatonin production you need B-vitamins, especially B1, B6 and B12, so take a B-complex with breakfast.

■ You also need adequate magnesium; take 400mg daily at bedtime.

Helpful Hints

■ Melatonin is released naturally during sleep. It is important therefore that you get around 7–8 hours of deep, satisfying sleep. REM sleep, when we dream, is particularly important for melatonin production. Note that REM sleep is not induced by sleeping pills.

■ It is vital to sleep in a properly darkened room. Even very low light levels can impair melatonin secretion. If your blinds and curtains are not adequate, consider a fabric-sleeping visor.

■ Electromagnetic radiation during sleep can also cause the reduction of melatonin production. Therefore turn off the bedroom TV at the mains, use a battery-operated clock, and don't sleep with the electric blanket on unless it's really cold. See *Electrical Pollution*.

■ Certain pain-relievers, such as aspirin and ibuprofen, cause the partial suppression of melatonin.

MEMORY   (see also *Alzheimer's Disease, Circulation* and *Parkinson's Disease*)

At the age of 56 I regularly forget people's names and where I left certain objects – we all do. And just because you forget a few things, it doesn't automatically mean that you have Alzheimer's or dementia, so don't panic. Most people think that once a brain cell dies, it's gone forever, but scientists in the US have now proven that brain cells can be regenerated. Just like our muscles, the brain needs regular use – and if you don't use it, you lose it. The secrets to improving your memory are to keep your brain active and to eat less junk food and more super-brain foods. There really is no need for your memory or brain function to decline with age. My mother-in-law is 91, and her brain is as sharp as a razor – she has spent 30 years regularly completing crosswords.

Temporary memory loss is not uncommon after drinking alcohol, if your blood sugar level is low, after a high fever, following surgery, after an epileptic fit, or when you are under stress. Depression and acute anxiety can also cause temporary memory loss. More serious memory loss can occur after an accident, brain injury, or stroke. Senile dementia involves progressive loss of short-term memory until the individual is unable to remember what they did or saw only a few moments before. Many prescription drugs, such as long-term use of statins or sleeping pills, and/or the long-term use of drug 'cocktails' (as in people who might be taking pills for high blood pressure, cholesterol, and so on), affect memory. External influences, such as poor eyesight and hearing, can also inhibit our ability to learn – thus affecting memory.

However, the vast majority of cases of poor memory are caused by years of eating too many of the wrong foods, especially saturated fats, which clog the arteries until the small capillaries are affected, preventing sufficient fresh, red blood reaching the brain and depriving it of oxygen. Simply taking a *deep* breath more regularly – even every 20 minutes or so – can help improve brain function.

Lead is well known to affect memory, which is why lead-free petrol was introduced on both environmental and health grounds. Mercury fillings are also linked to memory loss (see *Mercury Fillings*).

Foods to Avoid
- If you want to keep your memory sharp, you need to cut down on high-fat foods, such as meat and full-fat dairy foods. Also avoid mass-produced pies, cakes, biscuits, white bread, pizzas, burgers and so on, which not only deplete nutrients, but also contribute to clogging your arteries (most of these foods are usually high in fat, sugar and salt). Research shows that people who eat high-fat, nutrient-poor foods, such as burgers and chips, are less intelligent and have poorer memories than those who eat a low-fat, nutrient-dense diet.
- Alcohol depletes the body of vital nutrients – avoid it.
- Avoid excess sodium-based table salt, and don't add salt to food once it has been cooked.
- In some people excess wheat triggers 'brain fog'. In fact any food to which you have an intolerance can trigger this problem. See *Allergies*.
- Avoid too much sugar, which ages your brain.
- Avoid aspartame and monosodium glutamate (MSG).

Friendly Foods
- Always eat breakfast. Low-sugar cereals, such as muesli or porridge, are great as they are rich in B-vitamins, which are often lacking in dementia patients (especially B12).
- Low blood sugar levels can easily trigger 'foggy-brain' symptoms, such as memory loss. Make sure you eat small meals regularly to balance blood sugar (see *Low Blood Sugar*).
- Omega-3 essential fats, rich in EPA and DHA, are vital brain nutrients. They are found in oily fish, such as tuna, salmon, sardines, herrings, and mackerel.
- Use unrefined, preferably organic, olive oil, and sunflower, walnut and sesame oils for salad dressings and to drizzle over cooked foods (see *Fats You Need To Eat*).
- Fresh coffee is often criticised, but in terms of memory function it seems to help it, particularly in the elderly. Two cups a day is fine.
- Green leafy vegetables, particularly spinach, cabbage, pak choy, celery, broccoli and spring greens, as well as red and purple fruits, such as strawberries, blueberries, blackberries and cherries, are rich in antioxidants, which help to slow memory decline.
- Eat more apples, papaya, pineapple, grapes, prunes and raisins.

- Eat more wholegrain foods, such as brown pasta and rice, and wholemeal bread and flour, and barley and buckwheat.
- For those with a sweet tooth, use a little honey, brown rice syrup or fructose instead of refined sugar.
- Phosphatidyl choline is a vital brain nutrient found in egg yolks (ask for Columbus eggs – free range eggs from chickens that are fed on healthy essential fats) and fish (especially sardines).
- Take lecithin granules, a brain food that also reduces the amounts of LDL, the 'bad' cholesterol, in your body. Taking this brain nutrient during pregnancy can result in brainier children. Sprinkle a tablespoon of the granules over your breakfast cereal, or into salads or yoghurts. Make sure the brand you buy is a GM-free product with at least 30% phosphatidyl choline content, such as Cytoplan. **NC**
- Eat more ginger and live, low-fat yoghurt to aid digestion.
- Add freshly chopped sage to your salads and meals as it has been shown to improve memory and brain function.

Useful Remedies

- *As some of the supplements given below thin the blood naturally, if you are on blood-thinning drugs, speak to your doctor before trying those marked with a * – in time your prescription drugs dose could be lowered.*
- Take a good all-round combination formula that contains vitamins, minerals, antioxidants, brain nutrients and essential fats all in one powder, such as Kudos 24 (see details in *General Supplements*; p.160).

- The Siberian herb rhodiola has been shown to greatly improve concentration and memory. In Siberia where rhodiola tea is drunk regularly, many people live until well past 100. It also reduces the negative effects that stress hormones have on our body and mind. Kudos makes a high-strength, one-a-day capsule. Take it for 1 month, then leave it for 2 months, and then start again. **KVH**
- The herb ginkgo biloba is proven to increase memory as it improves blood-flow to the brain. **SHS**
- An extract of the periwinkle called *Vinpocetine, like ginkgo, is a herb that helps improve circulation. It is especially useful when blood-flow to the brain is diminished, as in the hardening of the arteries or minor strokes, and it also helps some people with tinnitus (ringing in the ears). Take 20–40mg daily. **NC**
- Phosphatidyl serine – 100mg up to 3 times a day – has been shown to improve mental function. Take it early in the day, as at night this can increase dreaming and delay you getting to sleep.
- Co-enzyme Q10 – 100mg a day – can improve energy-production within the brain
- Include a vitamin B-complex, as B-vitamins are essential for normal brain function (these should already be in your multi).
- The amino acid L-glutamine also makes a great brain food as it is the most abundant amino acid in the fluid that surrounds the brain. Take 250mg daily.
- Acetyl L-carnitine – an amino acid – helps slow progression of early dementia and slows deterioration in the brain. Take 500mg x 3 times daily before meals.
- Glutathione is a vital brain nutrient. See *Liver Problems*.

Helpful Hints

- Regular exercise is vital for aiding memory, the more oxygen you get to the brain, the less likely you are to lose your memory.
- Common sage contains considerable amounts of thujone (a naturally occurring substance that gives sage its flavour), which if used as sage essential oil can trigger fits in sensitive individuals. However, Spanish sage contains almost no thujone. Regular head massage with this Spanish sage essential oil (diluted in a base oil) has been shown by Dr John Wilkinson at Middlesex

University to increase memory functioning. For details of Spanish sage oil call Essentially Oils Ltd, Chipping Norton, Oxfordshire. Tel: 01608 659544. Website: www.essentiallyoils.com (All sage is great and safe for cooking.)

- Chelation therapy helps to unclog your arteries, which increases the amount of blood and oxygen that reaches the brain. Chelation therapy helps to remove all deadly metal toxins from the body. I give full details of this treatment in my book *500 of the Most Important Ways to Stay Younger Longer* (Cico Books). There are several chelation clinics in the UK. For details, call 01942 886644; or log on to www.chelation.com. Dr Robert Trossell also gives this treatment in London at 4 Duke Street, London W1U 3EL. Tel 020 7486 1095; or call Dr Wendy Denning on 020 7224 2423
- Keeping the brain active is a crucial aspect for improving memory. Play more word games and do crosswords. During car journeys or when on a train or when queuing in a supermarket, add or multiply varying numbers in your head.
- Minimise aluminum exposure – this includes many deodorants, cooking pans, some cheeses and so on (see *Alzheimer's*).
- Meditation helps to improve memory – see *Meditation*.
- Minimise exposure to mercury (see *Mercury Fillings*).
- Avoid using a mobile phone for more than 20 minutes at a time and avoid using them in cars and trains, which amplifies the negative effects. (See *Electrical Pollution*).
- If, after trying these remedies for 3 months, you are still experiencing memory problems, consult a nutritionist who is also a doctor (see also *Helpful Hints* in *Alzheimer's Disease*).
- Rubbing the essential oil of basil and/or rosemary, diluted in a base of almond oil, into the scalp will help to increase circulation to the scalp and clear your mind, thus aiding concentration.
- For further help read *Optimum Nutrition for the Mind* by Patrick Holford (Piatkus).

MÉNIÈRE'S SYNDROME   (see also *Tinnitus* and *Vertigo*)

This is a little-understood problem of the inner ear, which causes recurrent attacks of vertigo, nausea and ringing in the ears, and progressive deafness. People with this problem tend to feel unsteady and suffer headaches and neck pains. Causes are suggested as being linked to salt retention, food intolerances, nutritional deficiency as a result of poor absorption, or even a spasm in the walls of small blood vessels. See also *Leaky Gut*.

Foods to Avoid
- Many people with this problem react to soya, wheat, corn and yeast foods.
- Avoid sodium-based salt.
- Generally avoid any foods containing gluten, salt, caffeine, fried foods and alcohol.
- Reduce full-fat milk and dairy produce.
- See also *General Health Hints*.

Friendly Foods
- Eat more ginger, garlic and onions, which are very cleansing.
- Papaya and pineapple contain digestive enzymes, which aid absorption.
- Add 2 tsp of cider vinegar to water and sip – the mixture is rich in potassium, levels of which may be low in this condition.
- See *Friendly Foods* under *Leaky Gut* and *Vertigo*.
- Cherries, blueberries, blackberries and plums are all rich in flavonoids, which help to support ear function.

Useful Remedies

- Take a high-strength multi-vitamin and mineral.
- The herb ginkgo biloba helps to increase circulation in the ears. Take one high-strength daily. **KVH**
- Take a digestive enzyme capsule with main meals.
- 5–10mg of manganese may be useful. A deficiency in this mineral has been linked to Ménière's Syndrome. Most multi formulas will contain this amount.

Helpful Hints

- See a chiropractor or osteopath who can check for any cranial, spinal or neck misalignments.
- Acupuncture has shown to be very useful for this condition (see *Useful Information*), because it helps to increase circulation to the ears.

MENOPAUSE

(see also *Osteoporosis*)

At the age of 56, I am writing from a place of experience on this subject. Many women believe that the menopause is an illness for which you need a drug (orthodox HRT) – it's not. In formal terms, the menopause is part of the normal cycle of a woman's hormonal life when the menstrual cycles cease. In more informal terms, it's a time of great potential. The children have grown up, you are wiser and more mature, and it's a time when you can begin a new and exciting chapter in your life.

In the meantime, the menopause generally occurs between the ages of 45 and 55, though it can occur as early as 35 or as late as 65 years of age. Chemotherapy and excess exposure to hormone-altering chemicals, such as pesticides and herbicides, can also trigger an early menopause.

Dr Marilyn Glenville, an expert on the menopause, says, "At the time of menopause, a woman still produces oestrogen but not sufficient to prepare her womb for pregnancy. Levels of progesterone plummet or disappear completely. The ovaries continue to produce small quantities of oestrogen for at least 12 years after the onset of the menopause."

For most women the menopause happens in 3 phases. First comes peri-menopause – when you still have periods, but they may become heavier or lighter, and symptoms such as hot flushes can appear. Then comes menopause, when ovarian function declines and periods stop. The last phase is called post-menopause, which begins 12 months after your last period.

Throughout this time, many signs associated with ageing can appear, as the hormonal balance alters with the drop in oestrogen and progesterone levels. Skin is more likely to wrinkle, there can be an increased growth of facial hair, and a thinning of hair in the temple region. Muscles lose some strength and tone, and many women suffer hot flushes and insomnia. Your joints may begin to ache and bones can become more brittle, increasing the risk of osteoporosis. Vaginal dryness often results from these hormonal changes. The vaginal wall also becomes thinner and blood-flow is restricted. Dryness can make sexual intercourse painful or uncomfortable and can lead to irritation and increased risk of infection. You will be happy to note that regular sexual intercourse increases blood flow into the vagina.

Loss of bladder-tone, which can result in stress incontinence (leaking urine when you cough, sneeze, laugh or exercise), can also result (see *Incontinence*). HRT has now been linked to an increase in urinary incontinence, and studies have shown that conditions such as Alzheimer's and memory loss may also be speeded up by orthodox HRT. Also, no significant difference has been found between the quality of life in those women taking HRT against those who were given a placebo.

You may also experience a whole host of emotional ups and downs – one minute feeling on top of the world and the next in the pits of despair. The good news is that by eating the right diet and taking the right supplements, and through exercise and using natural hormone replacements, virtually all the symptoms of the menopause can be avoided or alleviated.

I do not advocate taking orthodox HRT because of the increased risk of high blood pressure, weight gain, and gall-bladder and liver problems, not to mention breast and endometrial (uterine) cancers. The increased health risks of orthodox HRT have now been shown to far outweigh the benefits. Yes, it slows the rate of bone loss, but only while you are taking it. Also, if you are under a lot of stress at this time, adrenal function is greatly affected. Healthy adrenal glands continue to supply post-menopausal women with oestrogen. But if you are stressed, then your adrenal glands are kept busy pumping the stress hormone cortisol and they make less oestrogen.

On the subject of oestrogen, most women are also becoming aware of the condition known as oestrogen dominance. This occurs when the amount of oestrogen in the body is not balanced by the proper amount of progesterone. This can occur from failed ovulations, or by over-exposure to environmental chemicals found in herbicides, pesticides and plastics, called 'xenoestrogens', which have an oestrogen-like effect on the body. These chemicals accumulate in our fatty tissue and greatly increase the risk of cancers.

When you have too much oestrogen activity compared to progesterone, you can suffer symptoms such as water retention, bloating, and menstrual irregularities. Globally we are living in a dangerous ocean of hormone-disrupting chemicals, which are triggering lowered sperm counts and causing animals and fish to change sex – and we too are seeing sexual mutations.

One problem with conventional HRT is that the drugs do not use progesterone, but synthetic hormone-like substances, called progestins (or progestogen) – essentially, these are artificial hormones. These have side-effects such as irritability, liver dysfunction, vaginal bleeding, blood clots and so on, and they reverse the positive effects of oestrogens on the heart. Conventional HRT also uses much higher levels of oestrogen than natural HRT. For this reason, I prefer to use natural HRT (see *Useful Remedies* on page 248).

If you have had a partial hysterectomy (that is, your ovaries are remaining) before menopause, you will still have hormonal changes similar to the normal menstrual cycle. If you need supplemental hormones and are told that you need only oestrogen because you do not have a uterus, you should also take real (natural) progesterone with any oestrogen supplementation. If you have had a total hysterectomy and need HRT, use the lowest dose of oestrogen possible for you, and always use real (natural) progesterone with it.

Some women go through early menopause, which can happen for many reasons, ranging from oestrogen-like chemicals in the environment or smoking, drinking heavily, or being severely malnourished. Whatever the cause, it is important to make sure that the bones remain healthy, therefore have a bone scan periodically and a urine – deoxypyrodinoline – test to measure bone breakdown. If bone loss is occurring then you need to take the appropriate measures (see *Osteoporosis*).

Foods to Avoid
- In general avoid the typical Western diet of white flour, full-fat dairy and fatty meats.
- Avoid chemicals that mimic oestrogens (xenoestrogens) found in pesticides or herbicides by eating organic foods.
- Intensively reared animals have often been treated with antibiotics and hormones, another reason to eat organic meat and chicken.
- Minimise your exposure to foods stored in plastic containers and never heat or microwave food

in plastic containers – the containers will leach xenoestrogens into your food.

- Cut down on all caffeine, fizzy cola-type drinks, sugar and chocolate, and avoid drinking too much alcohol, which all act as stimulants and trigger blood sugar problems. Caffeine and/or alcohol can trigger a hot flush on their own.

Friendly Foods

- Increase your intake of fresh, locally grown and preferably organic fruits and vegetables.
- Fermented soya-based foods are truly one of the best foods for managing the symptoms associated with the menopause. Soya contains isoflavones (phyto-oestrogens), which have oestrogen-like effects on the body and block the harmful effects of oestrogens and xenoestrogens. But there has been much misinformation written about about soya, and Dr Glenville says, "Soya foods in their traditional forms of miso, soya sauce and tempeh (a fermented form of soya) are all rich in isoflavones, which have been proven to reduce the risk of developing cancers. But they are best eaten cooked."
- Isoflavones are also found in chickpeas, soya beans, lentils, alfalfa, fennel, kidney beans, and sunflower, pumpkin and sesame seeds, Brazil nuts, walnuts and linseeds (flax seeds). All seeds and their unrefined oils are rich in essential fatty acids, which also help to reduce joint pain and risk of heart disease, and help to lubricate the vagina (see *Fats You Need To Eat*).
- Foods from the brassica vegetable family help to protect against oestrogen-sensitive cancers, including breast cancer and cancer of the cervix, balance hormones and can greatly alleviate menopausal symptoms. These include cabbage, watercress, broccoli, pak choy, Brussels sprouts, cauliflower, kale, kohlrabi, mustard, rutabaga and turnips.

- Brazil nuts and sesame seeds are good sources of calcium.
- Live, low-fat yoghurt increases healthy bacteria in the gut, which aids absorption of nutrients from your diet.
- Vitamin B12 has been shown to reduce the irritability, bloating and headaches associated with the menopause and is found in oily fish, eggs and meats.
- Potassium and pantothenic acid (vitamin B5) help support adrenal function – they are found in whole grains, such as brown rice, amaranth, barley, and quinoa, as well as salmon, tomatoes, broccoli, cauliflower, avocado, dried apricots, banana, cantaloupe melon, oranges and fish.
- Use dried seaweeds, such as kombu, in your cooking (particularly in stir-fries), as seaweed is rich in iodine (which supports the thyroid) and calcium (see also *Thyroid*).
- Eat organic foods, including lean meat, chicken, vegetables and fruits, to avoid ingesting too many toxins from herbicides and pesticides.
- Folic acid found in wheat germ, eggs, leafy greens, calves' and chicken liver, dried yeast and beetroot is very important during the menopause to protect the bones.
- Include garlic in your diet, which helps to keep cholesterol levels in check.
- Drink more spring water, which helps to regulate body temperature.
- Avoid very hot drinks and hot spicy foods.
- If you have trouble sleeping, try valerian and passionflower teas.

Useful Remedies

- Try the Menopause Programme, which includes herbs such as blessed thistle, sqaw vine, Siberian ginseng, cramp bark and raspberry leaf, which all help to cleanse the reproductive organs and balance hormones. **SHS**
- If you dislike the taste of soya foods, then try soya isoflavone capsules. Most of the health companies on pages 13–15 make them. Take 50–100mg daily.
- Natural HRT can reduce many of the symptoms of menopause. It consists of natural progesterone made from wild yam and/or natural oestrogens from soya. The natural progesterone most often comes as a cream that you rub on the skin, Pharm West's is called Pro Body Cream. **PW**

- Natural oestrogens are mostly available in a combination formula with the 3 types of oestrogens found in a woman's body mixed with natural progesterone. The one I use is called Phyto-Estrogen Cream, which contains bio-identical hormones (meaning the exact same molecule that is found in the human body). Natural HRT supplementation can be used in place of orthodox HRT under the direction of a gynaecologist. If you are suffering low level hot flushes, insomnia, vaginal dryness or mood swings you may only need natural progesterone.

- Don't use hormones unless you have been tested by your doctor and if you have no hormonal symptoms and good bone density there is no need for extra hormones. Natural HRT creams are available only on prescription in the UK, but you can order them for your own use from Pharm West in the US. Use the natural progesterone (Pro Body Cream) for 2–3 months, but if there is not sufficient improvement then switch to the Phyto-Estrogen cream. For an information sheet on these creams Tel: 00 353 46 943 7317; or visit the website: www.pharmwest.com.

- Take a good-quality woman's multi-vitamin and mineral such as BioCare's FemGuard or Lambert's Gynovite. Dr Glenville also has her own formula especially for before and after the menopause. For details call The Natural Health Practice on 01892 515905. Any women's multi that you choose should contain boron, vitamin K, selenium, folic acid, vitamin D, vitamin E, calcium and magnesium to support you through the menopause.

- A remedy extracted from a Peruvian root vegetable called *maca* has been used for centuries to help alleviate hormonal-type symptoms. The root is rich in protein, minerals, vitamins, fibre and essential fats. Research shows that *maca* helps to stimulate the pituitary gland into producing hormone precursors, which eventually raises oestrogen and progesterone levels naturally, as well as balancing the adrenal glands, the thyroid, and the pancreas. Taken regularly this root has been shown to reduce the hot flushes, depression and palpitations associated with the menopause. Take 1 capsule daily. **KVH**

- Full-spectrum, natural-source vitamin E – 400iu per day – can help to reduce hot flushes.
- Take an EFA-formula containing omega-3 and -6 oils; at least 1 gram daily. See *Fats You Need To Eat*.
- Indolplex, by Phytopharmica, is a nutritional supplement made from extracts of the brassica vegetables, which contain indole 3 carbinole and diindolymethane, which increase the 'good' oestrogen (2-hydroxyestrone) and decrease the 'bad' oestrogen (16-a-hydroxyestrone). Take 2 tablets per day. To order call The Society for Complementary Medicine on 020 7487 4334.
- Vitamin K x 100mcg per day can reduce the heavy menstrual bleeding that is common in the peri-menopausal years. Vitamin K is also needed to keep minerals like calcium in the bones and out of the arteries.
- Vitamin B-complex – 100mg per day – helps to relieve stress, depression and mood disorders and is needed for energy production. (This should be included in your multi.)
- Black cohosh can effectively relieve hot flushes and other menopausal symptoms after 4 weeks of use. Additional herbs that are great for reducing menopausal symptoms include agnus castus, hops, liquorice root, dong quai and wild yam. These herbs can be taken individually or in combination formulas. Dr Glenville has an excellent organic formula containing all these herbs. One teaspoonful can be taken twice daily (also available in capsules). Call 0845 8800915 for details or log on to www.marilynglenville.com
- See also details of the hormone DHEA below.
- The hormone pregnenolone is also important after the menopause – see below, under *Hormones*.

Helpful Hints

- If your doctor suggests that you use orthodox pessaries for a dry vagina, then avoid ones containing oestradiol, which is a stronger oestrogen and can increase the risk factors for hormone-related cancers. Ask for oestriol-based creams and pessaries, which are a weaker form of oestrogen. Also discuss with your doctor which type of oestrogen they might prescribe for your HRT patches and so on.

- If you are suffering heavy bleeding, you must have this checked by your doctor or gynaecologist.
- Regular weight-bearing exercise not only helps raise levels of DHEA, a vital anti-ageing hormone (see below), but also reduces stress, which makes symptoms and hormone imbalances worse. Also in mid-life our waistlines tend to expand. Exercise keeps you trim and increases bone density. It also makes you feel more positive and cheerful about life, and women who exercise regularly tend to suffer fewer hot flushes.
- Use relaxation techniques such as meditation or yoga (see *Meditation*).
- Add essential oils of geranium, chamomile and jasmine to your bath to aid relaxation.
- If you suffer from night sweats, wear loose-fitting cotton nightwear and have a change of nightwear ready. Use cotton blankets and keep the room cool.
- Homeopathic Sepia 30c x 1 daily for a week, has been found to reduce hot flushes.
- To further help prevent vaginal dryness and painful intercourse, avoid using deodorant soaps or scented products in the vaginal area.
- Use a water-soluble lubricant to facilitate penetration during intercourse.

- Dr Glenville recommends a great vaginal lubricant called SYLK, which is made from kiwi fruit. It is available from most health stores or on online from www.naturalhealth.practice.com. Or try a soya pessary from Arkopharma, which can be inserted to help lubrication. There are many creams containing wild yam available in health food stores, which can be used topically as a vaginal lubricant. Contact The Perfect Woman range for wild Mexican yam on 0117 968 7744, or contact them at www.natural-woman.com; or for more information on these creams look at www.wildmexicanyam.co.uk.
- Read *Natural Alternatives to HRT* and *Healthy Eating for the Menopause* both by Dr Marilyn Glenville (Kyle Cathie).
- Marilyn's website www.marilynglenville.com is packed with useful information; or to visit her practice call 08705 329 244. You can email the practice on health@marilynglenville.com
- If you require further information on natural progesterone and a list of doctors who use it, send £1 in stamps plus a large SAE to The Natural Progesterone Information Service (NPIS), PO Box 24, Buxton SK17 9FB. Tel: 07000 784849. Website: www.npis.info/contactus.htm

Hormones associated with the menopause

NB: you should never self-medicate with hormones – consult a qualified doctor or health practitioner who can prescribe the correct balance for your individual needs.

- *Cortisol:* You can find out more about this hormone and how it affects the menopause and contributes to osteoporosis in *Stress*.
- *DHEA, the menopause and ageing:* Around the time of menopause, women often undergo rapid age-transformation, and whilst most doctors suggest some kind of HRT, very few prescribe DHEA. DHEA helps reverse many of the unfavourable effects of excess cortisol, creating subsequent improvement in energy, vitality, sleep, premenstrual symptoms and mental clarity. This hormone is produced by the adrenal glands and is the most abundant steroid hormone in the body. It is made from cholesterol and can be converted into oestrogen or testosterone. By the age of 65, we make only 10–20% of the amount of cortisol we made at 20.

    One 20-year study found that DHEA levels were far lower in men who died of heart disease than in healthier men. Low levels of DHEA have also been found in Alzheimer's patients. In fact, there is now little doubt that DHEA helps prevent the ravages of brain-ageing. It protects against Alzheimer's and dementia and brings an improved overall sense of wellbeing, which scientists have identified as being due to increased levels of endorphins (the chemicals we make naturally when we are happy and during exercise).

Tests have shown that DHEA can help prevent cancer, heart disease, and bone and skin degeneration. It helps maintain brain function and gives powerful support to the immune system. It helps protect against infections, autoimmune disorders, obesity, diabetes and stress.

DHEA has also been shown in numerous studies to improve mood and energy levels in both men and women, and is therefore a valid treatment for depression and long-term negative stress. *This effect was found to be particularly noticeable for post-menopausal women.* One German study showed that DHEA considerably increased the libido and sexual satisfaction in the women taking part.

Fortunately, DHEA is easy to supplement in tablet form and serum levels can be controlled with ease. But, as always, before you begin to take hormones, have a blood test and find out what your natural hormone levels are. If DHEA is lower than 300mgm/dl, you would need to take a supplementary dose. Men should consider 25–50mg daily and can go as high as 100mg until levels normalise. Then they can take a maintenance dose of 50mg, which should be fine. Adjust the dose until you get a definite beneficial response.

In women, anything more than modest dosages may trigger increased facial hair growth, and spots and greasy skin. To avoid such undesirable side-effects, women should take no more than 25mg daily. Generally, 10–15mg is adequate and still provides the benefits. When I was very stressed a few years ago, a blood test showed that my DHEA levels were almost nil and I began taking 10mg daily. Within 2 months I felt as though I had been reborn. After 4 months I started to suffer spots on my forehead, which are a common side-effect of taking DHEA.

These days I take another form of DHEA called '7 Keto DHEA', which is not converted into oestrogens and testosterone within the body. You would have to purchase this at a US health store.

NB: Because it can be metabolised into testosterone and oestrogen, DHEA use should be avoided by anyone who currently has prostate cancer or breast cancer. Having said this DHEA helps prevent cancer in those who do not have it. Also do not take this hormone if it you are pregnant, nursing, or have prior ovarian, adrenal or thyroid tumours. Women should avoid DHEA just prior to menopause, because their levels typically increase around that time anyway.

- DHEA is not available over the counter in health stores in the UK, although it is in the US. You can purchase it for your own use from Pharm West by calling freephone 00 353 46 943 7317. Website: www.pharmwest.com
- For more information, read *DHEA – Unlocking the Secrets to the Fountain of Youth* by Ley and Ash (BL Publications). To order from The Nutri Centre Bookshop, log on to www.nutricentre.com; or email bookshop@nutricentre.com
- *Pregnenolone:* Pregnenolone is manufactured in the body from cholesterol and is a precursor to the production of DHEA, testosterone, oestrogens, cortisol and aldosterone (a kidney-control hormone). Probably because of its involvement with many hormone pathways, pregnenolone tends to decline less dramatically in later years. By the age of 75, our bodies produce 60% less pregnenolone than the levels produced in our mid-30s. For this reason pregnenolone levels are one of the important biomarkers of ageing. Also, strict cholesterol-controlled diets, vegan diets and the medical use of cholesterol-lowering drugs could impair your natural production of pregnenolone.

However, the best news about pregnenolone is its mind-enhancing function. Studies have shown that this hormone increases memory, improves concentration, gives you quicker reaction times, helps protect the all-important myelin sheath around nerve fibres, increases resistance to stress and reduces depression. Pregnenolone is, therefore, an ideal supplement for helping to reduce many conditions associated with ageing – such as, confusion, forgetfulness, loss of energy, apathy, decreased sense of worth, and depression.

Another positive point is that pregnenolone converts directly to progesterone. Therefore, if you suffer from oestrogen dominance, try supplementing pregnenolone before you try DHEA.

There are no dietary sources of pregnenolone and supplemental pregnenolone is made from substances found in soybeans. A safe starting dose is 30mg daily.

Pregnenolone is not available over the counter in health stores in the UK as it is in the US.

MERCURY FILLINGS

There is now a huge body of evidence to show that mercury fillings are detrimental to health. Mercury is one of the most toxic substances known to man and is an accumulative poison. Originally, it was thought that the mercury vapour could not escape as it was locked into solid metal fillings: but we now know this is not the case. Mercury vapour is now proven to pass through the blood–brain barrier; it deposits in the brain affecting structure and function. The British Dental Association state that about 3% of the population are estimated to suffer from mercury sensitivity (when the same ratio of people have, say, flu, this is considered to have reached epidemic proportions) – that is, around 1.8 million people. Amalgam fillings are still widely used in the UK and the US. Between 15 and 20 million amalgam fillings a year are carried out on the NHS in the UK alone. David Hefferon, a holistic dentist practising in London, says, "There is now good evidence from research at the University of Calgary in Canada showing that mercury causes brain cell degeneration. This research and many more facts on mercury are available via www.iaomt.org – The International Academy of Oral Medicine and Toxicology."

Dr Jack Levenson, a dental surgeon who has now passed away, spent almost 20 years investigating the effects of the potential dangers of dental amalgam, and told me a few years ago, "There is a strong body of research linking mercury to heart disease, Alzheimer's, Parkinson's, multiple sclerosis, motor neurone disease, migraines, chronic fatigue, digestive disorders, infertility in men and women, antibiotic resistance, joint and muscle pain, impaired immune function, hair loss and excessive hair growth, visual disturbances, numbness, tingling and tremors."

Are you nervous? When Jack tested my teeth, two of my amalgam fillings were 10 times over the supposed safe limit of mercury emissions. I had them removed on the spot. It would seem that the government continues to refuse NHS patients safer, composite white fillings in order to save millions of pounds. If they admit that amalgam has poisoned millions of people the litigation bill would be huge and health insurance companies would then be forced to pay for the fillings' removal and replacement. Money, not health, it seems is once again the bottom line here.

Friendly Foods
- Eat organic vegetables, as mass-produced fruits, grains and vegetables are often treated with a mercury-based fungicide.
- Coriander detoxifies mercury from the body.

Foods to Avoid
- If you have mercury fillings, avoid larger fish such as cod, haddock, tuna and swordfish, which often contain high quantities of mercury. (Around 20 tons of mercury plus lead, cadmium and copper is dumped into the North Sea annually from industry.)

Useful Remedies
- If you have mercury fillings, take a good-quality multi-vitamin and mineral to help support your

immune system. See details of Kudos 24 in *General Supplements* on p.160.

- Mercury depletes the mineral selenium, which is known to reduce the incidence of cancer and heart disease. Take between 100 and 200mcg daily.
- Vitamin E increases the effectiveness of the selenium – take 400iu daily.
- Vitamin C – take 2 grams daily with food.
- It is important that you are re-assessed by your dentist every 2–3 months as the mercury can take up to a year or so to be eliminated.
- NAC – N-acetylcysteine – an amino acid, really helps to detoxify the liver. Take 500mg twice daily 30 minutes before food.
- See also *Liver Problems*.
- You need a full spectrum of B-vitamins – as mercury greatly affects the liver and the B is needed to help detoxify its negative effects.
- Organic chlorella – www.theellaclinic.co.uk supply a very pure form. David Hefferon suggests taking 5 tablets twice a day – as the chlorella binds to heavy metals, which helps eliminate them.

Helpful Hints
- Many vaccines use mercury as a preservative.
- If you would like a free mercury information sheet, plus a list of dentists in the UK who specialise in safe removal of amalgam fillings, send a large SAE with 3 1st-class stamps to The British Society for Mercury Free Dentistry, 221, Old Brompton Rd, London SW5 OEA. Or call their information line on 020 7373 3655. Jack Levenson has sadly passed away, but Adele Wright has now taken over this practice.

- David Hefferon – who still removes mercury fillings – now has a specialist Holistic Dental Practice at the Ella Clinic, 12 Upper Wimpole Street, London. Tel: 020 7935 5281.
- Contact IAOMT – The International Academy of Oral Medicine and Toxicology – at 30 Bournemouth Road, Lower Park Stone, Poole BH14 OES. Tel: 01202 741622. Visit their website to view the latest research on mercury: www.iaomt.org. The Academy gives lots of information on mercury fillings and holistic dentistry.
- Otherwise contact the British Dental Society for Clinical Nutrition, Welbeck House, 62 Welbeck Street, London W1N 1AE. Send an SAE for information on mercury.
- You can also contact Patients Against Mercury Amalgam on 020 7256 2994. They publish a newsletter about dentists practising mercury-free dentistry.
- www.melisa.org also carry the latest research into links between mercury and Parkinson's and mercury and multiple sclerosis.
- The Henry Spink Foundation at www.henryspink.org contains great fact sheets about mercury.
- Read *Toxic Bite* by Bill Kellner-Read (Credence); or *The Toxic Time Bomb* by Sam Ziff (Aurora).

MIGRAINE

(see also *Allergies, Low Blood Sugar* and *Liver Problems*)

One in every 8 people in the UK suffers regular migraines – which affect twice as many women as men. Twenty per cent of women and 7% of men experience migraine with an average of 3 attacks per month, each requiring 6 hours of bed rest. In Britain alone, the cost of migraines has spiralled to more than £1 billion a year. Migraines usually occur on one side, at the back or front of the head and an attack can be precipitated by flashing lights or partial blindness. Others suffer tingling sensations, sensitivity to light or noise, vomiting, and so on. Some people are debilitated for a few hours, others several days and in addition an attack can often be accompanied by nausea and vomiting.

Migraines are linked to food intolerances, internal toxicity and sometimes to the menstrual cycle. In fact, says nutritionist Gareth Zeal, "Almost 90% of migraine cases I see are linked to food intolerances." In addition 40% of migraine patients also have the bacteria *Helicobacter Pylori* – see *Stomach Ulcers*. Migraines can also be a sign of liver congestion, so you really need to cut down on alcohol, caffeine and fats – and keep the diet clean. (See also *Leaky Gut*, *Constipation*, *Liver Problems* and *Low Blood Sugar*.) Weather changes, stress or lack of sleep can also trigger migraines.

Foods to Avoid
- The foods most commonly known to trigger an attack are cheese, red wine, peanuts, corn, coffee, wheat, and citrus fruits and juices.
- Avoid refined sugars, which are found in most cakes, biscuits, pastries, snacks and fizzy drinks.
- Avoid food additives, colourings, preservatives, alcohol and caffeine as much as possible.
- Avoid hard margarines, shortenings, and any foods containing hydrogenated fats and oils.
- Cut down on red meat, full-fat dairy produce and eggs. Cut down on eggs only if you have an intolerance.
- Some sufferers have problems with fish such as tuna, so keep a food diary and note which foods cause the reactions.
- In one study when 54 migraine patients followed a low-fat diet the incidences of headaches were reduced from 9 monthly attacks to 3.
- If you are constipated on a regular basis, certain bacteria in the bowel can convert tyrosine (high in peanuts) to tyramine, which again is thought to be a trigger. Cheese is also high in tyramine.

Friendly Foods
- Eat more fresh pineapple, which aids digestion, and has anti-inflammatory properties.
- Include more turmeric (curcumin) in your diet, as it has great anti-inflammatory properties. You can also take this in capsule form.
- Eat more linseeds (flax seeds), and sunflower, pumpkin and sesame seeds to keep your bowels regular. Sprinkle them over a low-sugar breakfast cereal.
- Drink at least 6 glasses of water daily. Dehydration can trigger a migraine especially in summer.
- Eat more healthy grains, brown rice, lentils and barley, and try amaranth, oat and rice crackers as a change from wheat.
- Eat plenty of fruits and vegetables, preferably organic.
- Make sure you eat quality protein, such as fresh chicken or cooked tofu once a day.
- Use unrefined walnut, sesame, sunflower and olive oils over salad dressings.
- Live, low-fat, non-dairy-based yoghurt contains healthy bacteria, which aid digestion and keep the bowel healthy.
- Oily fish is rich in omega-3 fats, which naturally thin the blood and reduce the severity of migraines – if you eat 3 portions a week.
- Drink vervain tea to help reduce head pain, and add the essential oil to your bath.

Useful Remedies
- Ginkgo biloba helps to prevent the blood vessels constricting. Take 120mg of standardised extract daily.
- As all the B-vitamins are vital for preventing headaches, particularly folic acid, B2, and B6, take a high-strength B-complex daily.
- Include 1 gram of vitamin C daily in your supplements.
- Take calcium, 1000mg with 400iu of vitamin D, plus 500–1000mg of magnesium for 2 months – a lack of these minerals (especially magnesium) is associated with migraine and they act as muscle relaxants. Many companies make combination formulas.

- As digestive problems are heavily associated with migraines, take a digestive enzyme with main meals.
- If you crave sweet foods take 200mcg of the mineral chromium for at least 1 month to reduce food cravings.
- Omega-3 fatty acids (fish oils) – 500mg taken twice daily – should help relieve migraine headaches.
- Migraine Relief Formula contains vitamin B6, magnesium citrate, willow bark (a natural painkiller) plus ginger and feverfew – a herbal anti-inflammatory with natural calming effects. Take 2 tablets daily.
- The herb butterbur has been shown to help reduce the duration of migraines. Take 500mg twice daily during an attack. You can also use it as a preventative.

Helpful Hints

- Low blood sugar can trigger an attack, so eat healthy meals regularly.
- Migraine is often triggered by food allergies, liver congestion or hormonal problems, so keep a food diary to see if you can identify foods that trigger an attack. See *Allergies* and *Useful Information*.
- Regular aerobic exercise has been shown to reduce migraine attacks and yoga helps to reduce stress levels.
- Taken regularly, rosemary or fresh ginger tea can help bring relief from some of the symptoms.
- Grinding the teeth over many years often causes the jaw to slip out of alignment. This causes blood-flow to the head to be restricted, triggering regular headaches and/or migraines. Problems with vertebrae in the neck can also disrupt blood-flow to the brain. See a chiropractor or a cranial osteopath who can re-align the neck and head (see *Useful Information*).
- Many people have found that by wearing magnetic jewellery pain is relieved.
- Call The Migraine Trust Helpline. Tel: 020 7436 1336. Website: www.migrainetrust.org
- Empulse is a pulsed electromagnetic treatment – the setting is governed by an analysis of the brain's electrical activity. It is a non-invasive, non-drug-based preventative treatment. Contact Julian Campbell, Electromagnetic Therapy Services on Freephone 0800 542 0724. Website: www.empulse.com
- Further information can be obtained from the Migraine Action Association. Tel: 01536 461333. Website: www.migraine.org.uk

MOUTH PROBLEMS   (see also *Bad Breath*)

Burning mouth syndrome

This is most common in women especially after the menopause and may be triggered by decreased hormone production, nerve damage, stress, or sensitivity to certain foods. It may also be linked to digestive problems. In rare cases it can be due to a lack of vitamin B12 and folic acid. Symptoms can include a swollen tongue, metallic taste, soreness and a dry mouth and tongue even when the tongue looks normal. It can also be triggered by low stomach acid (see *Low Stomach Acid*). If you have a cold or flu, symptoms are usually worse. This condition also denotes that your liver is under stress. Excessive talking can exacerbate the problem.

Foods to Avoid

- Burning mouth syndrome is usually made worse by highly spiced or acidic foods, such as vinegar, oranges or pineapple.

- Avoid too much alcohol, and black tea and coffee, which are all acid-forming in the body
- Meat, cheese and chocolate are especially acid-forming, and could make symptoms worse.

Friendly Foods

- Keep your diet clean (see *General Health Hints*) and drink plenty of water.
- Eat more organic nuts, seeds and fish, which are high in zinc.
- Cereals, oats, alfalfa, eggs, liver, brown rice, skimmed milk and fish are all rich in B-vitamins.

Useful Remedies

- A swollen tongue can be a sign of iron deficiency – have a blood test.
- A dry mouth is a specific sign of potassium phosphate deficiency – take 75 mg daily. **BLK**
- Take vitamin C – 1 gram per day – to prevent deficiency.
- Take vitamin B6 – 30mg per day.
- Take vitamin B12 – 800mcg sublingual tablet daily – to prevent deficiency.
- Take folic acid – 400mcg per day.
- As all the B-vitamins work together, take the B6, B12 and folic acid in a B-complex.
- Take zinc –30 mg per day – as lack of zinc is linked to this problem. As zinc depletes copper, make sure your zinc supplement contains about 1–2mg of copper.
- GLA is an essential fat found in evening primrose oil – take 250mg of GLA per day to prevent deficiency. **BC**

Helpful Hints

- Mouth problems often reflect problems in the gut and digestive system. See a nutritionist who can re-balance your diet and suggest supplements to boost your immune system (see *General Health Hints*).
- Suck ice cubes if the pain is severe.
- This problem is exacerbated by stress, so learn to meditate, and practice some form of relaxation.
- As nitrates and other chemicals found in drinking water are known to make symptoms worse, install a good water filter. Contact The Pure H2O Company on 01784 221188. Email: info@purewater.co.uk. Website: www.purewater.co.uk

Cracked lips

Lips that are sore and cracked especially at the corners of the mouth are usually a sign of a deficiency of B-vitamins, especially vitamin B2 which is found in milk, eggs, liver, green vegetables and most other fresh vegetables. The problem is also linked to lack of vitamin E and essential fats found in wheat germ, avocados, oily fish, seeds and their unrefined oils. Dehydration is a major cause.

Rarely, cracked lips can be a sign of vitamin-A toxicity. You would need to have taken thousands of units of vitamin A for over a month for this to happen, but nevertheless if you have been taking extremely high doses of vitamin A, have a blood test.

Useful Remedies

- Take a high-strength vitamin B-complex.
- Take a multi-vitamin and mineral that contains at least 30mg of zinc, 1–2mg of copper, 200iu of full-spectrum vitamin E and 500mg of vitamin C. See details of Kudos 24 in *General Supplements*; p.160.
- Rub pure vitamin E cream onto the lips at night.

Helpful Hints
- Use a lip balm made from vitamin E and aloe vera. Body Shop makes a great range.
- Take homeopathic Nat Mur 6x twice daily for 3–4 days.

Mouth Ulcers

Mouth ulcers are quite common and usually occur on the inside of the cheek, tongue or gums. They denote that the body is run down or under stress, but can also be caused by accidentally biting the side of mouth, excessive tooth brushing, eating food that is too hot, eating acidic and spicy food, or cigarette smoke. Many people suffer mouth ulcers after eating oranges, pineapple and/or tomatoes, while others find ill-fitting dentures or braces are the problem. Any chronic dental problem can trigger an outbreak. If the ulcers do not clear within 3 weeks, see your doctor.

Sodium lauryl sulphate, a foaming agent used in quite a few cosmetics, particularly toothpaste, can also trigger this problem. You might also be deficient in B-vitamins and iron, so a blood test would be useful to confirm this.

Foods to Avoid
- Sugar, vinegars, pickles, tomatoes and tomato sauces, peanuts, strawberries, pineapple, plums, rhubarb, kiwi fruit, oranges and grapefruits are problem foods for those who suffer from mouth ulcers.
- Avoid really hot and spicy foods.
- Reduce your intake of sugary treat foods and white-flour-based breads, cakes and biscuits, all of which lower immune function.
- Avoid really salty foods, such as crisps, peanuts and salted meats and fish.

Friendly Foods
- Liquorice tablets or sticks can be chewed to speed up the healing of the ulcers. You can also drink liquorice tea.
- Eat more Manuka honey with an activity level of 10+ as this honey is very healing.
- Drink more camomile tea or green tea. Green or white tea helps to boost immune function.

Useful Remedies
- Vitamin C and zinc are often deficient in people who suffer mouth ulcers. Take 1 gram of C daily plus 30mg of zinc.
- Take a good multi-vitamin and mineral – ask at your health shop or see details of Kudos 24 in *General Supplements*; p.160.
- Vitamin B-complex helps to prevent and heal mouth ulcers.
- *Lactobacillus/Acidophilus* contains healthy bacteria, which help to improve the health of the digestive tract. Take 3 capsules daily. **BC**

Helpful Hints
- Stop smoking.
- Rinse your mouth out with a warm salt solution several times a day. Add 1 tsp of salt to a glass of cooled, boiled water. Add a few drops of goldenseal or liquorice tincture to aid healing.
- If stress is the culprit, exercise and relaxation may be the long-term answer.
- Try a herbal mouthwash containing bee propolis, calendula and St John's wort – and the homeopathic remedy Merc Sol, all of which are great for mouth ulcers. **OP**
- Tea tree oil is a natural antiseptic and makes a marvellous mouthwash when a few drops are mixed with warm water. Some people have found they are allergic to the material that false teeth are made from. Ask your dentist to test you for an allergy – porcelain is used as an

alternative material.
- I find that if I use a toothpaste containing fluoride, I get mouth ulcers. Try to avoid all fluoride.
- Mouth problems often reflect problems in the gut and digestive system. See a nutritionist who can re-balance your diet and suggest supplements to boost your immune system (see *General Health Hints*).

MRSA AND SUPERBUGS

(see also *Antibiotics* and *Immune Function*)

One of the unhealthiest places you can find yourself these days is in certain hospitals, where the worst infectious microbes are unavoidably found. In recent years this elementary truth has taken on a bizarre and frightening new dimension with the emergence of strains of pathogenic bacteria that are resistant to all known antibiotics, including methicillin – giving rise to the conditions technical name MRSA, standing for 'methicillin-resistant *Staphylococcus aureus*.

MRSA produces symptoms no different from any other type of *Staphylococcus aureus* ('Staph') infection. Confined to the skin, a patient may experience redness and inflammation around wound sites. But once it enters the body, symptoms can be more serious and include fever, lethargy, headache, urinary tract infections, pneumonia, toxic shock syndrome, and even death.

Staph infections, including MRSA, occur most frequently among persons in hospitals and healthcare facilities (such as nursing homes and dialysis centres), who have weakened immune systems. Where the infection has been acquired by someone who has had no hospital contact or medical procedure, it is known as CA-MRSA – community-associated MRSA.

The media term 'superbug' has distracted from the fact that MRSA is a manmade problem and was entirely avoidable. Overuse and abuse of antibiotics has led inevitably to the emergence of resistant strains. The advice that follows here – on combating bacteria without the use of antibiotics – will become increasingly important as the problem spreads.

The key to fighting any infection is to support and enhance the process of natural immunity and not rely on medication. This can be done through proper diet, supplements, and specific safe remedies, such as herbs and homeopathy. Make sure you boost your immune system *before* going into hospital for any reason. MRSA rarely affects really healthy individuals (see *Immune Function*).

Foods to Avoid
- Eliminate sugar, which has been scientifically shown to slow the performance of white cells needed to isolate and destroy the invader. This means stay off all manufactured and "junk" foods, because sugar is often an unsuspected ingredient, and limit your intake of sweet fruit juices, and fruits such as dates, grapes and mangoes (berries, on the whole, contain less sugar than most other fruits).
- Also avoid artificial sweeteners such as aspartame.
- Keep in mind that honey, brown rice syrup, and maple-type syrups are all sugar – but healthier.
- See also *Food Poisoning*.

Friendly Foods
- See also *Immune Function* and *General Health Hints*.
- Garlic is especially useful as it has anti-bacterial and anti-viral properties.
- You can eat small amounts of Manuka pure honey with a UMF level of 15, which has been shown to kill MRSA bacteria. The higher the UMF, the more antiseptic the honey. If the MRSA

causes open sores, then Comvita also make a high-strength Manuka dressing. From all good pharmacies.

- If you are desperate for sugar, try Slim Sweet, a low Glycemic Index sweetener from the lo-han fruit. From all health stores.

Useful Remedies

- See also *Antibiotics*.
- Bee propolis is a substance that bees manufacture to sterilise their hives, which has been shown in three studies to kill MRSA bacteria. You would need to take 3 grams a day before any stay in hospital and for at least a month afterwards. Bee Health make a potent formula – call them on 01262 607890. Website: www.beehealth.co.uk
- *Astralagus membranaceous* or Chinese root is widely used throughout the Orient. Scientific studies from the University of Texas Medical Centre in Houston have shown conclusively that it boosts immune performance by enhancing white-cell activity, stimulating interferon and reducing infection times (*Astralagus* could also therefore be beneficial for cancer and AIDS patients). It is non-toxic for normal cells and in tests actually enabled them to live longer than untreated cells. For more details of the pure herb, contact The Specialist Herbal Supplies on 0870 774 4494. **SHS**
- Herbs such as pau d'arco and St John's wort have been shown to help destroy MRSA. You would need 3–4 grams of St John's wort daily and 1–3 grams of pau d'arco. If you are taking blood-thinning medication, avoid St John's wort.
- Reishi mushrooms (*Ganoderma lucidum*) have known immune-boosting properties. For details call the Nutri Centre or Sloane Health Foods. **NC SL**

- Or try Host Defense by New Chapter, a mushroom supplement with a blend of reishi, maitake, and shiitake mushrooms, which has been shown to increase human Natural Killer (NK) cell activity. From all good health stores.
- If you are placed on high doses of antibiotics, make sure that you take a course of healthy bacteria afterwards. See *Antibiotics*.

Helpful Hints

Professor Keith Scott-Mumby, who has helped write this section, says, "If you or a loved one find you are battling an intractable infection of any sort, you may like to know about two important treatments. You'll need to find a specialist physician who understands and is willing to use these unusual approaches. Expect opposition but when conventional medicine has little to offer, it's time to ignore the criticisms of other approaches and strike out for yourself."

- **First – you can try intravenous Vitamin C** In the 1930s and 40s a US physician named Frederick R. Klenner began treating a variety of serious infections with high doses of intravenous vitamin C. These included polio (none of his cases developed infantile paralysis, at a time when hundreds were being afflicted), measles, mumps, chicken pox and pneumonia. Klenner even used this magnificent natural detox compound to treat snake bites. Others following his work, notably Thomas E. Levy, have found remarkable benefits treating malaria, hepatitis, staphylococcal infections, Rocky Mountain spotted fever, and amoebic dysentery. In the UK vitamin and mineral infusions are becoming more commonplace. Dr Wendy Denning offers this treatment in London (Tel: 020 7224 2423); or Dr Robert Trossell on 020 7486 1095.
- **Second – you can try hydrochloric acid injections** Faced with a desperate situation you may be glad of some comfort from another successful historic idea. In 1927 Dr Burr Ferguson, MD of Birmingham, Alabama, began injecting patients with severe infections using very dilute (1:1,000 concentration) of hydrochloric acid. This is a substance that occurs naturally in human stomachs in far higher concentrations. Ferguson's results were published in the journal *Medical World* in 1932. One of the most sensational cases was a woman at the point of death from puerperal

sepsis. Rather nervously (he knew he would be criticized if it went wrong), Ferguson injected the woman with hydrochloric acid. Within an hour her temperature had dropped from 106°C to 103°C and the woman said she felt much better. Save for weakness, the following day all trace of the infection had disappeared! These were dramatic pioneer days. But it seems that after decades of foolishly abusing antibiotics, doctors may be driving us back to the time when these humbler (and far cheaper) remedies will once again become necessary (read more on http://www.tldp.com/issue/11_00/martin.htm). (For more details of Dr Keith Scott-Mumby's work log on to www.alternative-doctor.com.)

- In the UK Dr Patrick Kingsley offers this treatment at his Leicestershire practice – call 01530 223622. Also Dr Wendy Denning on 020 7224 2423.
- Above all make sure that if any nurse or doctor – or anyone else – has contact with you in hospital, you ask them to thoroughly wash their hands in warm soapy water before touching you. You can also take anti-bacterial wipes with you – and wear sterile gloves, available from all chemists. Keep your visitors to a minimum, and as much as possible make sure that your room or the area around your bed is cleaned really thoroughly. If a relative will take your towels and so on to wash, have them boiled to thoroughly clean them. Simple measures can save lives.
- You can buy oregano essential oil as a spray, or coat any surfaces with this oil, which has potent anti-viral and anti-bacterial properties. You can also inhale steam with added oregano. Or, apply a little of the pure oil to the spine; or dilute it in a base of almond oil for massage. One of the best brands of therapeutic oils I have found is Young Living Oils from the US.

In the UK these are available from PSA Life Mastery on 01749 679900. Website: www.psalifemastery.com (see the *Resources* page). Their combination formula, which includes cloves, lemon, eucalyptus and rosemary is called Thieves' Oil. This name stems from the days when 15th-century thieves rubbed these oils on themselves to avoid contracting the Plague while they robbed the bodies of the dead and dying. The formula has been scientifically tested and found to have a 99.996% kill rate against all airborne bacteria. With 'Bird Flu' threatening, this is a great oil to use regularly.

MULTIPLE SCLEROSIS (MS)

Multiple sclerosis (MS) is an inflammatory progressive neurological disease that affects the central nervous system – the brain and spinal cord. Inside your brain and spinal cord there are two types of matter – grey and white, which are made up of millions of nerve cells. The white matter contains nerve fibres that are coated with myelin (like an electrical cable with a white outer-insulating case). The job of the myelin is to speed nerve transmission and allow the easy passage of electrical signals. When the myelin breaks down or becomes inflamed, nerve transmission is disrupted, thus resulting in the damage seen in MS.

MS is also an auto-immune disease, which means that the body's own immune system attacks the myelin. Initial symptoms may be tingling, numbness, or weakness affecting a hand, foot, or one side of the body; double vision; or a loss of sensation in various parts of the body. More women than men suffer MS, which can begin at virtually any age – but the average seems to be around 35.

There are four main types of MS, but each sufferer has a unique set of symptoms and disease pattern making it very difficult to diagnose. For this reason it is often missed by doctors for many years leading to considerable frustration for the MS sufferer.

Type 1 – Benign MS This starts with a small number of mild attacks followed by complete recovery. It does not worsen over time and there is no permanent disability. The first symptoms are usually sensory. It is only possible to classify people as having benign MS when they have little sign of disability 10–15 years after the onset of the disease. Around 20% of people with MS have the benign form.

Type 2 – Relapsing Remitting MS This is the most common form of MS. Periods of remission are interrupted by periods of attacks. The attacks can range from mild to quite debilitating. In the early stages of disease, complete recovery between the relapses is common, but over time remissions may result in residual symptoms caused by the damage to the myelin at the time of the attack. Around 25% of people with MS have the relapsing-remitting type.

Type 3 – Secondary Progressive This type starts out as relapsing-remitting MS, but after repeated attacks the remissions stop and the condition moves into a progressive stage. The time it takes to move into the progressive phase varies, but it usually happens within 15–20 years from the first onset of MS.

Type 4 – Primary Progressive Some people with MS have no distinct relapses and periods of remission. From the beginning they experience steadily worsening symptoms and progressive disability. This may level off at any one time, or may continue to get worse. Around 15% of people with MS have this type, which is also known as 'chronic progressive'.

The general medical profession is still looking for a 'cause' for this disease. In addition, the major drug companies are investing a lot of money in finding a 'treatment'. However, there are a number of factors known to affect disease progression that are worth investigating. The onset of MS has been attributed to viruses and having a weak nervous system that is then aggravated by trauma, shock, infection, or toxic metals, especially mercury. Dr Patrick Kingsley, one of Britain's leading alternative nutritional physicians specialising in cancer and MS, says, "Many of my patients have high levels of mercury in their spinal fluid, and the first thing I recommend is that they have the emissions measured from any mercury fillings." Dr Kingsley also says that "MS symptoms can also mimic those of candida, so this possibility needs to be eliminated." Parasites are another consideration as is a leaky gut. (See also *Candida*, *IBS* and *Leaky Gut*.)

Up to 70% of people with MS have problems absorbing nutrients properly so deficiencies are common, especially of B-vitamins, vitamin D, and the essential fats (EFAs) that are needed to make up myelin. EFAs play a critical role in MS (see the 'Swank' diet below) – for this reason therapeutic doses of some supplements are needed. Many patients also have multiple sensitivities to certain foods, the most common being cow's milk and products, plus gluten. In fact, these foods are now considered a major trigger. However, individual patients may react to almost any food, which needs to be identified on a personal basis. Many patients benefit when they follow a proper anti-candida and gluten-free diet. (See also *Allergie*s.)

Specialist Diets
Nutrition is seen as by far the single most important factor in managing MS. The most common diets used are:

The Swank low-saturated-fat diet
Professor Swank started his research in the 1940s in North America. He noticed MS was higher in countries in which the diet was rich in animal fats and where lots of dairy was consumed. Therefore, he recommended a low-saturated-fat diet (see *Fats You Need To Eat*).

The Omega Factor – Essential fatty acids (EFAs)
Following an article in the *Lancet* back in the 1970s, a lot of interest was directed towards the omega-6 oils, particularly GLA from starflower, evening primrose or borage oil, which is more

easily metabolized by the body than the linoleic acid that comes from sunflower oil. Again see *Fats You Need to Eat*.

Stone Age Diet 'Best-Bet Diet'

A Canadian scientist Ashton Embry's research has resulted in the 'Best Bet Diet'. The thinking behind this diet is that some people are especially sensitive to 'modern foods' so he came up with a Stone Age diet that excludes all 'new' foods – or foods that may have been around during the Stone Age, but have changed significantly. For example, modern wheat is bred to increase its gluten capacity so that cakes, breads and pastries can feel soft and fresher for longer. The Best Bet Diet excludes all gluten grains, dairy produce, beans and legumes, eggs, margarine, refined oils, yeasts, refined sugar and saturated fat. Ashton Embry has succeeded in getting some proper scientific trials under way in Canada on diet and MS. He has an excellent website at www.direct-ms.org

Foods to Avoid

- Cut down on saturated fats. Especially reduce or avoid those from animal origin – meats, and all full-fat dairy produce; butter, cheese, milk and cream. Be careful of curries as these are generally cooked using ghee, a clarified butter. Especially avoid cow's milk, yoghurt and even quark.
- Avoid all hydrogenated and trans fats and oils, found in many meat-substitute meals, margarines, biscuits, cakes, pastries and most processed vegetable oils. (See *Fats You Need To Eat*.)

- Do not eat fried food, crisps, chips, samosas, onion bhajis, burgers and so on as this can lead to inflammation. Instead grill, stew, poach, steam and bake.
- Avoid all refined carbohydrates, such as white bread and rice, pies, pastries, pizza, cakes and biscuits.
- As sugar also triggers inflammation in the body, avoid it as much as you can – look out for hidden sources in many sauces and processed foods.
- Avoid caffeine found in tea, coffee, colas, chocolates, some pain killers and many energy drinks.
- Avoid alfalfa sprouts. Although these are an excellent food source for most people, they should be avoided by those with auto-immune diseases.
- Avoid alcohol, which can cause nerve damage and depletes essential B-vitamins known to help MS.
- Identify and eliminate any food intolerances – see *Allergies*.

Friendly Foods

- Great alternatives to caffeine drinks are Barley Cup, No Caf, herbal and fruit teas, diluted fruit juice, Caro, vegetable juices, slippery elm tea, Yannoh, dandelion coffee and bamboo coffee.
- Instead of cow's milk choose oat, rice, nut, almond or skimmed goat's milk
- Juices, soups and salads contain lots of nutrients in an easily absorbable and nourishing form without creating great demands on our digestion.
- Eat plenty of oily fish. Choose from wild salmon, mackerel, herring, sardines and anchovies. These help to reduce inflammation and also provide the raw materials for making myelin. Deep sea fish are known to have high levels of mercury so need to be limited to once per week – this includes tuna and swordfish
- Eat plenty of fresh and preferably organic leafy green vegetables, full of B-vitamins and antioxidants, which help to protect the good fats from damage.
- GLA (gamma linolenic acid) is found in sunflower seeds and safflower oil and helps to nourish the nerve-endings. Use unrefined, organic seeds and oils. Keep them in the fridge.
- Pumpkin, sunflower and sesame seeds and linseeds (flax seeds) and their unrefined oils are all

rich in essential fats, which are vital for people with MS.

- Use cold-pressed sunflower, olive, hemp, linseed (flax seed) oil, or a mix of these oils, for salad dressings.
- Eat organic food as much as possible.
- People on vegan or gluten-free diets often experience some relief from symptoms – but the diet would need to be kept up for at least two years. Vegan diets are rich in essential fats needed for nerve function and low in saturated fat.
- Eat more brown rice, quinoa, kamut, spelt, lentils, barley and whole grains.
- Eat seaweeds that are rich in kelp and iodine, available from all health shops.
- Eat plenty of GM-free, organic lecithin granules, which are important for the structure of the myelin sheath that surrounds and protects the nerves.
- Blueberries are a particularly good source of antioxidants, which protect myelin from free-radical damage. Eat some daily; in winter buy them frozen.
- Add more curcumin – from the spice turmeric – to foods. This helps to slow the erosion of the myelin sheath.

Useful Remedies

- Take a good-quality multi-vitamin and mineral to cover your basic needs.
- Take a total of 10,000iu per day of vitamin A. Newborn infants fed a diet low in this vitamin have an increased risk of developing MS. Take only 3000iu if you are pregnant.
- Take 100mg of vitamin B1 (thiamine) daily, which is an essential component of myelin; as is vitamin B12 – take 1000mcg per day. Also take 50mg of vitamin B6.
- If you prefer not to take 3 pills, and as all the B-vitamins work together, instead buy a high-potency B-complex and take one daily.
- You can take up to 3 grams of vitamin C daily. Take it with meals in an ascorbate formula.
- If muscle aches are a problem, take 600mg of magnesium at bedtime, as magnesium helps to relax the muscles.
- Omega-3-rich fish oils help to support nerve-endings and are needed for normal functioning of the brain and nervous system, and the production of myelin. Take 1 gram per day.
- Star flower oil is rich in omega-6 GLA, which is anti-inflammatory and helps regulate the immune system. Take from 1 gram daily. Or you can order GLA itself from BioCare. **BC**
- Alternatively you could take Omega Plex powders, which contain a perfect blend of omega-3 and -6 fats in an easily digestible form. Dr Kingsley says the balance of 2 parts omega-3 to 1 part omega-6 is an ideal ratio for people with MS. **BC**
- Take a digestive enzyme with main meals to help increase the absorption of nutrients from your food. **BC**, and all good health stores.
- Co-enzyme Q10, a vitamin-like substance, is a potent protective antioxidant and also plays an important part in energy production. Take 60mg daily.
- Take a good probiotic (healthy bacteria) supplement daily to help keep digestion and bowel in top condition. Try Nutri's Ultra Probioplex. **NC**
- Studies have shown Acetyl L-carnitine to be more effective and better tolerated than the medication Amatadine, which is given to improve energy. Take 1000mg twice a day 30 minutes before meals. Available from www.positivehealthshop.com; or Tel: 01275 846664.

Helpful Hints

- Get any possible food allergies checked out. IWDL (Individual Wellbeing Diagnostic Laboratories) do a comprehensive test. Contact IWDL on 08704 190435 or check out their website at www.iwdl.net
- Vitamin D helps to regulate immune function and lift mood. Ask your GP to run a 25 (OHD) test to look at your levels. Optimal levels are 45–50 ng/ml or 115–128 nmol/l. If your levels are out

of this range contact a nutritional therapist who can help you to address this. Any levels below 20 ng/ml are considered serious-deficiency states and will increase the risk of auto-immune diseases. Contact the Institute for Optimum Nutrition to find a practitioner. Tel: 020 8614 7800.

- Check the possibility of excess mercury in your diet or environment.
- Consider having a hair mineral analysis to check your body levels of mercury. This is a non-invasive test that requires a small sample of hair. Contact The Analytical Research Laboratories on 0131 229 1077 for details.
- Dr Kingsley has found that vitamin-B12 injections help some patients. If you need to reach Dr Kingsley in the UK, call his practice. Tel: 01530 223622.
- Make sure your body knows what rest and exercise both feel like: take three 10–20 minute rest periods every day, spaced throughout the day, and do some form of fairly vigorous exercise every day, such as walking, press-ups or weight-lifting. Start slowly and build up gradually.
- Cranial osteopathy is a whole-body treatment that works with the central nervous system and the rhythmic pulsation that it produces. It has been very beneficial for some people with MS, as it helps to raise the vitality of the whole body. Find a practitioner at www.cranial.org.uk
- Among practitioners of alternative medicine, there is a degree of consensus – not generally shared by conventional doctors – that MS can be controlled. This type of approach involves nutritional, environmental, and lifestyle changes. It is important that treatment be followed under the guidance of a qualified practitioner. Because MS affects each patient differently, treatment programmes are individualised within the same overall plan. Dietary and nutritional needs are often addressed, as are food allergies, digestive health and environmental toxins. Recommendations may be made for detoxification therapy, as well as for the removal of mercury amalgam dental fillings. Consult a doctor who is also a nutritional physician (see *Useful Information*).

- Have a look at www.melisa.org – a medical network that gives the latest research linking mercury fillings to MS (see also *Mercury Fillings*).
- *New Pathways* is a magazine that provides information on all aspects of complementary and orthodox therapies found to be useful in MS. Subscriptions to *New Pathways* are £10 a year, available from The Multiple Sclerosis Resource Centre, which also has an excellent website: www.msrc.co.uk. Their information line and 24-hour telephone counselling service is on Tel: 0800 783 0518.
- The Multiple Sclerosis Society also has a Helpline on 0808 800 8000.
- Under Pressure is the UK's leading MS Clinic, giving advice and treatment for all levels of MS. Susie Cornell, sufferer and author of the book *The Complete MS Body Manual*, is the director of the clinic. Susie leads the field with a revolutionary approach in the natural treatment of MS. For more information telephone 01245 268098.
- For more help read *Multiple Sclerosis* by Judy Graham, the founder of the Multiple Sclerosis Resource Centre. She has also written a very informative book called *Multiple Sclerosis and Having a Baby*.
- There is now some exciting work going on in the Netherlands in which doctors are injecting umbilical-cord-derived stem cells from natural births into MS and chronically ill patients. Two ladies from the UK are walking again thanks to this pioneering treatment. Both my husband and I have had stem-cell therapy – which had a profound effect on our health. Dr Robert Trossell, whom I have known for several years, heads the team in the Netherlands. For more information look at www.pmc-rotterdam.nl

■ Dr Trossell also consults for one week a month in London at 4 Duke Street, London W1U 3EL. Tel: 020 7486 1095. However, the stem-cell therapy is administered in the Netherlands.

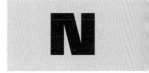

NAIL PROBLEMS *(see also Absorption and Low Stomach Acid)*

Nails are made up mostly from keratin, a protein-like substance also found in your hair. There are fat and water molecules in-between the keratin, which help to keep nails healthy and supple.

Your nails are a great barometer of your health. For example, if you are stressed or have poor digestion, then stomach acid levels often fall, in which case you may experience longitudinal ridges in your nails, which denotes low stomach acid. Ridges across the nails (from top to bottom) can denote a lack of calcium and/or magnesium, and stress.

White spots can denote that you are either ingesting too much sugar, alcohol, and junk foods, or have insufficient zinc in your body.

Brittle, transparent and flat-looking nails that curl up at the edges, are a common problem, associated with low iron levels. However, as excessive iron after the age of 50 is linked to heart disease, don't take too much iron unless a blood test shows you need it.

Brittle, splitting nails are a sign of silica deficiency; while soft peeling nails indicate a calcium deficiency. Excessively curved nails (like an upside down spoon) can indicate a potassium deficiency.

Anyone who has their hands in water for long periods usually has weaker nails; and biting the nails is an obvious cause for poor nails. Fungal infections turn the nails white, or at the very least they cause a discolouration and deformity in the nails. Nails can thicken if you eat too much protein, or when the immune system is at a low ebb. If your nail beds are red, your liver may be congested from too much fat and alcohol and you should have your cholesterol levels checked.

Foods to Avoid
■ Avoid junk foods, fizzy drinks, white bread, biscuits and pastries – all these foods deplete the body of nutrients, especially B-vitamins.
■ Reduce your intake of caffeine and alcohol.
■ Keep sugar to a minimum.
■ Hard thick nails can denote that you are eating too much fat and excess protein. Avoid hydrogenated or trans fats, and avoid too much fat from animal sources, including from full-fat milk, cheeses, chocolates, pies, desserts and so on.

Friendly Foods
■ Make sure that you eat good-quality protein at least once a day as nails are made from protein. Try chicken, fish, cooked tofu, or a little organic lean red meat. However, don't overeat protein, which can make the nails hard and thick, 6oz (150g) daily is fine.
■ Eggs, blackstrap molasses, almonds, red meats and spinach are rich in iron.
■ Oily fish, and unrefined nuts and seeds (especially hazelnuts, Brazil nuts and walnuts, and

sunflower, pumpkin and sesame seeds, and linseeds/flax seeds) are rich in zinc and essential fats. Use their unrefined oils over salads and cooked foods to nourish your nails.

■ Drink 6 glasses of water daily.

■ Eat more pumpkin, apricots, green leafy vegetables, cantaloupe melons and sweet potatoes for their vitamin-A content.

■ Cereals, brown rice, oats, organ meats, eggs, lentils, peas, nuts, and leafy green organic vegetables are all rich in B-vitamins, which are vital for healthy nails.

■ Eating a small amount of pineapple and papaya before or after meals aids digestion.

■ Eat one avocado a week and sprinkle organic wheat germ over cereals and desserts, as they are rich in vitamin E.

■ Silica-rich foods are lettuce and all high-fibre foods, vegetables and whole grains.

Useful Remedies

■ Take a comprehensive multi-nutrient vitamin and mineral powder that includes essential fats, such as Kudos 24 (see *General Supplements* for details; p.160).

■ Take a B-complex plus 2.5mg of biotin, a lack of which is linked to brittle nails. Vegetarians and vegans often also have low levels of B12 found in meat, fish and eggs, therefore make sure that your B-complex contains at least 50mcg B12. (Most multi formulas will include all the B-group.)

■ The mineral silica is important for healthy nails. Take 75mg daily.

■ If you have fungal infections, as well as following a low-sugar diet, the herbs pau d'arco (2 x 500mg capsules twice daily) and cat's claw (2 x 500mg capsules twice daily) will reduce fungus in the body and nails.

■ New Era Tissue Salt Combination K helps reduce brittle nails, and Combination L helps reduce fungal problems.

■ MSM, an organic form of sulphur, helps to strengthen nails. Take 200mg daily.

■ White blobs (more than tiny spots) on the nails can denote a lack of selenium. Take 200mcg daily.

Helpful Hints

■ Massage jojoba, neem and lemon oil into your nails to nourish and prevent splitting. **OP**

■ Nail-polish remover contains solvents, which are notorious for drying out nails and making them more brittle. Most nail salons and beauty counters sell oils specifically for the nails, which can be used after polishing. Always use a base coat.

■ To remove yellow stains from nails, soak them in a cup of warm water that contains the juice of 1 lemon for 15 minutes daily.

■ Massage your nails regularly with jojoba, olive or almond oil.

■ If you have a fungal infection, soak your nails in white distilled vinegar for at least 10 minutes twice a day. You can also use diluted tee tree oil or neem oil on the nails. The Organic Pharmacy makes a neem and tea tree cream, which can be used on hands and nails. **OP**

■ Bacteria, viruses and superbugs can breed under the nails and being in close contact with someone who has dirty nails is a great way to pass on infections. Also if you shake hands with someone who has a cold, this too will spread the virus. Keep your nails clean.

■ If your nails are constantly in water, then wear surgical or rubber gloves. Wear gloves when gardening.

■ Only use nail salons that keep their instruments scrupulously clean.

NAUSEA

(see *Vomiting*)

NUMBNESS/TINGLING SENSATIONS – FINGERS AND TOES

These types of symptoms are usually a sign of poor circulation (see *Circulation*), but can be caused by pressure on a nerve. These sensations are common if you sleep or sit in an awkward position, but may also be a symptom of cervical spondylosis (pressure on nerves in the neck, causing numbness in the hands, a stiff neck, or headaches) or carpal tunnel syndrome (numbness in the thumb-side of the hand, and sharp pain at night). If you suffer continually with really cold fingers and toes during the winter, you may well be suffering from Raynaud's Syndrome (see *Raynaud's Syndrome*). Any conditions that reduce circulation to the nerves in the skin will produce these types of symptoms. If symptoms continue have a check-up, as numbness is also linked to MS and ME.

Foods to Avoid
- See *Circulation*.
- Generally avoid caffeine, animal fats and smoking.

Friendly Foods
- See also *Circulation*.
- You are likely to be lacking in essential fats, which are found in oily fish, linseeds (flax seeds), and sunflower and pumpkin seeds and their unrefined oils. See also *Fats You need To Eat*.
- Eat more blueberries, blackberries, sweet potatoes, cherries, apricots, spinach, and leafy green vegetables. These are all rich in flavonoids, which strengthen capillaries.
- Wheat germ and avocados are rich in vitamin E, which thin the blood naturally.
- Garlic is great for circulation, while ginger will warm you.
- Lecithin granules aid repair of the nerve endings – sprinkle them on breakfast cereal or in yoghurts.

Useful Remedies
- Take a high-strength vitamin B-complex daily. A deficiency of B-vitamins can cause tingling in the nerve endings.
- Older people may also benefit from a B12 injection or a 1mg B12 tablet; a lack of this vitamin is linked to tingling in the extremities.
- Take 1–2 grams of vitamin C with bioflavonoids daily, to help repair nerve endings.
- Essential fats are needed for good circulation and well-toned blood vessels. Omega-3s (found in fish oils) have been shown to reduce blood-vessel spasms, omega-6s (in nuts and seeds) inhibit blood-vessel constriction.
- Fish oil is a great source of omega-3 fatty acids (EPA and DHA). A pure fish oil is more beneficial than linseed (flax seed) oil. A good, clean fish oil is Eskimo-3 (comes in capsule and liquid form). Good-quality omega-6 fatty acids (GLAs) are found in evening primrose and borage (starflower) oils. See *Fats You Need To Eat*.
- As this problem can denote a deficiency of calcium, take 600mg of calcium daily, plus a multi-mineral that includes 400mg of magnesium.
- Herbs such as horse chestnut and butcher's broom help increase circulation – V Nal is an excellent formula.

Helpful Hints
- If, after taking these supplements for 6 weeks, you still have numb and tingling fingers or toes, see your GP.
- Walking for half an hour each day, and skipping, rebounding and swinging your arms full circle regularly will help to get your circulation moving.

- It is also helpful to massage your hands and feet. Obviously it is easy to massage one's own hands, however if you find it difficult to massage your feet, ask your partner, a relative or a friend to do it for you. Use essential oils of geranium, ginger, black pepper and lavender in a base oil. If you have no one to massage your feet, pop a few drops of the oils in the bath and soak your feet for 10 minutes. For details of pure therapeutic oils – contact PSA Life Mastery on 01749 679900 or log on to www.psalifemastery.com and look under the Resources page.
- Reflexology and acupuncture often help reduce or eliminate this type of problem (see *Useful Information*).
- You may have a trapped nerve, in which case consult a chiropractor or osteopath.
- If the tingling and numbness is in the feet, wear magnetic insoles to increase circulation. These are available from all good sports shops and pharmacies.

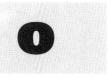

OBESITY
(see Weight Problems)

OSTEOARTHRITIS
(see Arthritis)

OSTEOPOROSIS   (see also *Acid–Alkaline Balance, Menopause* and *Stress*)

When I had my bone-density checked two years ago, it was fine. And then I spent a year writing another book, and was remiss about going to the gym as much as I should, and was under considerable stress. My diet was (and is) fine, and I have taken the right supplements for years. However, as my mother suffered severe osteoporosis – and I am the classic shape for osteoporosis (tall and thin) – I now have borderline osteo. Needless to say I am horrified, after doing so many right things, that my bones are not brilliant – but obviously it was not enough right things! Cause and effect. So, take heed – prevention is better than cure, and I hope by the time this book is published, with all the right actions I have taken, my bones will be much improved. After all, osteoporosis is not necessarily inevitable. The ageing process causes a gradual reduction in bone-density, but fractures should still be a rare occurrence. When osteoporosis develops there is a greater than normal decrease in bone mineral density, which leads to the bone fragility that can result in fractures, especially in the hips, wrists and spine.

One in 3 women and 1 in 12 men will develop osteoporosis during their lifetime. It is estimated that 3 million people in the UK alone suffer this condition, but many cases go undiagnosed. The occurrence increases with age, especially after 50, and women are at greater risk of developing osteoporosis after menopause, when the reduction of hormonal protection causes accelerated bone loss, which increases to 3–5% per year for 3 to 5 years and then continues at the rate of 1–1.5% per year.

Although osteoporosis is thought of as a disease of old age, recent research suggests that its roots lie in adolescence. A poor diet, lacking in vitamins and minerals such as calcium, magnesium and boron, during the teens can sow the seeds for brittle bones. This was definitely right in my case.

Phosphorous is a vital mineral, but high levels in the diet can deplete bone. Unfortunately, high levels of this element are found in fizzy, canned drinks, which are undoubtedly contributing to the growing numbers of young people with brittle bones. Junk foods, alcohol, and too much caffeine and sugar also deplete minerals.

Osteoporosis is also associated with a lack of weight-bearing exercise, excess animal protein in the diet, low body weight, and lack of skin exposure to sunshine (being out in the daylight increases vitamin-D levels in the body). My mother suffered osteoporosis, partly due to her poor diet, but also, she never exposed her skin to the sun. When she died at 78, her skin was amazingly wrinkle-free, but her bones were in a dreadful state. Hence I firmly believe that women who are fanatical about staying out of the sun, would definitely benefit from exposing their skin regularly to 15 minutes of early morning or late-afternoon sun to boost their vitamin-D levels.

A family history of osteoporosis, premature menopause, some cancers and long-term use of certain drugs, such as tranquillisers and steroids, also increase the risk for osteoporosis.

Other risk factors are a thin body-frame and smoking. Women who suffered anorexia when they were younger are also at risk. Women who exercise to the point where their periods stop are also at risk because of low hormone levels. As always a sensible balance is needed.

The hormones adrenaline and cortisol, when produced to excess, such as in long-term stressful situations and lifestyles, can thin bone, hence keeping yourself stress-free encourages healthier bones (for more details about cortisol, see *Stress*). Lack of absorption of nutrients within the gut is another contributing factor to thinning bones (see *Absorption*).

Traditionally, osteoporosis is prevented and treated by hormone replacement therapy (HRT). But naturopath Bob Jacobs says, "Women who have taken HRT for 10 years or more may have a greater bone density than those who have not taken it, but they lose any increased bone density rapidly when the HRT is stopped, and end up with only 3.2% higher bone density than women who took nothing. HRT can prevent osteoporosis only if women take it for the rest of their lives. When women exercise regularly, eat a healthy diet and take the right vitamins and minerals, bone density can be maintained and even increased, without having to endure the potential side-effects of conventional HRT, which are an increased risk of breast and endometrial (womb) cancers, thrombosis and strokes. Far better to use natural hormone therapy." (See *Useful Remedies*.)

Foods to Avoid

- Generally cut down on caffeine-based foods and drinks. More than 3 cups of strong coffee a day can increase your risk of developing osteoporosis by as much as 80%.
- Our Western diets tend to be very high in acid-forming foods, which cause more calcium to be excreted in urine. These include all the usual suspects of 'white' foods: breads, cakes, croissants, biscuits, white pasta and rice and so on (see *Acid–Alkaline Balance* for more information).
- Reduce sodium-based table salt, which increases calcium loss.
- On average we eat 50% too much animal protein, which increases acidity of the blood and promotes calcium loss from the bones. Women should avoid eating more than 3oz (68g) of animal protein a day, unless they are weight-training.
- Avoid fizzy drinks, because the artificial carbonation creates carbonic acid, which dissolves bone, and the excess phosphates force more calcium to be excreted.
- Avoid excess alcohol. Consuming more than 2 alcoholic drinks daily decreases calcium absorption from your diet. It also interferes with the synthesis of vitamin D, which helps the bones absorb calcium.

Friendly Foods

- Vegetarians tend to suffer less osteoporosis as their diet usually contains far more vegetables, grains and fruits.
- Ideal foods for strong bones – that is, foods that are high in calcium *and* reduce calcium loss – are green leafy vegetables, such as kale, alfalfa, kelp, cabbage and spring greens. In contrast, all dairy foods increase the loss of calcium, but also provide calcium – 4oz (100g) of kale, or spring greens will have at least as much beneficial effect on calcium balance as 8oz (200g) of milk or 4oz (100g) of Cheddar cheese.
- Eat more fermented soya-based foods, which are high in phyto-oestrogens (see *Menopause*).
- Calcium is found in green leafy vegetables, fish and sesame seeds, which contain as much calcium as many milks.
- Magnesium is found in brown rice, buckwheat, lentils, peas, corn, almonds, cashew and Brazil nuts, sunflower, sesame and pumpkin seeds, wheat germ, and whole-grain cereals.
- Vitamin D is found in egg yolks, oily fish, organ meats and milk. It allows the body to absorb the calcium and phosphorous needed for healthy bones.
- Vitamin K is vital for healthy bones, as it keeps calcium in the bones and out of the arteries where calcium deposits add to arterial plaque. Vitamin K is found in broccoli, green cabbage, lettuce and especially kale.
- As low stomach acid is often a factor in osteoporosis, eat more pineapple or papaya before meals to aid absorption.
- Silica is another vital mineral for healthy bones, found in lettuce, celery, millet, oats and parsnips.

- Boron is a trace mineral needed for healthy bones and is found in raisins, prunes, nuts, non-citrus fruits, and vegetables.
- Add 1 tbsp of organic cider vinegar and honey to a glass of warm water daily. Sip throughout the day. This helps the body to assimilate more calcium.
- Drink mineral waters in preference to tap water. Fiji water is rich in silica.

Useful Remedies

- Natural plant phyto-oestrogens and soya-based oestrogen supplements promote a positive calcium balance, they help make bone more resistant to releasing calcium, and reduce urinary calcium loss. Oestrogen levels decline with age in both men and women, with a particularly dramatic drop in women at menopause. All health shops sell such supplements.
- Natural Phyto-Estrogen Cream contains natural (meaning the exact molecule that is found in the human body) progesterone made from wild yam and oestrogen from soya beans, which helps to prevent osteoporosis and can, with proper nutrition help, increase bone density. To find out if you are at risk of osteoporosis, have a bone-density scan via your doctor and also ask for a urine DPD test to show if you are currently losing bone. If the bone scan is OK and the urine test shows no bone loss, then you don't need extra hormones. But if your density is low and the urine test shows excessive bone break down, then the use of natural hormones, the right diet, supplements, and exercise can be very useful. For a free information sheet on Phyto-Estrogen Cream call Freephone 00 353 46 943 7317 (between 10am and 5pm), or log on to www.pharmwest.com
- Most doctors recommend that you take twice the amount of calcium to magnesium, but some research has shown that in fact we need more magnesium than calcium. Dr Robert Trossell, a nutritional physician based in Europe and London, says, "We have found that a greater majority of women need more magnesium than calcium and I recommend at least equal amounts, or more magnesium than calcium. An optimum dose would be 1000mg of magnesium and 600mg of calcium taken in a chelated (or citrate) form, as they are more easily absorbed. These

minerals are known as nature's tranquillisers and are better utilised if taken at night."

- Vitamin K x 100mcg daily is very important for gluing the calcium into your bone matrix. Research has shown that vitamin K can reduce fracture risk by 65%. The beneficial effect of vitamin K is particularly noticeable in post-menopausal women who are not receiving oestrogen treatment. Most bone formulas contain some vitamin K.
- Vitamin C – 1000–2000mg per day with meals in an ascorbate form – promotes the formation of proteins required in bone and is also involved in the synthesis and repair of all collagen, including cartilage and matrix of bone.
- Zinc – 15mg per day – is necessary for bone-building.
- Vitamin D – 400iu – is essential for calcium and phosphorus absorption.
- Boron – 3mg per day – is necessary for the conversion of vitamin D into its active forms. It also helps the body produce natural oestrogen. This mineral is vital for healthy bones. In the US more women die from complications of a fracture of the femur than from breast cancer. Researchers also conclude that people living in countries with lower boron levels in the soil suffered much more arthritis.
- Vitamin B-6 – 100mg per day – is a necessary co-factor for many enzyme reactions involved in bone-building.
- All the companies listed on pages 13–15 make multi-vitamin and mineral and bone formulas that contain a balanced supply of most of these nutrients, which also includes HCl (stomach acid) to aid absorption. Don't be afraid to call and ask a nutritionist for help.

Helpful Hints

- Do not smoke. Women who smoke generally experience menopause up to a year and a half earlier than non-smokers, and thus face a longer period of oestrogen deficiency and accompanying bone loss. Smoking also hampers efficient processing of calcium. Smokers have a higher rate of spinal fractures than non-smokers.
- Chelation reduces the chances of developing osteoporosis (see *Helpful Hints* in *Heart Disease*).
- Osteoporosis is a largely preventable disease and there are some commonsense things you can do to reduce the risk. The most important is weight-bearing exercise. Swimming and cycling are great exercises, but they don't increase bone density as they are not weight-bearing. Skipping, jogging, walking, using weights, aerobics and rebounding (mini-trampolines) are great exercises to beat osteoporosis. Tennis players have a 30% higher bone density in their serving arm compared with their non-serving arm. For anyone already suffering osteoporosis, join a local gym and begin exercising with a professional.
- Weight training also increases bone density. In an ideal world begin weight training in your 20s and 30s before your bones start to thin, but it is never too late.
- Some clinics and doctors' surgeries in the UK have regular visits from mobile bone-screening services. All you have to do is place your foot in a small ultrasonic device, which measures the bone density in the heel of the foot, and you have a full read-out within 15 minutes. This simple and inexpensive test, while not as accurate as a full bone-density scan from a hospital, is a great way to know where you stand! For details call 01923 857616; or visit: www.mssuk.org
- Sunlight is needed to make active vitamin D in the body, so even if you are not a keen sunbather, then at least expose your skin to 15 minutes of sun regularly – but not between 11am and 3pm. Vitamin D helps us to absorb calcium.
- Dr Marilyn Glenville is one of the UK's leading experts on natural ways to cope with the menopause and osteoporosis. For more information log on to: www.marilynglenville.com. She has also written an excellent book *Osteoporosis, The Silent Epidemic* (published by Kyle Cathie).

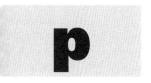

PALPITATIONS

(see also *Heart Disease* and *Tachycardia*)

This is a fairly common problem that just about everyone experiences at one time or another. If you are under stress, if you have suffered a shock, or if you are anxious, in response your heart begins to beat faster. Once the anxiety has passed, your heart rate should calm down, but if it doesn't then you have a problem. Palpitations occur when the heart beats irregularly; it can skip a beat or feel like a fluttering in the chest. If you find that you regularly suffer any of these symptoms and that they do not recede when you are calm, or if you are regularly short of breath, then you definitely need to see your doctor. Palpitations can also indicate that there is some problem with the electrical circuitry in the heart.

Foods to Avoid
- Avoid heavy alcohol intake, which can damage the heart muscle.
- Avoid stimulants, such as tea, coffee, chocolates, fizzy drinks and anything containing caffeine, which in itself can make you palpitate, as it stimulates the release of adrenaline into the blood-stream. My mother and brother suffered this problem if they touched *any* caffeine – once it was eliminated the problem disappeared.
- Food additives can trigger an attack in sensitive individuals.
- Generally don't eat large, heavy meals, which place an added strain on the body.
- Avoid hard fats and fried foods, and eating too much meat and full-fat dairy produce.
- Avoid any energy drinks containing the plant extract guarana, which is basically neat caffeine. Same for drinks like Red Bull.
- Any foods to which you have an intolerance may also cause palpitations. The most common are wheat, eggs, dairy from cows, and citrus fruits.

Friendly Foods.
- See *Angina*, *Heart Disease* and *General Health Hints*.

Useful Remedies
- L-theanine, extracted from green tea, helps to calm down the whole system without making you sleepy. Take 100mg 3 times daily.
- A pinch of cayenne pepper swallowed with a little water in most cases helps regulate the heart beat very quickly.
- An irregular heartbeat is linked to a calcium, magnesium and potassium imbalance or deficiency. Take 99mg of potassium daily for 1 month.
- Also take a calcium/magnesium formula containing 100–400mg of magnesium, 200mg of calcium.
- Folic acid – 600 mcg – daily helps to stabilise the heart beat.
- Niacin – 50 mg daily – helps stabilise the heart beat. Make sure you buy the **No-Flush** variety, as niacin can cause flushing of the skin, which can be scary if you are not aware of this effect.
- Also take a B-complex, as all the B-group vitamins work together to calm the nerves.
- Take a good-quality multi-vitamin and mineral containing 400iu of natural-source vitamin E. This helps the heart muscle to receive more oxygen.
- Co-enzyme Q10, a vitamin-like substance that is made in the body, helps to regulate heartbeat. As we age we manufacture less, so try 60mg daily – and then increase to 100mg daily.

Helpful Hints

- As palpitations can be linked to an overactive thyroid, ask your doctor to do a blood test to check thyroid function.
- Learn to meditate, which reduces stress, as worrying about this condition can precipitate an attack. See *Meditation* and *Stress*.
- To combat worrying, which only exacerbates the condition, learn how to breathe properly by taking yoga lessons.
- If you feel an attack beginning, splash your face with cold water, lie down, close your eyes, and breathe deeply and slowly for a few minutes until the attack passes.
- Essential oils of lavender and ylang ylang have a calming effect, try a few drops in your bath. You can also inhale the ylang ylang directly from the bottle to help slow your breathing. Try regular aromatherapy massage, which is very relaxing.
- Go for leisurely walks breathing deeply.
- Avoid eating large meals if you are anxious.

PANIC ATTACKS (see also *Low Blood Sugar, Palpitations, Phobias* and *Stress*)

Panic attacks occur during periods of acute anxiety and in Britain there are approximately 10 million sufferers. Feelings of intense panic lead to the person hyperventilating, which can produce feelings of light-headedness and tingling in the fingers and toes caused by too much oxygen. Panic attacks have a huge variety of causes, most of them based on fears or phobias. Obviously if a loved one dies suddenly, such as in a car accident, and you are with them, a panic attack would be triggered by acute shock. Some people have panic attacks if they see spiders or, if a person has had one heart attack or stroke, at the least pain they panic, believing another attack is imminent. When I had my near-death experience in 1998, for almost 2 months I suffered panic attacks, and believe me if someone tells you to pull yourself together, they are wasting their time. Reassurance and patience are what are needed. Panic attacks are also linked to low blood sugar.

Foods to Avoid

- Avoid stimulants, such as caffeine, sugar and alcohol, which can cause severe mood swings and disrupt blood sugar levels. Sugar substitutes such as aspartame are just as bad, so read labels carefully.
- Cut down your intake of animal fats, burgers, pies and processed foods.
- Tinned and pre-packaged foods are high in salt. Combine this with a panic attack and up goes your blood pressure.

Friendly Foods

- Eat calming foods that will also help to balance your blood sugar, such as brown rice, couscous, noodles, jacket potatoes, porridge, quinoa, whole-meal bread and pasta, lentils, and rice and corn pastas. These slower-release carbohydrates are essential to stabilise blood sugar levels.
- Eat small meals regularly.
- Snack on bananas, pears, apples and low-fat yoghurts.
- Eat at least one portion of quality protein, such as fish, chicken, lean meats or tempeh, daily.
- Don't skip meals.
- There are plenty of low-sugar and low-fat seed bars and snacks available from good health stores.
- Cut down on sodium-based salts; use a magnesium/potassium-based salt.

- Generally include more fruits and vegetables in your diet.
- Eat more oily fish rich in omega-3 fats, and seeds such as sunflower, sesame and pumpkin, as well as walnuts, almonds and Brazil nuts, which are all rich in omega-6 essential fats. (See *Fats You Need To Eat.*)
- Low levels of serotonin are linked to feelings of depression. Serotonin is made from a constituent of protein called tryptophan. Fish, turkey, chicken, cottage cheese, beans, avocados and bananas are all rich in tryptophan, which helps to keep you calm.
- Sprinkle wheat germ over a low-sugar breakfast cereal. My favourite is Nature's Path, who make great cereals from amaranth, quinoa and kamut, which are sweetened with a little apple juice. Available worldwide. Cereals are rich in B-vitamins, which help to keep you calm.
- Porridge is a very calming food.
- Eat more lettuce, mushrooms, peppers and root vegetables, which are also calming foods.

Useful Remedies

- Homeopathic Argent Nit, Gelsemium and Aconite taken in a combination helps reduce anxiety. Very potent – the Organic Pharmacy make them in one mixture. Take one pill as soon as you feel onset of symptoms. **OP**
- Take a good-quality B-complex daily to help support your nerves.
- Take **no-flush** niacinamide, which acts like a natural tranquilliser. **Make sure this is a no-flush variety**, as this amount would cause an extreme skin-flushing effect. You can take up to 500mg 4 times daily if symptoms are severe. **SL**
- Inositol, one of the B-Group vitamins, has been shown to reduce panic attacks. A good source is lecithin granules. Sprinkle liberally over yoghurts, fruit and so on.
- Take up to 2 grams of vitamin C daily with meals, as mild to moderate deficiency is associated with nervousness.
- Take 400iu of vitamin E, 1000mg of calcium and 400mg of magnesium daily. Many people who suffer panic attacks are lacking in these minerals.
- Take potassium – 99mg per day. Low levels can increase susceptibility to anxiety.
- Try L 5-Hydroxy Tryptophan (L 5-HTP), 50–200mg per day. This is the precursor to serotonin, which is called the 'happy brain neurotransmitter'. Panic attacks can be reduced by increasing serotonin levels in the brain. **HN**
- Take the herb rhodiola, which helps the body cope with physical and emotional stress. Really excellent. Kudos make a high-strength one-a-day. **KVH**

Helpful Hints

- Bach Flower Remedies are helpful for reducing panic attacks. Try Star of Bethlehem, Rescue Remedy, or Jan de Vries Emergency Essence, and if you feel an attack coming on, treat the flower remedy as your medicine. Say to yourself as you place it under your tongue, "This will calm me down in under 3 minutes." Keep repeating this phrase and it will help.
- Regular exercise reduces stress and builds confidence. A regular aromatherapy massage with lavender oil helps you to stay calm and balances the emotions. A warm, relaxing bath, and sound, restful sleep do wonders to ease stress.
- Learn how to control the attacks; fighting them will make them only worse. Tell yourself that this is just the body's way of getting you to take care of yourself. Speak to yourself gently, as you would to comfort a child.
- Hypnotherapy and self-hypnosis called Neuro-Linguistic Programming have proven very successful for reducing panic attacks and phobias. See *Useful Information* for details.
- If you know you are hyperventilating have a large paper bag at the ready and breathe slowly and calmly into the bag to help calm you down and to stop you fainting.
- Homeopathic Aconite 200c taken upon onset of an attack is a great remedy if you have intense fear.

■ First Steps to Freedom, a self-help group, have a helpline for people with phobias. Fact sheets, self-help booklets, audio/video tapes, books and online support groups are available. For further information write to First Steps to Freedom, 7 Avon Court, School Lane, Kenilworth, Warwickshire PV8 29X Tel: 0845 120 2916. The helpline is open 10.00am–10.00pm every day. Website: www.first-steps.org

PARASITES   *(see Irritable Bowel Syndrome)*

PARKINSON'S DISEASE

Parkinson's Disease is a degenerative disorder of the central nervous system. It affects some 120,000 people in Britain, including 1 in every 100 people over the age of 60. It affects men more often than women. Although Parkinson's tends to affect people over 50, it sometimes occurs in younger people if they have suffered any type of brain inflammation, carbon-monoxide poisoning, over-exposure to toxic metals, or certain drugs.

The condition triggers deterioration of the nerve centres in the brain responsible for controlling movement. As the condition progresses, muscular movement is affected. Eventually co-ordination can become a nightmare and it's common for patients to experience tremors, rigidity and muscular spasms in different limbs to varying degrees. Other symptoms include unsteadiness, chronic constipation, impaired speech, a fixed facial expression and a shuffling gait. The person knows what they want the muscle to do, but the messages received by the muscle group are not properly coordinated to allow smooth movement.

The reason for this impaired muscle control is a lack of the brain chemical dopamine. No definitive cause has yet been proven, but nutrient deficiencies, heavy metal toxicity, especially from mercury and aluminium, pesticides, over-consumption of the artificial sweetener aspartame, viruses and carbon-monoxide poisoning are all suspects. Some prescription drugs can cause Parkinson's-like symptoms.

To replace the dopamine most patients take a synthetic form of the amino acid L-dopa, which the body then makes into dopamine, helping restore proper brain function. Many of the drugs used to treat Parkinson's can cause lethargy and extreme mental confusion, or completely uncontrolled jerky movements if there is too much L-dopa in the body. As every case is unique, I strongly recommend that anyone with Parkinson's consult a nutritional physician who is trained in PD (Parkinson's Disease) management, as this condition needs highly specialised care (see *Useful Information*).

Foods to Avoid
■ Reduce stimulants, such as coffee, colas, tea and alcohol, as these foods can affect tremors.
■ Cut down on all animal fats, which impair the metabolism of essential fats (see *Fats You Need To Eat*).
■ Avoid sugar in any form, highly refined and processed foods, and especially additives and preservatives, such as monosodium glutamate and aspartame, because of their negative affect on the brain.
■ With professional guidance you may also need to eliminate gluten-containing grains, such as wheat, rye, oats and barley – as the gluten can prevent absorption of nutrients and medication.
■ Cut down on peanuts, bananas and potatoes, yeasty foods, liver and meat, which contain vitamin B6. This vitamin can interfere with the medication L-dopa. If you are not taking L-dopa,

vitamin B6 is important for Parkinson's.

■ Don't fry food and avoid all hydrogenated and trans fats, often found in margarines and pre-prepared foods. These fats are also found in most mass-produced cakes, biscuits, pies and so on. Always check labels.

Friendly Foods

■ Ensure an adequate dietary intake. Because chewing can become difficult, loss of appetite is common and then nutrient deficiencies can speed the progression of the disease. Foods can be liquidised or meal replacements used.

■ As much as possible eat only organic foods, which contains fewer pesticides and herbicides. A University of Miami post-mortem study in 1994 found pesticides more often than in those who had died of Parkinson's Disease than in those who had died of other causes.

■ Research has shown that restricting protein intake is helpful and that 90% of the daily intake should be eaten with the evening meal, when you are not having your L-dopa medication. This is extremely important advice not always given to patients on L-dopa. Protein competes for absorption with the L-dopa, so eating protein during then day, when most sufferers take their medication, can block the efficacy of the medication.

■ Protein can be found in lean meats, fish, eggs, beans, dairy foods, nuts and seeds, lentils, fermented soya foods and whole grains. The best sources for Parkinson's sufferers are small amounts of soya, eggs, oily and white fish, and poultry

■ Eat more corn-based foods and corn pasta.

■ Include apples, pears, mangoes, kiwi fruit and vegetables, such as cabbage, cauliflower, carrots and broccoli, in your diet.

■ Use unrefined, organic sunflower, sesame and olive oils for salad dressings and to drizzle over cold foods. These oils are rich in essential fats, which are vital for healthy brain function as they enhance brain cell wall stability (see *Fats You Need To Eat*).

■ Get into the habit of juicing. Use organic carrots, beetroots and artichokes, which are high in vitamins and minerals and help to cleanse the liver (see *Liver Problems*).

■ If you have mercury fillings, eat lots of seaweed, apples and coriander, which detoxify metals from the body. See *Mercury Fillings*.

■ Dried or ready-to-eat fruits such as prunes, figs and apricots, help to ease or prevent constipation, as does drinking at least 8 glasses of water daily.

■ Begin drinking green or white tea, rich in antioxidants.

Useful Remedies

■ It is vital to take various nutrients in specific amounts for each individual case, and the supplements you take also depend on the time of day and which medication you are taking. Again I strongly recommend that you see a qualified nutritionist or nutritional physician who can devise a programme specifically for you. Your own GP will need to refer you to a nutritional physician and they will be able to find the address of your nearest practitioner by contacting: British Society for Allergy, Environmental and Nutritional Medicine (BSAENM). Website: www.bsaenm.org Tel: 0906 3020010 (information line).

Meanwhile here are some general guidelines:

■ Studies from the Birkmayer Institute for Parkinson's in Vienna has shown that NADH, a co-enzyme form of vitamin B3, can help increase energy levels, reduce depression and stimulate the body to produce more L-dopa. 5mg should be taken on an empty stomach at least 40 minutes before food. Professor Birkmayer's highly absorbable NADH is called Springfield Enada and is available worldwide. Anyone who is very stressed and suffers from palpitations should avoid this supplement. However, in some cases the intravenous form of this nutrient is more effective in Parkinson's – speak to your doctor about the intravenous form.

- Antioxidants – such as vitamin C, up to 1 gram daily with food – and 400iu of full-spectrum, natural-source vitamin E, in addition to an antioxidant complex may help to slow the progression.
- L-methionine – an essential sulphur amino acid, which readily crosses the blood-brain barrier where it can be converted into the vital nutrient S-adenosyl methionine (SAM-e). L-dopa supplementation reduces brain SAM-e levels. **NC SL**
- The amino acids tyrosine and phenylalanine help to ensure that the brain has sufficient raw materials for the synthesis of dopamine. Dosages would need to be set by a qualified doctor or nutritionist – see above.
- Phosphatidyl Serine (PS) is another vital brain nutrient that improves nerve-cell health. The body can manufacture PS, but only if you tend to eat lots of organ meats. 100mg can be supplemented 2–3 times a day.
- For extra fibre to ease constipation and cleanse the bowel, try psyllium husks daily in warm water. They taste dreadful, but do help reduce constipation. Also available in capsules.
- The herb St John's wort can ease depression, but should not be taken by people with Parkinson's as it can interfere with medication.
- If you have mercury fillings take vitamin C x 500mg daily, which chelates with heavy metals and carries them out of the body, plus mercury antagonists: calcium x 450mg a day and zinc x 15mg twice daily.
- When we are young the body makes a vitamin-like substance called Co-enzyme Q10, but as we age levels fall. CoQ10 seems to offer protection against certain degenerative brain functions. Take around 100mg daily – under advice.
- Chlorella helps to rid the body of unwanted heavy metals – take 500mg twice daily. Ask for an organic-source chlorella.

Helpful Hints

- Mercury fillings are linked to Parkinson's – have them checked by a holistic dentist and removed if necessary (with all the necessary protection during removal – otherwise you can become even more contaminated). See *Mercury Fillings* for more information.
- As many of the world's oceans are heavily polluted, high levels of mercury are also being reported in some coastal fish.
- Aluminium and mercury have been linked to Parkinson's, therefore avoid all aluminium cookware or aluminium foil. Read labels carefully as cake mixes, antacids, buffered aspirin, self-raising flour, pickles, processed cheeses, and most deodorants and toothpastes contain aluminium.
- Monosodium glutamate (MSG), the food additive, and aspartame the artificial sweetener, have been linked to Parkinson's; therefore avoid all additives and preservatives whenever possible. More than 3,000 foods and drinks contain artificial sweeteners.
- Reduce stress. At times of stress the body uses dopamine to make the stress hormones nor-adrenaline and adrenaline, using up your already short supply. Tools for reducing stress, apart from removing any obvious sources, include exercise, massage, relaxation techniques, meditation or enjoyable hobbies (see *Stress*).
- If tremors are worse at or after meal times, avoid protein (meat, fish, beans, nuts, seeds) at meals where you take your medication, as protein competes with the L-dopa for absorption.
- Constipation is a major symptom that must be dealt with to ensure the proper elimination of toxins. In addition to the dried fruits, linseeds (flax seeds) and water are recommended; and try abdominal massage in a clockwise circular motion to massage the bowel. Take walks after meals, or supplement with magnesium (150mg x 3 times per day) to relax the bowel. See *Constipation*.

- As organophosphates (OPs), from pesticides and herbicides, are now found in drinking water, use a good-quality water filter, such as Watersimple from The Fresh Water Filter Company (Tel: 0870 4423633. Website: www.freshwaterfilter.com) or The Pure H2O Company (01784 221188. Website: www.purewater.co.uk).
- A book well worth reading is *Parkinson's Disease, The Way Forward* by Dr Geoffrey Leader and Lucille Leader (Bath Press). To order call 020 7323 2382. This user-friendly book presents an integrated approach to the management of Parkinson's Disease.
- Dr David Perlmutter, a neurologist in Naples, Florida, has pioneered the use of intravenous glutathione, which has had a dramatic effect on most of his Parkinson's patients. His book *The Better Brain Book* (River Head Books) makes fascinating reading. Available from the Nutri Centre bookshop (NC), or log on to Dr Permutter's website: www.BrainRecovery.com. In the UK doctors who administer chelation therapy usually work with glutathione – for more details of chelation see *Helpful Hints* in *Heart Disease*. For more details on glutathione, see *Liver Problems*.
- Stem Cell Therapy holds great promise for Parkinson's Patients – for more details of where you can find treatment, see *Multiple Sclerosis*.
- For further help contact The Parkinson's Disease Society. Helpline: 0808 800 0303. Website: www.parkinsons.org.uk. Or the European Parkinson's Disease Society. Tel/Fax: 01732 457683. Website: www.epda.eu.com

PCOS – Polycystic ovarian syndrome

(see also *Infertility*)

One in 5 women who has a scan during gynaecological investigations has polycystic ovaries. About 80% of these women experience a variety of symptoms and are then classed as having PCOS. Symptoms may include, irregular or no periods, erratic or no ovulation, sub-fertility, recurrent miscarriages, excess facial and body hair, fatigue, acne, weight gain that is hard to shift, hair loss, mood swings, abdominal pain, aching joints, and dizziness. Long term there is a sevenfold increase in the risk of cardiovascular problems and diabetes. Depression, anxiety and low self-esteem are also problems with this condition .

The job of the ovaries is to produce hormones, ripen and release eggs ready for fertilisation, and prepare the lining of the womb for pregnancy. If no fertilisation occurs, then the lining is shed, leading to a period. This whole process is governed by the sex hormones. Follicle stimulating hormone (FSH) and luteinising hormone (LH) are made by the pituitary in the brain, and in response to these hormones the ovaries then produce progesterone, testosterone and oestrogen. PCOS occurs when there is an imbalance in these hormones, namely high oestrogen, testosterone and LH. High levels of the hormone insulin needed to balance blood sugar levels are also produced. The body's insulin receptors on the surface of cells seem to switch off and stop listening to the signal from insulin, and so to compensate, the body overproduces insulin, which further disrupts the sex hormones. Research shows that by enhancing the body's ability to register the insulin, all hormone levels can become normalised.

Foods to Avoid
- Sugar in all its forms, as sugar affects hormone levels in the body. Avoid it in breakfast cereals, cakes, biscuits, sweets, and chocolate; and look out for it hidden in many sauces, such as ketchup and salad dressings.
- Alcohol exerts an oestrogen-like action in the body, so is best avoided. If you must indulge, keep to a minimum and drink red wine as this helps to protect against cardiovascular disease.

- Cut right back on caffeine, which can disrupt hormone levels – coffee, tea, cola drinks, and some painkillers contain it.
- Eat less red meat, beef, pork, dairy products and fried foods. Excess consumption of the wrong kinds of fat can lead to weight gain and cardiovascular problems (sufferers of PCOS have a higher risk of developing cardiovascular problems). When preparing foods grill, bake or stir-fry with olive oil.

Friendly Foods
- Eat small regular meals that contain complex carbohydrates – brown rice, pasta, rye bread, millet and quinoa – as this will help to keep blood sugar levels in the body more even and hence reduce insulin which disrupts hormone levels.
- Eating protein – lentils, beans, eggs, lean chicken and turkey, nuts and seeds – with all meals and snacks helps to make insulin more effective and hence reduce levels.
- Omega-3 essential fatty acids, found in linseeds (flax seeds), hemp seeds and oily fish (salmon, mackerel, fresh tuna, herring and anchovies), have an important role to play in helping to control insulin resistance and hence hormone disruption.
- Go organic, as many of the pesticides liberally sprayed onto foods can have a hormone-disrupting action
- Fibre is known to bind to excess hormones and help to remove them from the body. Eat more wholegrains, brown rice, millet, beans, lentils, oats and lots of fresh fruit and veggies.
- Have some live, sugar-free yoghurt daily to feed the good bacteria in the gut as this helps to break down excess hormones. Add some berries for flavour as these have a cardiovascular protective action.
- Phyto-estrogens help to reduce high oestrogen levels. Therefore eat foods such as miso and tempeh (a fermented form of soya), plus linseeds (flax seeds), beans and lentils.

Useful Remedies
- Take a good-quality B-complex providing between 50 and 100mg. B-vitamins are essential for balancing sugar levels in the body and help with oestrogen-related hormonal problems. Most multi-vitamin and mineral formulas contain B-vitamins.
- If your PCOS is causing you a lot of stress and upset, consider taking 5-HTP – known to lift mood. 100–300mg per day, taken at bed time with a small carbohydrate snack – oat cakes are ideal. (Do not take this alongside St John's wort or antidepressant medication.)
- Agnus castus has been used for centuries to balance female hormones. Bioforce do a great tincture – use 15–20 drops twice a day. Tel: 01294 277344. Website: www.bioforce.co.uk
- Take a phyto-estrogen supplement (one a day), such as Novogen Red Clover (available from the Nutri Centre). **NC**
- Add in a milk-thistle complex to support the liver's ability to break down excess hormones. Milk Thistle Plus, available from BioCare, is a tea that also contains liver-supporting dandelion and liquorice. **BC**

Helpful Hints
- If you are overweight, lose weight. Studies at St Mary's Hospital in London found that moderate weight loss helped to correct hormonal abnormalities, reduced body hair, and improved chances of conception.
- Exercise not only helps with weight loss and strengthens the heart, but also releases feel-good hormones in the body, so it can give you a lift if you are feeling blue. Aim for three 20-minute sessions per week. Start with a gentle walk outside, as daylight is also known to lift low moods and depression.
- Use a water filter. Millions of women currently take the contraceptive pill and pee it into the water cycle; if you drink it, this is known to have an effect on hormone levels.

- Food wrapped or cooked in plastic or cling film will have negative effect on hormone balance. The risk is increased when these plastics are heated. If you do have to buy food that is wrapped in plastic, transfer these foods to a glass container as soon as you get home.
- Women with PCOS have found acupuncture useful in helping to kick start non-existent cycles and regulating cycle length.
- Learn to relax and tackle your stresses, both physical and emotional. Stress contributes to high insulin levels and hormonal imbalances.
- Essential oils of vitex agnus castus, geranium and rose may be beneficial to balance hormones; whilst sandalwood, neroli, ylang ylang and mandarin are good for relaxation. Add to a relaxing bath or use in an oil burner.
- www.verity-pcos.org.uk is a great, informative website with lots of practical information and fact sheets. They also run conferences about PCOS 3 times a year.

PHLEBITIS

(see also *Circulation* and *Leg Ulcers*)

Phlebitis is caused by inflammation of the walls of the veins, usually near the surface of the skin. It is often combined with the formation of small blood clots on the area of the inflammation. It may be caused by a sensitivity to external irritants such as washing powders or by food allergies. The condition can occur after injections or intravenous infusions and is common in intravenous drug abusers. It is more common in people who have varicose veins and also in blood vessel disorders such as Buerger's disease. Symptoms include swelling and redness along and around the affected segment of vein, which can become very tender when touched. The best way to prevent this condition is to keep your circulation in good condition by eating the right foods.

Foods to Avoid
- Identify and avoid foods to which you have a sensitivity, the most common being wheat and dairy from cows.
- Use a good-quality reverse osmosis water-filter system. Try The Pure H2O Company on 01784 221188. Email: info@purewater.co.uk. Website: www.purewater.co.uk. As organophosphates (OPs) are now found in drinking water, many sufferers find some relief when they switch to pure water.
- Cut down on all saturated fats, found in animal produce, sausages, meat pies, full-fat cheese, milk, chocolate and hard margarines.
- Don't fry food and never use mass-produced, refined, hydrogenated oils. See *Fats You Need To Eat*.
- Reduce your intake of cakes, burgers, biscuits, and white breads and pastas.
- Many of these foods are packed with fats, salt and sugar. Sugar converts to fat in the body if not used up during exercise (see also *General Health Hints*).

Friendly Foods
- Increase your intake of oily fish, which is rich in the omega-3 essential fats that help to thin blood naturally.
- Sprinkle wheat germ and lecithin granules over cereals and desserts. They help to emulsify the bad fats, which aids circulation.
- Buy a packet each of organic, unsalted walnuts, Brazil nuts, almonds, sunflower and pumpkin seeds, sesame seeds and linseeds (flax seeds), which are high in omega-6 essential fats. Whiz them all in a blender and keep in an airtight jar in the fridge. Sprinkle over any foods you like.

These add healthy fats, fibre and minerals, such as zinc, to your diet, which are vital for skin- and wound-healing.

- Eat more wholemeal bread, pasta and noodles. Try lentil, corn, spelt and rice pastas, which are freely available in supermarkets and health shops.
- Use skimmed milk or try organic rice milk or low-fat goat's milk, which are both low in fat.
- Include garlic in your diet, which thins blood naturally.
- Olive oil and avocados are rich in monosaturated fats, which are healthy and aid healing.
- Eat more fresh fruits and vegetables, especially pineapple and papaya, which are rich in digestive enzymes that aid healing.

Useful Remedies
- Take 400iu daily of natural-source vitamin E to help thin the blood naturally.
- Take a high-strength multi-vitamin and mineral made specially for men and/or women over 50.
- Some people find relief by placing raw papaya on the affected area for an hour a day.
- Bromelain, extracted from pineapple, has good anti-inflammatory effects. Take 2000–3000mcu daily. **FSC**
- Use Circulation Tincture – containing witch hazel, horse chestnut, ginger and bilberry, which all help to increase circulation and reduce swelling associated with this condition. Available in one liquid formula from the Organic Pharmacy. **OP**
- Rutin is an excellent bioflavonoid for helping to strengthen the artery and vein walls. 300 mg daily.

Helpful Hints
- Basically, you need to get moving. Begin by walking for 15 minutes daily and gradually increase over a 1-month period to 1 hour a day.
- When applicable, use stairs instead of lifts.
- An extremely gentle and easy exercise regime, such as swimming, yoga, Qigong or T'ai chi, would also be helpful; as would reflexology and acupuncture (see *Useful Information*). T'ai chi can be practiced by people of any age – well into the 80s and 90s.

PHOBIAS

(see also *Panic Attacks*)

A phobia is an extreme or irrational fear attached to a specific object or situation that is basically not life-threatening – but for the person with the phobia, the fear is often overwhelming and their lives can become a nightmare. Most common phobias are fear of confined spaces, or various animals and insects, such as birds or spiders. Certain social situations provoke anxiety in some people, who fear that they will become trapped or embarrassed. Low blood sugar can contribute to this problem (see also *Low Blood Sugar*).

Foods to Avoid
- As much as possible, avoid stimulants, such as coffee, tea, alcohol and sugar, and cut down on foods or drinks containing caffeine or sugar.
- See also *Panic Attacks* and *General Health Hints*.

Friendly Foods
- Low levels of serotonin are linked to feelings of depression. Serotonin is made from a con- stituent of protein called tryptophan, so include more foods such as fish, turkey, chicken, cottage cheese, beans, avocados, bananas and wheat germ in your diet to raise your mood and help keep you calm.
- Calming foods also include brown rice and pastas, noodles, couscous, potato, lettuce,

mushrooms, peppers and root vegetables.

- Oats are a great food for helping to re-build nervous tissue – have oat-based porridge for breakfast daily.
- Sprinkle wheat germ over breakfast cereals or fruit whips. There are plenty of cereals available made from amaranth, quinoa and kamut, sweetened with a little apple juice. Cereals, including porridge, are rich in B-vitamins, which help to keep you calm.
- Drink more green tea and liquorice tea.

Useful Remedies

- The amino acid L-theanine – found in green tea – really helps to keep you calm without making you feel in any way sleepy. 100mg taken 4 times throughout the day. **NC SL**
- The herbs ashwagandha, Siberian ginseng and gotu kola are adaptogenic herbs, which help the adrenal system to normalize. These are all included in the Advanced Stress Formula by Holos Health www.holoshealth.com. **NC**
- Niacinamide, vitamin B3 (500–800 mg daily) acts as a natural anti-anxiety agent, **but you must ask for the no-flush variety**, otherwise you will find your skin looks like a cooked lobster.
- 1000mg of calcium, 500mg of magnesium and 30mg of zinc will help keep you calmer. **SVHC**
- 5-Hydroxy Tryptophan (5HTP) is a supplement that helps to raise serotonin levels in the brain naturally, which helps to improve mood and calm you down. Start with 25mg and increase over 10–14 days to 75mg 3 times daily.

Helpful Hints

- Learn to meditate (see *Meditation*). People who practice regularly have lower blood pressure, are less anxious, and are more able to cope during stressful situations.
- First Steps to Freedom, a self-help group, have a helpline for people with phobias. Fact sheets, self-help booklets, audio/video tapes, books and online support groups are available. For further information write to First Steps to Freedom, 7 Avon Court, School Lane, Kenilworth, Warwickshire PV8 29X. Tel: 0845 120 2916. The helpline is open 10.00am–10.00pm every day. Website: www.first-steps.org
- Hypnotherapy is an excellent way to find the root cause of your problem and to learn how to let it go so you can lead a normal life (see *Useful Information*).
- Paul McKenna, the world-renowned hypnotherapist, has made some great self-hypnosis CDs and tapes that help to remove phobias. Tel: 0845 230 2022. Website: www.paulmckenna.com
- Homeopathic Aconite 200c is a good remedy when you are experiencing intense fear or terror.
- Get some more exercise, which helps to produce more mood-boosting chemicals in the brain.

PILES (HAEMORRHOIDS) (see also *Constipation*)

Piles are basically varicose veins formed inside the anus when veins become enlarged. If you suffer chronic long-term constipation, then the veins can break through the anus and protrude externally. If you feel this happening and the vein is still soft and pliable you can carefully ease the swollen vein back inside the anus. But if the pile becomes hardened and forms a clot and remains outside the anus, this calls for immediate medical attention. When you go to the loo, if you have piles or an anal fissure, you can often see blood in the stools and experience extreme discomfort and itching in that area. Also, if your liver is congested – which is common in this problem – it can place more pressure on your back, which in turn adds pressure to your venous system, which can make piles worse.

Piles can also be caused by persistent coughing, pregnancy and childbirth, standing and sitting for long periods, overuse of laxatives, and travelling long distances sitting on heated car seats – all of which raise pressure in rectal veins. If you bleed from the anus at any time, you should seek medical attention immediately.

Foods to Avoid

- Generally you need to avoid eating too many foods based on flour – cakes, white breads, refined biscuits, pies and desserts – as flour gunks up the bowel. If you mix flour and water together you get a very sticky paste and this does not change consistency in the bowel!
- Melted cheese and full-fat cheeses can also cause constipation.
- Red meat takes a long time to digest. If you must eat meat, have only small portions.
- Coffee, canned fizzy drinks, and alcohol all dehydrate the bowel.
- Avoid mass-produced foods, such as burgers and high-fat take-aways.
- Reduce your intake of full-fat dairy products from cows.
- Avoid sodium-based salt.
- For some people, eating citrus fruit and tomatoes makes the situation worse.

Friendly Foods

- Drink at least 6 glasses of water daily even if you are not thirsty.
- Eat far more fresh, lightly cooked vegetables and salads – especially green leafy vegetables such as celery, spinach, spring greens and cabbage.
- Figs, prunes, apples, pineapples, apricots, bananas, mangos, papaya, avocados, grapes and melons will all help reduce the constipation. Strawberries, raspberries, peaches, sultanas, raisins and dates should be eaten regularly.
- Eat good-quality protein, such as skinless chicken, and fish, tempeh, beans, peas and pulses.
- Eat more wholemeal bread, pastas and noodles.
- Enjoy low-sugar, high-fibre cereals for breakfast. Try cereals made from kamut, spelt and quinoa, which are less likely to irritate the gut than wheat bran.
- Use oat and rice bran.
- Try blackstrap molasses, Manuka honey and unsweetened jams instead of sugar.
- Replace cow's milk with low-fat goat's milk and organic rice milk, which are both low in fat and the rice milk is non-dairy.
- Almonds, sunflower, pumpkin, sesame seeds and linseeds (flax seeds) are all rich sources of fibre.
- Drink coffees made from rye and chicory, herb teas such as rose hip, and unsweetened fruit juices.
- Use more unrefined organic olive, sunflower and walnut oils for salad dressings.
- Eat live, low-fat yoghurt, which is rich in friendly bacteria that encourage healthy bowels.

Useful Supplements

- The herb butcher's broom helps to improve circulation in the lower body and helps tone the veins. Take 500mg twice daily.
- Horse chestnut capsules help to strengthen the capillaries – take 50–75 mg of standardised aescin (the active ingredient) twice daily.
- Take 2 grams of vitamin C, 1 gram of bioflavonoids, and 400iu of full-spectrum, natural-source vitamin E daily with food, which help to strengthen the blood-vessel walls.
- Vitamin A, 20,000iu per day for a month, will help to repair tissue damage. Take this dose for only 1 month and take no more than 3,000iu if you are pregnant. Note that if you eat a lot of liver, this is very rich in vitamin A and you would not then need to take extra vitamin A as a supplement.
- Vitamin B-complex aids digestion, which in turn aids bowel function.
- Zinc is vital for soft tissue healing, take 30mg daily with 1–2mg of copper.

p

■ After 3 months on this regimen, switch to a good-quality multi-vitamin and mineral. Rutin (found in buckwheat) helps to strengthen vein walls. Take 300mg daily.

Helpful Hints

■ Insert Pilewort suppositories – which are best used before going to bed. They are made with olive oil, beeswax and pilewort, to help soften the pile and reduce any swelling.

■ Take one or two cayenne pepper capsules with main meals, which increases circulation and helps to reduce any bleeding. **SHS**

■ Apply combinations of zinc oxide, vitamin E, and aloe vera gel or olive oil to the affected area. This should help to soften the piles and make them less painful.

■ Apply cold witch hazel lotion frequently to haemorrhoids to shrink the swollen blood vessel. The Organic Pharmacy make a witch hazel, bilberry and horse chestnut cream. **OP**

■ In an emergency situation, or if you cannot see your doctor immediately, try dissolving 1 tbsp of Epsom salts into 6 tbsp of lukewarm water and apply with cotton wool to the affected area. This helps to reduce the swelling until you can see your GP.

■ Nelson's Homeopathic make the remedy 'Haemorrhoid', which is very effective.

■ Homeopathic remedies, such as Staphysagria or Aesculus Hippocastamum (horse chestnut) can also help. See a qualified homeopath for individual remedies.

■ Bathing the anus in cold water every morning can help prevent recurrence of piles. Bowel function can be affected by drugs such as antacids, anti-depressants, excessive iron tablets and laxative abuse. If you think these may be a factor, see your doctor.

■ Laxatives taken in the long term can make the bowel lazy, and can increase the need to strain.

■ Squat rather than sit to open your bowels to take pressure off the lower part of the bowel.

■ After you have opened your bowels, squeeze the cheeks of the bottom together several times. This action will encourage blood flow into that area, which helps stop piles forming.

PILL, THE CONTRACEPTIVE

The progestogen- (synthetic progesterone) only or mini-pill, provides contraception by thickening the mucus in the cervix and making it impenetrable by the sperm. The combined pill, which contains both oestrogen and progestogen, prevents pregnancy by thickening the mucus and suppressing ovulation. Potential side-effects from taking the pill are an increased risk of cancers of the breast and cervix, blood clotting in the legs, high blood pressure, increased risk of heart disease and stroke, weight gain, fluid retention and migraines. Women who took the pill for 10 years or more back in the sixties have a much higher risk of developing breast cancer. The pill depletes the body of vital nutrients, such as vitamins B and C, and magnesium, calcium and zinc. I took the pill for more than 10 years from the late 1960s to early 1970s, which I believe was the root cause of continual heavy bleeding, which at 31 caused me to undergo a hysterectomy. If you must take the pill, then have regular breaks of several months at a time. Taking the pill over long periods can increase the risk of developing candida (see *Candida*).

Foods to Avoid

■ Greatly reduce your intake of refined sugars, too much animal protein, dairy products from cows, saturated fats found in dairy and hard margarine, and cakes, pastries, burgers, sausages and so on.

■ Reduce your intake of sodium-based salt, caffeine, and tobacco.

■ Reduce alcohol intake.

■ See *General Health Hints*.

Friendly Foods
- Include organic raw wheat germ in your diet, as it is rich in vitamins B and E.
- Eat far more wholegrains, brown rice, quinoa, couscous, wholemeal breads and pastas, fruits and vegetables.
- Cereals and oats are also rich in B-vitamins.
- Cherries, kiwi fruits, cantaloupe melons, apricots, and most fruit and vegetables are rich sources of vitamin C.
- Eat more fish, plus sunflower, pumpkin and sesame seeds, which are high in zinc, as the pill raises copper levels which lower zinc levels.
- Eat more live, low-fat yoghurt, containing healthy bacteria, which are depleted by the pill.
- See also *General Health Hints*.

Useful Supplements
- Take a high-strength multi-vitamin and mineral such as Femforte 1 by BioCare or Solgar's Omium. **BC SVHC**
- Make sure any supplement you take contains at least 30mg of zinc.
- Take a B-complex, as the pill depletes all the B-vitamins.
- Take vitamin C in a magnesium or calcium ascorbate form. Taking 250mg–500mg with food daily helps to prevent any deficiency caused by the pill.
- Indole 3 Carbinol is an important nutrient extracted from broccoli, which helps to regulate hormones. Take 200mg daily. From all good health stores.
- Support your liver with 500mg of milk thistle twice daily (you should take the milk thistle only when you **stop** taking the pill).
- See also *Liver Problems*.

Helpful Hints
- Studies since the 1960s have consistently shown that women are at 9.6 times greater risk of a pulmonary embolism when taking the pill – even the lower oestrogen-containing pills. If you are on the pill you should not smoke, as this considerably increases the risk of some hazards, such as blood clots and heart disease. Call the Women's Nutritional Advisory Service for more information. Tel: 01273 487366 (Monday–Friday 9am–5.30pm)

POLYCYSTIC OVARIAN SYNDROME see *PCOS – Polycystic Ovarian Syndrome*

POLYMYALGIA RHEUMATICA

(see also *Rheumatoid Arthritis*)

This is an auto-immune-type condition in which the body begins to attack itself. Polymyalgia tends to affect twice as many women as men and is rare under the age of 50. It typically tends to last for 2 to 3 years and is characterised by aching and stiffness in the large muscle groups – especially in the neck, shoulders and pelvis. There may also be pain in the chest and ribcage, but pain in this area is more common in fibromyalgia. There is often stiffness in the morning, a feeling of nausea, there may be a low-grade fever, and anxiety or depression are common. Lack of sleep can make both polymyalgia and fibromyalgia much worse. Polymyalgia is similar in nature to rheumatoid arthritis. People who suffer chronic fatigue, such as ME also tend to suffer fibromyalgia. High homocysteine levels (a toxic by-product from digesting proteins) may be linked to these conditions – for more information on homocysteine see *High Blood Pressure*. Candida is especially linked to fibromyalgia (see *Candida*).

Foods to Avoid

- Avoid caffeine and alcohol, which are stimulants. These affect hormones in the body linked to pain receptors. Caffeine drinks includes cola-type drinks, chocolate, coffee and so on. Alcohol also acts like a depressant.
- Greatly reduce your intake of sugar, which can trigger inflammation in the body – and trigger low blood sugar and mood swings.
- Read labels and make sure you avoid hydrogenated and trans fats, which are found in most mass-produced meat pies, sausages, salami, margarines, cakes, biscuits and so on. See *Fats You Need To Eat*.

Friendly Foods

- Eat more cold-water fish, such as herrings, mackerel, and wild salmon and trout, as they are high in omega-3 essential fats, which help cell-membrane function.
- Eat more whole foods (preferably organic) including fruits and vegetables, especially squash, carrots, pumpkin, watermelon, watercress, cantaloupe melon, mango, sweet potatoes, cabbage and kale.
- Avoid white flour and wheat, which can irritate the gut. Try millet, buckwheat, quinoa and amaranth grains, which are now available in breads, biscuits, pastas and crackers from any good health store, and in numerous supermarkets. Eat more brown rice or kashi.
- Eat more fresh pineapple, which has anti-inflammatory properties.
- Use more turmeric in curries, as it is highly anti-inflammatory.
- Drink nettle leaf tea.
- As dehydration is often a problem, drink more water.
- See *General Health Hints* and the dietary advice given in *Rheumatoid Arthritis*.

Useful Remedies

- B-vitamins – especially B6, B12 and Folic acid – are needed to support the nerves and they help lower a high homocysteine level. Therefore, take a B-complex daily.
- Minerals such as magnesium help to relax the muscles – so does calcium. You can buy these minerals in a powdered formula – and you would need 600mg of magnesium and 400mg of calcium spread throughout the day. Of the two, magnesium is the most important – if you buy this in capsule form ask for magnesium citrate and take your last 200mg before bed. **BC**
- Ask at your health shop for an essential-fatty-acid formula containing omega-3 and -6 fats. You would need about 1–2 grams daily.
- MSM – a type of organic sulphur – really helps to reduce pain and inflammation, and is good for reducing muscle spasms. Take 2 grams daily spread throughout the day.
- The amino acid L-theanine extracted from green tea acts like a natural tranquillizer, but it does not make you sleepy. You can take 100mg three times daily to help calm the brain and reduce anxiety.
- Healthy bacteria – known as probiotics – often help, as sufferers from both these conditions tend to also suffer from a leaky gut (see *Leaky Gut*).
- Take a digestive enzyme with all main meals.

Helpful Hints

- People who don't get sufficient sleep tend to suffer more muscle pain; therefore, get more sleep. Sleep is **very** important for these conditions.
- Moderate exercise, such as swimming, walking, cycling and so on, will all help.
- Have a regular massage using therapeutic grade oils – such as wintergreen – which are anti-inflammatory. For details of Young Living oils see p.15.
- Regular acupuncture is wonderful for reducing pain and stiffness with these conditions.
- Soak in warm baths with Epsom salts or sea salt to help relax the muscles.

POST-NATAL DEPRESSION

Until recently many women have felt at times ashamed to discuss this subject, but since people like actress Brooke Shields have talked more openly about this subject, more women are being encouraged to get help. Although the birth of a child is, for most women, a time of great joy, some women feel extremely low immediately after giving birth. This can be due to hormonal changes. Extreme fatigue can be due to fluctuating blood sugar levels. In naturopthic terms post-natal depression can be linked to adrenal exhaustion, as hormones produced during pregnancy and the birth, such as cortisol and adrenaline, sap the adrenal glands, which can leave you feeling totally exhausted and emotionally drained. See *Stress*.

In addition anxiety about coping with a new baby, financial problems, and, of course, the realisation that life has changed for good can all add to this condition. For a few women, the feeling of depression lasts for much longer than a few weeks, which can seriously undermine their ability to cope. Most doctors offer anti-depressants and tell the mother the depression will soon pass. In fact this condition can be greatly alleviated by taking the right supplements for a few weeks. Symptoms vary from increased or decreased appetite, a feeling that one is a failure, and sometimes aggressive feelings towards the baby (see also *Low Blood Sugar* and *Depression*).

Foods to Avoid
- Reduce stimulating foods, such as sugar, caffeine and alcohol, which trigger the release of more cortisol.
- See Foods to Avoid in *Low Blood Sugar*.

Friendly Foods
- See Friendly Foods in *Depression* and *Low Blood Sugar*.

Useful Remedies
- The herb St John's wort is very useful for this problem, but not until you have finished breast-feeding.
- You can take the herb agnus castus to help re-balance your hormones even if you are breast-feeding – 5ml of the tincture daily.
- As low levels of B-vitamins are associated with this condition, take a B-complex daily for at least 2 months.
- Calcium 500mg, magnesium 1000mg and zinc 30mg can be taken as a formula once daily. Taking these minerals will greatly ease symptoms after a few days.
- Take a multi-vitamin and mineral that contains at least 500mg of vitamin C and 150mcg of selenium. See details of *Kudos 24* in *General Supplements* (p.160).
- Take Bach Rescue Remedy – Star of Bethlehem and Gentian also help to lift the depression.
- Try Femarone – a herbal formula containing raspberry leaf, squaw vine and uva ursi, which all help to balance hormones following childbirth. **SHS**
- Take homeopathic Caullophylum, Cimicifuga Pulsatilla and Sepia – 1 pill 4 times a day. This blend helps to balance the hormones and reduces feelings of doom and hopelessness, tears and so on. **OP**

Helpful Hints
- Taking all the above nutrients during your pregnancy (not the St John's wort) can help prevent depression, especially if you suffered after an earlier pregnancy.
- Post-natal depression is often caused by the sudden fall in progesterone levels just before birth in women whose bodies are slow to begin making progesterone again. You can use a natural progesterone cream, which is easily absorbed and will bring your progesterone levels up again

p

until your body takes over. If you require further information on natural progesterone and a list of doctors who use it, send a first-class stamp to The Natural Progesterone Information Service, PO Box 24, Buxton, SK17 9FB.

- In Britain, natural progesterone cream is available on prescription – but overseas and in Ireland it is freely available over the counter and it can be ordered for your own use. For an information sheet call 00 353 46 943 7317 between 10am and 5pm; or log on to www.pharmwest.com
- Homeopathic Ignatia 30c, taken twice daily for up to a week, is particularly good for mothers who thought that having a baby was going to be all roses.
- And for those who feel enveloped by a black cloud, try Cimicifuga 30c twice daily for up to a week.
- As much depression is linked to the liver, see also *Liver Problems* and *Depression*.
- Mild post-natal depression can be helped by getting more sleep, and by getting out of the house and away from the baby. Don't bottle up your feelings; talk things over with a friend. By letting your feelings out it really helps to put things in perspective and to realise how many women are in a similar situation.
- For more help and advice call the Women's Nutritional Advisory Service on 01273 487366 (Monday to Friday, 9am–5.30pm).

PRE-MENSTRUAL TENSION and PRE-MENSTRUAL SYNDROME (PMT/PMS)

PMS causes a variety of physical and emotional symptoms in the days prior to menstruation. They vary from mood swings, food cravings and depression to breast tenderness and enlargement, fluid retention and bloating. Changes in hormone levels cause some women to experience migraine-type symptoms. For 1 in 10 women pre-menstrual mood changes are extreme. PMS is associated with low levels of progesterone and excess oestrogen (see *Menopause* for details of natural progesterone cream). Low blood sugar is common prior to a period and once blood sugar is balanced symptoms often disappear (see also *Low Blood Sugar*). Many women with PMS also have candida (see also *Candida*). Congestion of the liver is also linked to PMS (see *Liver Problems*).

Foods to Avoid
- Generally you need to cut down on animal fats, burgers, sausages, and heavy, rich meat-based meals that usually contain high levels of saturated fat and salt.
- All high-salt foods, such as crisps and salted peanuts, and highly processed meat, such as salami, should be avoided as salt will add to the water-retention problem.
- Stimulants, such as alcohol, tea and coffee, caffeine in any form, fizzy drinks, chocolate, snacks, cakes, biscuits and fast foods (such as croissants and Danish pastries) will all play havoc with your blood sugar.

Friendly Foods
- Starting the day with an oat-based cereal, such as porridge, with a chopped apple and a few sunflower seeds and raisins, will help to balance blood sugar until lunchtime.
- Drink more water and try calming herbal teas such as camomile.
- Eat more quality protein, such as fresh fish, eggs, chicken and turkey without the skin, cottage cheese and cooked tofu.
- Foods such as tempeh or miso, sweet potatoes, broccoli, cauliflower, and Brussels sprouts all

help to balance your hormones naturally.

- Lentils, barley, brown rice, oats, peas, and sunflower, pumpkin and sesame seeds, plus all dried beans and pulses, are rich in fibre, protein and essential fats.
- Eat plenty of small snacks containing at least 55 grams of protein; include plenty of fruits and vegetables.
- Add organic sunflower and walnut oil to salad dressings.
- Snack on apples, pears and bananas, and try rice and oat cakes, spelt, amaranth crackers and wholemeal bread spread with a low-fat houmous, tahini or goat's cheese.
- Many health food shops now sell low-sugar snacks. If you were to eat these with a piece of fruit, again this will help reduce any cravings.

Useful Remedies
To be taken all the time, not only during a period:
- A B-complex containing at least 50mg of B6 per day, which is needed in the liver to process oestrogens.
- Natural-source, full-spectrum vitamin E, taken 300–600iu daily, which helps to reduce the symptoms of PMT.
- Take calcium at 400mg and magnesium at 600mg per day, to reduce the symptoms of PMS as these minerals help keep you calm. Most companies now make a two-in-one formula.
- Gamma linolenic acid (GLA) is the main ingredient of evening primrose oil, which helps to reduce breast pain. Take 100–500mg of GLA daily.
- Also take a multi-vitamin and mineral for women that contains a further 50mg of B6 to make your total daily intake 100mg per day.
- If your sugar/carbohydrate cravings are really bad, take 150mcg of chromium daily, which kicks in after a few days and really helps to reduce sugar cravings.
- The amino acid L-glutamine also helps to reduce cravings; it also helps heal the gut. Take 500mg twice daily 30 minutes before food.
- Try a herbal menstrual formula containing blessed thistle, squaw vine and barberry, and cramp bark – which all help to cleanse the reproductive organs and balance hormones. **SHS**

Helpful Hints
- Dr Marilyn Glenville, a leading nutritional physician and expert in women's health problems, has formulated drops containing blue cohosh, agnus castus, lady's mantle and cramp bark that help relieve breast pain, water retention, mood swings and headaches. For more information, log on to the website: www.marilynglenville.com
- When you are stressed, you produce too much adrenaline, which eventually exhausts your endocrine (hormone) system and depletes calcium from your bones. See *Osteoporosis* and *Stress*.
- Start taking more regular exercise to reduce stress, or learn to meditate. Find some time each day to call your own, even if it's only a relaxing bath for 30 minutes.
- Treat yourself to an aromatherapy massage each month, or add essential oils of rose, ylang ylang, neroli, jasmine or geranium to your bath. Clary sage is great for reducing cramping period pains.
- If you smoke, try to give up.

PRICKLY HEAT

This irritating and unsightly condition usually affects fair-skinned people, such as myself, in tropical or sub-tropical climates. It initially appears as an itchy red, raised rash of hundreds of tiny bumps anywhere on the body. It has been linked to food intolerances (see *Allergies*), and chemical levels in drinking water, but can just as easily be triggered by sun lotions, shower gels, and soaps, to which the individual becomes more sensitive in the heat and sun. I tend to suffer prickly heat on my shins if I stand for too long in tropical temperatures, which causes blood to 'pool' in my legs. Alcohol, antibiotics and aspirin can also trigger prickly heat. Many people who suffer these types of reactions have a leaky gut (see *Leaky Gut*).

Foods to Avoid

- Try cutting out cow's milk and products, as well as wheat, peanuts, tea and coffee – although the culprits could be something quite unusual like radishes or orange juice. See *Allergies*.
- Avoid really hot drinks and highly spiced foods.

Friendly Foods

- All foods that feed the skin from the inside out, such as apples, carrots, spinach (best raw), broccoli, pumpkin, cantaloupe melons, apricots, mango, papaya and figs.
- Artichokes, beetroot and asparagus cleanse the liver, which in turn aids healing in the skin.
- Onion and garlic are rich sources of quercetin, which is a natural anti-histamine.
- Avocados and oily fish are fabulous for the skin.
- Include more organic sunflower and pumpkin seeds, linseeds (flax seeds), almonds, and Brazil nuts in your diet, which are rich in essential fats.
- Use more organic, unrefined extra virgin olive, walnut or sunflower oils over salad dressings.
- Drink bottled or pure filtered water.
- Muesli and most cereals are high in B-vitamins, which help to prevent dry skin.
- Nettle tea will help reduce the inflammation.

Useful Remedies

- Take 2–3 grams of vitamin C in an ascorbate form with meals as vitamin C acts as a natural anti-histamine.
- Take a natural-source carotene complex for 7 days before travel and during your holiday. **HN**
- Take a high-strength B-complex.
- Take a multi-vitamin and mineral formula daily.
- Drink nettle tea.

Helpful Hints

- In most cases, prickly heat will clear up on its own in a few days if the affected area is kept cool and dry. Take regular cool showers and allow the skin to dry naturally.
- Avoid using any insect repellent on the affected areas.
- Once your skin is dry again, apply aloe vera gel.
- Don't use any type of oil-based product, which might block your sweat glands.
- If the prickly heat does not clear within 4–5 days and infection sets in, you must see a doctor.
- To prevent prickly heat, avoid situations that can lead to excessive sweating, such as hot, humid environments and strenuous physical activity.
- Wear loose-fitting cotton clothes.
- Buy products in their most natural and unadulterated state. For anyone who suffers dermatitis or skin allergies, The Green People Company makes organic skin, hair and body lotions, sun screens and toothpaste, and they also have an advice line. Tel: 01444 401444. E-mail: organic@greenpeople.co.uk Website: www.greenpeople.co.uk
- Many strong antibiotics and drugs make the skin very sun-sensitive. If you are taking antibiotics, stay out of the sun.
- Stay out of the midday sun and never allow your skin to go red.
- The homeopathic remedy Urtica 6c taken 3 times daily in-between meals helps to reduce the

redness. Discontinue once the rash begins to fade. Or try homeopathic Sol/Urtica 30c, which helps prevents prickly heat. You can also use Urtica Cream. **OP**
- Avoid hot baths and showers.

PROSTATE PROBLEMS

Approximately 50% of men aged over 55, and three quarters of men aged over 70, suffer from an enlarged prostate. That's more than 2 million men in the UK. In addition, 10,000 cases of prostate cancer are diagnosed in every year. Younger men are more likely to suffer from prostatitis, which is an inflammation of the prostate gland. Symptoms would be an urgency to urinate, a need to urinate more regularly, which could be painful, and there might be blood in the sperm. Treatment is generally by antibiotics.

The prostate is a walnut-sized gland that sits below a man's bladder. Its job is to secrete seminal fluids and contract strongly during orgasm to cause ejaculation. As men get older it is common for the prostate gland to gradually enlarge, up to 2–4 times its normal size, to about the size of a lemon. This is largely attributable to hormonal changes associated with ageing. After the age of 50 or so, a man's levels of testosterone decrease, while the level of other hormones, including oestrogen, increase. Unfortunately, older men will have had a lifetime of exposure to plastics, petrochemicals and pesticides, which all have hormone-disrupting (oestrogenic)-like effects in the body and are linked to hormonal cancers. Although testosterone levels decrease with age, some of the testosterone is converted into a far more potent form – dihydrotestosterone (DHT) – and the normal process by which it is broken down is inhibited by the excess oestrogens. The potent DHT collects in the prostate and causes the overproduction of prostate cells, which ultimately results in prostate enlargement.

The tube that takes urine from the bladder to the outside (the urethra) passes through the prostate, so the enlarged gland places pressure on the urethra, impeding the flow of urine and triggering the need to urinate more often. Many men get up 3 or 4 times during the course of the night. Other symptoms include difficulty in beginning urination, poor stream, dribbling at the end of urination and sometimes pain. An enlarged prostate can also trigger urinary infections, bladder stones and kidney damage.

The majority of prostate problems are a result of this gradual enlargement, termed benign prostatic hypertrophy (BPH), but occasionally the prostate can be affected by cancer. If you have blood in your urine, difficulty in passing urine, any swelling in your testicle area, **please, please** go to see your doctor.

Foods to Avoid
- Filter your main tap water supply before drinking. This is because hormone residues from the pill and HRT, are found in most water supplies and they have an oestrogen effect in the body. One of the purest waters you can drink is reverse osmosis de-ionised water, which can be bought in health stores or plumbed in under your sink. For details of reverse osmosis water contact The Pure H2O Company on 01784 221188, or visit their website at www.pureh20.co.uk.
- As pesticide and herbicide residues are now linked to prostate cancer, avoid non-organic foods as much as possible.
- Reduce your intake of animal fats found in meat, full-fat milks and cheeses, chocolate, hard margarines, and fatty take-aways. Dairy foods and too much non-organic red meat (usually full of chemical and hormone residues) increase the risk of prostate cancer.
- Don't eat processed meat pies and pastries.

- Avoid fried and barbecued foods.
- Reduce your intake of caffeine, alcohol and sugar.
- See also *General Health Hints*.

Friendly Foods

- The carotene lycopene is the most abundant nutrient stored in the prostate and studies have shown that men who eat 10 or more cooked tomatoes (in a little olive oil) weekly are 45% less likely to develop prostate cancer. The lycopene in tomatoes is released when they are heated in a small amount of oil. A great way to do this is to cut tomatoes in half, brush them with a little olive oil and add chopped garlic and basil. Grill or bake for a few minutes and serve. Lycopene is also found in guava and pink grapefruit.
- Eat organic foods as much as you can to avoid pesticide residues on fresh produce and hormones used in animal production. Additionally, locally grown fruits and vegetables in season contain more nutrients than those flown thousands of miles.
- Sprinkle plenty of pumpkin, sunflower and sesame seeds and linseeds (flax seeds) over cereals and yoghurt, or into soups. They are rich in essential fats and zinc, which are needed for a healthy prostate.
- Pumpkin seeds are rich in zinc, magnesium (a muscle relaxant) and essential fats, helping reduce the conversion of testosterone to the potent DHT – you should be eating 40–100g every day. Eat them raw or try lightly toasting them tossed in a little soya sauce to make a delicious and very prostate-friendly snack. Alternatively, blitz 2 tbsp each of pumpkin, sunflower and linseeds (flax seeds), keep them in the fridge, and sprinkle daily over cereals or salads.
- Eat more oily fish, which are rich in essential fats, and use unrefined organic walnut, sesame, sunflower and olive oils for salad dressings, or drizzle over cooked foods (see *Fats You Need To Eat*).
- Include plenty of fibre in your diet from fruits and vegetables, especially broccoli, kale, cauliflower and Brussels sprouts, which help to balance hormones naturally.
- Lentils, alfalfa, tomatoes, salad leaves, yellow peppers and organic carrots will help protect against cancers.
- Eat more brown rice, quinoa, spelt, millet, oats, cereals and oat and rice bran. The fibre helps remove excess hormones out of the body.
- Eat more pulses, such as barley, kidney beans, soya beans, plus lentils, and corn, rice and lentil pastas.
- Have one serving of cooked tempeh (a fermented form of soya), miso or soya sauce daily. There is currently much discussion about soya-based foods, such as tofu and soya milk. Whilst this argument is ongoing, it is generally accepted that fermented soya in the form of miso or tempeh is beneficial. Cooked tofu is OK, but if in any doubt avoid unfermented soya products, such as soya yoghurt and soya milk; or check with your health professional.

Useful Remedies

- The mineral zinc is more abundant in the prostate than any other organ in the body and its supplementation has been shown to reduce prostate overgrowth and symptoms of BPH. Zinc inhibits the conversion of testosterone to DHT, the primary hormonal trigger for prostate enlargement. Zinc deficiency is common in those with prostate problems. Take 20mg zinc 2–3 times per day. As zinc depletes copper levels, take a proportionate amount of copper, approximately 1mg of copper for every 15mg of zinc.
- The mineral selenium has been found to help prevent prostate enlargement and there is a significant inverse relationship between selenium levels in the body and prostate cancer. 200mcg per day can significantly reduce your risk of either.
- The herb saw palmetto has been proven effectively to reduce enlargement of the prostate gland

and dramatically improve the symptoms of BPH. Its active components reduce the production and activity of DHT. Take as capsules – 150–350mg of standardised extract twice a day. Or try Pros Formula containing saw palmetto, horsetail, couchgrass and hydrangea, which all help to normalise prostate function. Take 1 capsule 3 times daily. **SHS**

■ Another good herb for an enlarged prostate is pygeum. It is particularly good for relieving symptoms such as frequent or difficult urination and associated sexual dysfunction. Take 50–100mg of standardised extract twice daily.

■ One of the oldest remedies for enlarged prostate is nettle, taken either as a tincture or as tablets. 5ml of tincture, or 200–300mg of standardised extract 2–3 times per day in capsules. You can also try nettle tea with a little honey.

■ Essential fats, especially omega-3, found in fish oils, can also help prevent prostate enlargement. Take 1 gram of fish oil or 1 gram of linseed (flax seed) oil.

■ Many companies now make prostate formulas that include all these nutrients (see pages 13–15 for details).

■ Include a natural carotene source supplement that is rich in lycopene – 20–40mg daily.

■ If you do not like fermented soya foods then take an isoflavone extract – 50–100mg daily.

■ Take 2 grams of vitamin C with added bio-flavonoids daily, with food, because seminal fluid, which the prostate produces, requires vitamin C in large amounts.

Helpful Hints

■ An enlarged prostate is usually discovered via a rectal examination by a doctor. All men aged over 40 should have a yearly rectal examination. Early detection greatly increases your chances of a complete cure.

■ Ask your partner to see if they can feel any abnormalities, make this a fun thing, but try doing it once a month.

■ Regular exercise is vital as it boosts immune function and also naturally reduces levels of stress hormones. However, do not cycle as this will put pressure on the prostate. Swimming and walking are great exercises.

■ To help improve circulation to the area and reduce inflammation, lie on your back, bend your knees, bring the soles of the feet together and bring the feet as close to your buttocks as possible. Relax your legs, letting the knees fall outwards towards the ground. Hold this position for 5 minutes. Attempt this exercise only if you are fit and have no joint problems in your hips and legs.

■ Massage essential oils of cypress, tea tree and juniper berry mixed with a little jojoba carrier oil, into your lower back and groin areas to help strengthen the prostate.

■ See an osteopath or chiropractor to check that the pelvis and spine are not misaligned. In certain cases a major nerve connection from the lower part of the spine to the prostate becomes trapped and once this is released water can be passed normally (see *Useful Information*).

■ If you have prostate cancer see *Useful Remedies* under *Cancer*.

■ There is a test for prostate health called a PSA, or Prostate Specific Antigen test. If your levels of PSA are elevated, it can mean that your prostate is becoming enlarged, or it may possibly be an indication of prostate cancer. This is not a test for cancer per se, but it indicates prostate-cell activity. Other factors can raise the levels of PSA – for example ejaculation can raise it for 2 days, although in general, the higher the level the more likely it is to be a sign of cancer. Biopsies are needed to confirm this.

■ Enlarged prostate can be treated surgically with a procedure called a Trans Urethral Resection of the Prostate (TURP). This very common procedure is more effective than drugs, although it can have side-effects including impotence and incontinence, and 1 in 8 men who have the operation need another operation within 8 years. This highlights that surgery doesn't address the underlying cause – although if you've tried everything listed here and are desperate, discuss this and other options, including newer laser procedures, with your doctor.

- For further help and advice contact The Prostate Help Association, Langworth, Lincoln LN3 5DF. Website: www.pha.u-net.com. They also have informative self-help books and CD-ROMs for sale. Otherwise contact The Prostate Cancer Charity via their helpline (0845 300 8383) or website www.prostate-cancer.org.uk
- If your prostate is enlarged, be cautious about using over-the-counter cold or allergy remedies. Many of these products contain ingredients that can inflame the condition and cause urinary retention.
- Read *Prostate Health in 90 Days* by Larry Clapp (Hay House); or *Prostate Cancer* by Philip Dunn (Ostrich Publishing; and available through the Prostate Help Association website).

PSORIASIS

(see also *Candida*)

This is a chronic skin condition that can occur at any age. It is characterised by patches of red, raised, and scaly skin. Once it begins scaling the skin can take on a silvery, fish-like look. It does seem to have some hereditary links, but symptoms often don't appear until adulthood. It usually does not itch, but can cause discomfort and embarrassment. Areas most commonly affected are arms, elbows, behind the ears, scalp, back, legs and knees. It may be triggered by prolonged stress, a traumatic event, food intolerances, essential-fatty-acid deficiencies, low stomach-acid levels, constipation, liver congestion and vitamin B-complex deficiencies. It is also linked to the yeast fungal overgrowth candida. Many people with psoriasis may have poor liver function, as skin problems can denote that the liver is under stress – in which case you need to see a qualified nutritionist, who can modify your diet to help detoxify the liver. See *Liver Problems*.

Foods to Avoid
- Eliminate wheat and any food containing wheat for 1 month and see if this helps. Some people also have an intolerance to gluten.
- Citrus fruits and tomatoes aggravate the problem in some sufferers.
- Cut down on saturated and hydrogenated fats, especially red meat, mass-produced vegetable oils, take-aways, mass-produced burgers, red meat, cakes, pastries, pies and full-fat dairy produce.
- It is likely that you are eating too many of the above foods, which are all acid-forming in the body. See *Acid–Alkaline Balance*.
- Keep a food diary and note when symptoms become worse. Recall what you ate the day before and this may be your answer.
- As much as possible, eliminate alcohol.
- Cut down on sugary foods and drinks.

Friendly Foods
- Most people with psoriasis are deficient in essential fats. Therefore eat more salmon, sardines, mackerel, herring and tuna – at least twice a week And be sure to read *Fats You Need To Eat*.
- Eat as great a variety of fresh foods as possible.
- Eat more brown rice, millet and buckwheat, which are gluten-free.
- Eat more pectin-rich foods, such as apples and carrots. Greatly increase your intake of whole fruits and vegetables.

- Figs, prunes, kiwi, canteloupe melons, spinach, and papaya are all great for the skin.
- Add unrefined, organic walnut, sunflower, sesame and olive oils to salad dressings and drizzle over cooked foods.
- Use organic rice or low-fat goat's milks instead of cow's milk.
- Pumpkin seeds, linseeds (flax seeds) and sunflower seeds are all high in zinc and essential fats.
- Begin making fresh vegetable juices with raw beetroot, artichoke, carrots and apples or any vegetables you have to hand – add to this a teaspoon of green food powder (such as Dr Gillian McKeith's Living Food Powder, which helps to re-alkalise the body), 20 drops of dandelion and milk thistle tincture, and half a cup of organic aloe vera juice, which all help cleanse the liver – and drink immediately upon juicing.
- Celeriac and kale are also great for the liver

Useful Remedies.

- Evening primrose oil, 5–6 grams, or linseed (flax seed) oil capsules 3–5 grams per day, will help to reduce the inflammation of psoriasis. You take these mainly because they are high in GLA (Gamma Linolenic Acid) – therefore if you don't want to swallow high doses of evening primrose oil, take a 1 gram of GLA daily. **BC**
- Take a B-complex that contains 400mcg of folic acid and 100mg of B6, which are often low in people with this condition.
- B12 injections have proved helpful to many people who have low stomch acid (see *Low Stomach Acid*).
- Take vitamin C with bioflavonoids – 2 grams daily to help reduce the inflammation.
- Take a multi-vitamin and mineral that contains at least 30–40mg of zinc.
- Betaine hydrochloride (stomach acid) is often useful. 1 capsule with main meals aids digestion and the absorption of nutrients. If you have active stomach ulcers, take a digestive enzyme instead, which is free of HCl.
- Most psoriasis sufferers are deficient in vitamin A, therefore for 1 month take 25,000iu of vitamin A daily and then reduce to 5000iu daily (this amount should be in your multi). If you are pregnant do not take more than 3,000iu of vitamin A daily. If you eat liver, it is very high in Vitamin A – in which case you might not need the supplement, but I don't know anyone who eats liver every day!
- There has been extensive research into the healing properties of the plant *Mahonia aquifolium* for psoriasis sufferers. It is available as cream, ointment, shampoo, conditioner, scalp oil and body lotion. For details ask at your health shop or call Taylor Jackson Health Products on 0845 1081605.

Helpful Hints

- Regular colonic irrigation therapies help to detox the bowel. See *Useful Information* at the back of this book.
- Sea bathing is beneficial for psoriasis. Many sufferers find relief after bathing in Dead Sea salt because of its high mineral contents. Add 1kg to your bath and soak for 10 minutes.
- Homeopathic Ars-iod 6x taken twice daily for a few weeks is particularly good for dry, scaly, itching skin.
- Moderate sun exposure also helps psoriasis, but remember to wear a hypo-allergenic sunscreen.
- Smokers run a greater risk of psoriasis.
- Many people with this skin condition tend to be holding on to emotional issues – such as resentment, anger and bitterness. If emotions are repressed, in the long-term skin problems can result.
- For more help read *Healing Psoriasis: the Natural Alternative* by Dr John Pagano.

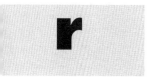

RAYNAUD'S DISEASE
(see also *Circulation*)

Raynaud's is 5 times more common in women than in men – and commonly begins between the ages of 18 and 30, although it can be later.

This condition is when constriction occurs in the blood vessels, which triggers intermittent spasms within the smaller blood vessels usually in the fingers and toes and occasionally in the nose and tongue. Initially, symptoms occur when the extremities are exposed to cold temperatures, especially if the person is stressed. The nerve receptors in these areas become particularly sensitive to the slightest chill, and fingers can become white, bluish or red, and tingling and numbness are common symptoms. This condition is linked to poor circulation, and a diet low in essential fats and other nutrients including iron. However, never take iron supplements unless you have had a blood test showing that levels are low, as iron is stored in the body and high iron levels are linked to an increased risk of heart disease. Another trigger for Raynaud's is smoking, which greatly affects micro-circulation. In rare cases the skin can ulcerate if it is starved of blood for too long (see also *Circulation*, *Fats You Need To Eat* and *Leg Ulcers*).

Foods to Avoid
- Cut down on saturated fats found in hard margarines, fatty meats, full-fat milk, dairy produce.
- Avoid coffee and caffeine, which constricts blood vessels.
- See also *Foods to Avoid* under *Circulation*.

Friendly Foods
- You need to eat foods that are high in vitamin E, such as raw wheat germ, and avocados, nuts and seeds.
- Rutin-rich foods help to strengthen the small blood vessels. These include buckwheat, the peel of citrus fruits, rose hips, apple peel, and cabbage.
- Make stews, soups and casseroles that are full of root vegetables – sweet potatoes, carrots, pumpkin and so on – as these types of foods warm you through and are rich in minerals.
- Eat plenty of iron-rich foods: lean red meat, liver, poultry, eggs, blackstrap molasses, fish, broccoli, and leafy green vegetables like spinach.
- Magnesium is a nutritional vasodilator, so include in your diet more low-sugar cereals, oats, honey, wholemeal bread and pastas, almonds, Brazil nuts, walnuts, mustard and curry powder. All leafy green foods are rich in magnesium – and foods like chlorella and green food powders are also high in iron.
- Cook with garlic and onions, which help to thin the blood naturally, plus fresh root ginger and cayenne pepper, which warm the body.
- Eat plenty of fruit high in vitamin C, such as cherries, kiwi and blueberries. If you hate cold food in winter, make berry-and-fruit compotes, or lightly glaze fresh fruit with a little honey and grill on kebab sticks. Serve with low-fat, live yoghurt and sprinkle with lecithin granules (which lower LDL-cholesterol levels).

Useful Remedies
- If you are not on blood-thinning drugs, take up to 800iu of natural-source vitamin E daily.

- Take vitamin C with bioflavonoids – 1–3 grams a day with food. These play a key role in the synthesis of collagen, which is the key component in the walls of blood vessels. Vitamin C is essential to ensure that the small arteries that supply the fingers do not become damaged during attacks.
- Take niacin (vitamin B3). Begin with 30mg and gradually increase to 100mg per day. Beware – this vitamin really boosts circulation and for about 30–45 minutes after swallowing, **it can cause a pronounced red flushing effect on the skin**.
- Take a high-strength multi-mineral that contains 250mg of magnesium, 500mg of calcium and 20mg of potassium, plus a trace of manganese.
- GLA is an essential fatty acid found in evening primrose, borage and blackcurrant oil, and is important for relaxing muscles. A recent study found that 12 capsules a day of evening primrose oil dramatically decreased the number of Raynaud's attacks. But as most people don't want to swallow 12 pills and the ingredient they need is the GLA, I suggest two Mega GLA capsules daily. **BC**
- Take a B-complex daily and if symptoms are severe ask your doctor for a B12 injection.
- Linseed (flax seed) and fish oils – 4–8 grams per day – contain essential polyunsaturated fatty acids, known as omega-3 and omega-6 fatty acids, which have been shown to lower the bad fats and thin the blood. Fish oils also improve one's tolerance to cold – hence the reason why the Inuits rarely feel the cold! See *Fats You Need To Eat*.
- The herb gotu kola really helps to increase circulation. Take 500mg twice daily during the winter or whilst symptoms are acute.
- Cayenne pepper in capsules helps to improve circulation and warm the body through. Start on 1 capsule 3 times daily and increase if desired. Take this with food – and you will see benefits after a month.
- If the cayenne pepper causes too much warmth in the stomach, then try Bl-Circ Formula containing a small amount of cayenne with ginger, hawthorn, low-odour garlic, ginseng, and parsley. **SHS**

Helpful Hints
- Take regular exercise to improve circulation. Swimming, skipping, and rebounding on a mini-trampoline are all wonderful ways to improve circulation. I used to suffer from this condition as a result of varicose-vein surgery. I was told that I had plenty of veins left, but the surgery reduced my circulation drastically. If you are thinking of having veins removed, you might like to keep this in mind. Wear warm socks for most of the year in bed. Never wear tight-fitting shoes, which restrict circulation.
- Make tea infusions with fresh root ginger, cinnamon twigs or angelica root.
- Try massaging hands and toes regularly with diluted essential oils of black pepper, rosemary, lavender or geranium, or add a few drops of each oil to your bath.
- Reflexology and acupuncture have helped many sufferers (see *Useful Information*).
- For further information contact Raynaud's and Scleroderma Association, 112 Crewe Road, Alsager, Cheshire ST7 2JA or call 01270 872776. Website: www.raynauds.org.uk

REPETITIVE STRAIN INJURY (RSI)

(see also *Carpel Tunnel Syndrome*)

Half a million people in the UK suffer from chronic pain in their wrists, shoulders or neck due to RSI. And thanks to the huge numbers of us that work on computers, numbers are on the rise. In typing this book I too have succumbed to RSI, but I keep it under control by wearing a wristband that goes through my thumb and around my wrist, which contains magnets. It's certainly helped me and you can find these bands in all good sports shops.

Meanwhile, an average of 4.7 million working days are lost each year to RSI, which obviously needs to be taken more seriously. Common symptoms include numbness, tingling pains, loss of grip, and restricted movement. Anyone who has a job or plays a sport regularly that involves repetitive movements is at risk of contracting RSI. The condition is basically inflammation of the tendons, known as tendonitis. Tendonitis usually heals within a few weeks, but if it becomes chronic calcium salts can deposit along the tendon fibres. The tendons most commonly affected are the Achilles, biceps, elbow, thumb, knee, inside of the foot, or shoulder joint.

Foods to Avoid
- Caffeine reduces the body's ability to cope with pain.
- Cut down on sugar and refined junk foods, which trigger inflammation in the body.

Friendly Foods
- Eat more oily fish, which is rich in vitamin A, which aids tissue-healing.
- Eat plenty of foods high in natural carotenes, which have anti-inflammatory properties. These include asparagus, French beans, broccoli, carrots, raw parsley, red peppers, spring greens, sweet potatoes, watercress, spinach, apricots, pumpkin, tomatoes and cantaloupe melon.
- Nuts (unsalted) and seeds, especially pumpkin, sesame, sunflower and linseeds (flax seeds), plus fish, are all high in zinc.
- Include more turmeric in food, which has highly anti-inflammatory properties.
- Pineapple, cherries and ginger all have anti-inflammatory properties.

Useful Supplements
- Take 2 grams of vitamin C as magnesium ascorbate daily, as vitamin C plays a major role in the prevention and repair of injuries. **BC**
- Vitamin A – 10,000iu per day – is necessary for collagen synthesis and wound-healing. If you are pregnant take only 3000iu daily. (If you eat liver keep in mind that 1 portion may contain 30,000 to 40,000iu of vitamin A).
- Zinc – 30mg per day. Zinc functions alongside vitamin A. An increased copper-to-zinc ratio is often found in individuals with chronic inflammatory conditions.
- Bioflavonoids are extremely effective in reducing inflammation. Take a 1-gram bioflavonoid-complex daily.
- Include a multi-vitamin and mineral in your regimen that includes 400iu of vitamin E, 200mcg of selenium, and 100–150 mg of vitamin B6.
- Glucosamine and MSM – 500mg daily. This is an organic form of sulphur and has proved useful for alleviating this problem. Most glucosamine supplements are derived from crab shells – if you have an intolerance to shellfish, ask for the vegetarian version made from corn. By Health Perception and available at all health stores.
- As fish oils – omega-3 fats – have an anti-inflammatory effect on the body, take 1–2 grams daily.
- Take 600mg of magnesium daily to help soothe the nerve-endings and repair muscles.

Helpful Hints
- Magnets really help to increase circulation, which brings more oxygenated blood to the problem area.
- Proper stretching and warming-up before exercise are important preventive measures.
- Rest the injured area as soon as it hurts to avoid further injury.
- Wrap some ice or a bag of frozen peas in a towel and apply to the painful area for 10 minutes every hour whilst symptoms are acute. Do not wrap so tightly that circulation is impaired.

- Compress the area with an elastic bandage to limit swelling.
- Elevate the injured body part above the level of the heart to increase drainage of fluids out of the injured area.
- You can also massage with essential oil of wintergreen, which has anti-inflammatory properties.
- If you sit for long hours at a desk, take regular breaks and really stretch out.
- Higher Nature makes an organic sulphur (MSM) and boswellia muscle balm that really helps to ease pain. **HN**
- The Alexander Technique helps individuals learn about healthy posture and, therefore, how to reduce or even eliminate RSI problems. Acute problems may benefit from treatment with osteopathy, chiropractic or acupuncture (see *Useful Information*).
- If after trying all these ideas for 6 weeks you are no better, consult a specialist in sports injuries or at least have an x-ray or scan.

RESTLESS LEGS

(see also *Circulation*)

This is a very distressing condition, which causes tickling, burning, or pricking sensations, or an irresistible urge to kick the legs about with involuntary twitching in the muscles of the lower legs. It can greatly affect sleep patterns. Also known as Ekbom's syndrome, restless legs is more common in pregnant and middle-aged women, smokers, diabetics, people with low blood sugar (see *Low Blood Sugar*), and those who drink too much coffee. It could also be partly hereditary. Common causes are lack of iron, vitamin E and the mineral magnesium (see also *Circulation*).

Foods to Avoid

- Cut down on your alcohol intake.
- The biggest trigger is caffeine in any form, so avoid coffee, tea and fizzy drinks. Eliminate any foods containing caffeine, including chocolate.
- Avoid too many foods containing sugar, which can cause your blood sugar to fluctuate and make symptoms worse.
- Reduce refined pastries, cakes, mass-produced pies and biscuits.
- See *General Health Hints*.

Friendly Foods

- You need to eat quality protein from chicken, fish, eggs, low-fat cheeses, pulses, beans peas, cooked tofu and so on – at least once a day.
- Eat more brown rice, quinoa and couscous. For snacks, eat rye crisp breads, or amaranth or rice crackers, which are delicious spread with a little low-fat homous or tahini.
- Eat more leafy green vegetables, fruits and honey, which are rich in magnesium.
- Iron-rich foods are liver, lean red meat, eggs, cereals, blackstrap molasses, and game meats, such as hare, venison and pigeon.
- As essential fats are vital, include oily fish in your diet at least twice weekly, and sprinkle organic unsalted sunflower and pumpkin seeds over cereals and salads.
- Eat raw wheat germ and avocados, which are rich in vitamin E and healthier monounsaturated fats.
- Eat more blueberries and bilberries when in season.
- Drink herbal teas, such as camomile, lemon balm or vervain.
- As you need plenty of B-vitamins with this condition, eat more porridge and low-sugar oat-based cereals and oat bran.

Useful Supplements

■ If you are deficient in iron take a liquid formula such as *Spatone* that is easily absorbed and does not cause constipation. Available from health stores worldwide.

■ Take a B-complex to calm the nerve endings. Folic acid (5mg) and B6 (100mg) are the most important.

■ Natural-source, full-spectrum vitamin E – 400iu twice a day – can be extremely effective in alleviating this condition. (If you are on blood-thinning drugs, vitamin E thins the blood naturally, so tell your doctor and have regular blood tests so that you can reduce your drugs.)

■ The mineral magnesium is very important for relaxing muscles, so take a good-quality multi-vitamin and mineral that contains 500mg of magnesium and also 400mg calcium. Take just before going to bed.

■ Cayenne pepper capsules really rev up the circulation and have an anti-cramping affect. Take 3 a day with meals.

■ See also *Useful Supplements* under *Circulation* and *Raynaud's Disease*.

Helpful Hints

■ A simple blood test will tell you if you are anaemic and actually need to take extra iron (see *Anaemia*).

■ Get plenty of exercise.

■ Massage your legs and feet (especially before bed) with essential oils of rosemary in a carrier of almond or olive oil – using kneading movements from the ankle upwards towards the knee. The legs can be bathed in alternate hot and cold water to improve circulation.

■ Use cramp bark cream before going to bed.

■ Try reflexology, acupuncture or regular aromatherapy massage to rev up the circulation.

■ Take all the suggested supplements for at least 3 months.

■ Wearing magnets in your shoes or in bed socks greatly aids circulation, which can reduce the symptoms considerably at night. Magnets are available at all large pharmacies.

■ If it's practical go for a walk for at least 30 minutes in the evenings.

RHEUMATOID ARTHRITIS
(see *Arthritis*)

ROSACEA
(see also *Low Stomach Acid*)

This is a common skin disorder in adults between the ages of 30 and 50, and women are 3 times more likely to be affected than men. It's thought that hormones play a role in this condition, and naturopaths state that lymphatic congestion is often a factor. Symptoms are a chronic acne-like eruption or flushing of the face, which usually affects the area around the nose and chin. Rosacea can be inherited, but it is more commonly associated with drinking too much alcohol, stress, coffee, tea, spicy foods, the menopause, and lack of stomach acid and B-vitamins. It can also be triggered by food intolerance and the most common triggers are wheat, cow's milk and oranges. Many people who suffer rosacea also suffer from migraines (see *Migraine*). A leaky gut is also implicated (see *Leaky Gut*). You also need to take care of your liver (see *Liver Problems*). Some nutritional physicians are also seeing links between rosacea and the *Helibactor pylori* bacterium, which can also cause stomach ulcers.

Foods to Avoid

- Generally cut down on coffee, tea, alcohol, hot drinks and hot spicy foods, which increase blood-flow and hence flushing.
- Keep a food diary and note as the flush appears what you were eating, drinking or feeling prior to the onset of symptoms.
- Don't eat heavy, rich meals, which place a strain on the digestion and liver.
- Don't eat too much food made from flour – these tend to be pies, cakes, and so on, which are often high in salt, sugar and saturated fats.

Friendly Foods

- Bitter foods, such as radicchio, fennel, chicory, celeriac and young green celery, stimulate stomach acid.
- Take a teaspoon of apple cider vinegar or lemon juice in warm water before a meal.
- Drink plenty of water even if you are not thirsty.
- Eat more pineapple and papaya to improve your digestion.
- Eat plenty of leafy greens especially spinach, cauliflower, broccoli, cabbage and celery.
- Eat more beetroot and artichokes to help cleanse your liver.
- Include plenty of live, low-fat yoghurt to help replenish healthy bacteria in the gut.

Useful Remedies

- If you are not suffering active stomach ulcers take one Betaine Hydrochloride (stomach acid) capsule with main meals. If this causes a slight burning sensation then switch to a pancreatic digestive enzyme capsule that is free from HCl. **BC**
- Rosacea sufferers often have a decreased secretion of the pancreatic enzyme lipase. Take 1 Lipozyme with main meals. **BC**
- As B-group vitamins are often depleted, also take a B-complex.
- There is a skin regime called Sher, which has helped many sufferers. For full details, contact The Sher System, 30 New Bond Street, London, W1S 2RN. Tel: 020 7499 4022. Website: www.sher.co.uk

- Apply a cream containing pine bark and blackcurrant leaf – which has potent anti-inflammatory properties and helps reduce redness and inflammation. There is one called Rose Plus. **OP**
- Try a herbal tincture made specifically for rosacea, which includes milk thistle, red clover, bilberry and gingko. **OP**
- Mix 1 tsp of fenugreek seeds in a cup of boiling water – allow to cool, strain and drink twice daily. This really helps to clear lymphatic congestion

Helpful Hints

- Sipping diluted lemon juice with main meals can help to treat low stomach acid, which is a factor in this condition.
- Homeopathic Arsenicum Brom 6c taken twice daily for 2 weeks helps to reduce symptoms.
- Try regular rebounding (buy a mini trampoline), which again helps clear any lymphatic congestion.

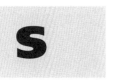

SAD SYNDROME – SEASONAL AFFECTIVE DISORDER

(see also Depression)

Approximately half a million people suffer this problem in the UK mainly between September and April, and 75–80% of sufferers are women. SAD syndrome is a condition that induces feelings of depression, low moods, increased appetite, PMS-type symptoms, difficulty concentrating, lack of energy and an increased desire to sleep during the winter months. Symptoms usually begin in late autumn or early winter and tend to disappear in late spring and early summer. During the winter months, the brain produces more melatonin, a hormone secreted by the pineal gland, which regulates glandular function and makes us feel more sleepy. In countries where sunshine is rare during the winter months, suicide rates increase. Not everyone experiences the same symptoms, but other common symptoms of SAD syndrome include cravings for sweet or starchy foods, weight gain, irritability, and an increased feeling of being of 'no use' to anyone. See also *Melatonin*.

Foods to Avoid
- During the winter months, reduce your intake of stimulants such as tea, coffee, chocolate, caffeine and sugar-based foods and drinks.
- Alcohol lowers brain levels of the neurotransmitter serotonin, which helps to keep us positive.

Friendly Foods
- Eat foods that help the body to produce more serotonin – fish, turkey, chicken, cottage cheese, beans, avocados, bananas, whey protein, and wheat germ.
- 60% of the brain is made up of fat, so eat plenty of oily fish, which is rich in omega-3 fats. Add linseeds (flax seeds) to your breakfast cereal as they are also rich in essential fats.
- Include more organic tempeh, miso soup, and beans in your diet. Kidney, canellini and black-eyed beans are a rich source of fibre and protein to help raise your mood.
- During the winter make rich stews with plenty of green and root vegetables, add brown rice and pastas.
- Low-sugar, oat-based muesli and cereals are rich in B-vitamins, which are great mood foods. Eat porridge for breakfast – sweeten with a chopped apple and a few raisins.
- Reduce your intake of refined, sugary foods, and if you crave sugar use a little honey or brown rice syrup as a sweetener, both of which are rich in magnesium.

Useful Remedies
- First, take a good-quality multi-vitamin and mineral supplement that contains at least 200mg of magnesium plus 30mg of zinc – see details of *Kudos 24* in *General Supplements*(p.160).
- Add to this a B-complex, as lack of vitamins B3, 6, 12 and folic acid are all linked to depression. (All the Bs are in Kudos 24 – see above). B6, B3 and inositol are necessary to convert tryptophan into serotonin.
- 5-Hydroxy Tryptophan (5-HTP) is derived from an African plant griffonia, and helps boost serotonin levels. This supplement has been shown to be as effective as orthodox antidepressants, without the negative side-effects. 100mg can be taken twice daily.

- St John's wort has proven very effective and you will need 500–1000mg a day. Not to be taken with blood-thinning drugs. If you are on any drugs check for contraindications with your GP.
- Cod liver oil is rich in vitamin D, a lack of which is associated with SAD syndrome – take 2 capsules or a teaspoon of the oil daily; or take 400iu of vitamin D daily.
- Try using organic rice, almond or oat milk or low-fat goat's milk instead of cow's milk.
- Amaranth, rye, rice, spelt or oat cakes make a good alternative to wheat-based breads.
- Take one gram of fish oil daily.

Helpful Hints
- Tanning beds should not be used to treat SAD. The light sources in tanning beds are high in ultraviolet (UV) rays, which harm both your eyes and your skin. Light boxes emit full-spectrum light. Use Biolight's full-spectrum lightbulbs – available from most good health stores.
- Exercise as much as possible during daylight to increase the production of serotonin – the feel-good hormone.
- Take a winter holiday in the sunshine.
- The SAD Association (SADA) have a support network, and by sending a large SAE to PO Box 989, Steyning BN44 3HG you will receive an information sheet. If you want a full SADA information pack, containing full details of SAD treatments, where to obtain light-therapy equipment, how to adapt your lifestyle, clinics, meetings and books then send £5. Tel: 01903 814942. Website: www.sada.org.uk
- For more help contact Outside In at www.outsidein.co.uk run by Angela Young – an expert in light therapies.

SCALP PROBLEMS

Dry, flaking, itching scalp (dandruff)

This condition occurs when the tiny cells in the outer layer of skin are shed at a faster rate than normal. Dandruff usually results from a malfunction of the sebaceous glands, affecting the amount of sebum or oils they produce. If too little sebum is secreted, the hair becomes brittle and dandruff appears. Dry skin on the scalp is also linked to eczema and psoriasis. An itchy scalp can also be linked to candida (see *Candida*). Dandruff is also associated with food intolerances.

Foods to Avoid
- I'm afraid it's the usual culprits of highly refined foods, high in animal fats; full-fat diary products; and sugar. See also *General Health Hints*.

Friendly Foods
- You need to increase your intake of essential fats found in oily fish, and sunflower, pumpkin and sesame seeds.
- Use organic walnut and olive oils, not only for salad dressings, but also drizzled over cooked dishes. Udo's Choice Oil is a perfect blend of omega-3 and -6 fats, which will help to feed the skin from the inside out. See *Fats You Need To Eat*.
- Eat more whole foods, brown rice and bread, barley, quinoa, millet, and brown bread and pasta.
- Greatly increase your intake of fresh fruits and vegetables, especially organic carrots, spinach, apricots, melon, guava, mango, pumpkin, sweet potato and squash, which are rich in natural source carotenes.

- Eat pineapple and papaya with main meals to aid digestion.
- Include more low-fat, live yoghurt in your diet to aid digestion.
- Eat more wheat germ and avocados, which are rich in vitamin E.
- Dry skin denotes dehydration, so drink at least 6 glasses of water daily.

Useful Remedies
- Take a good-quality multi-vitamin and mineral that contains 30mg of zinc as zinc is vital for skin healing – see details of *Kudos 24* in *General Supplements* (p.160).
- Take a B-complex (usually included in any multi).
- Vitamin E aids healthy skin, take 300iu daily.
- Omega Plex is a powdered formula containing a perfect blend of omega-3 and -6 fats. Mix half a teaspoon daily in a small glass of water. **BC**
- Your multi will contain some vitamin A – but make this up to 10,000iu per day. If pregnant take no more than 3,000iu altogether. And avoid taking extra vitamin A if you eat a lot of liver.
- The plant extract *Mahonia aquafolium* made into a cream, really helps to moisturize the scalp. Look at www.taylor-jackson.com

Helpful Hints
- Use natural-based shampoos that contain no chemicals and colourings. Aveda and the Organic Pharmacy both make great ranges.
- For organic shampoos and hair products try products from the Green People Company. To find your nearest stockist call 01444 401444. Website: www.greenpeople.co.uk
- Massage the scalp with pure rosemary oil mixed with jojoba or olive oil and leave on overnight.
- Homepathic Ars-alb 6x can be taken once or twice daily for a week.
- For more help see *Hair Loss*.

Greasy scalp

Greasy hair and scalps are usually caused by overactive sebaceous glands, which produce a waxy natural oil known as sebum, which keeps hair supple. This problem is more common during the teenage years, because as we age for most people the scalp becomes drier. It is far more common in men and teenagers and is linked to acne and hormonal changes. (See also *Acne*.) Greasy scalp can be aggravated by frequent washing with strong shampoos, which destroy the acid balance of the scalp. Always use a pH-balanced shampoo or add a little vinegar or lemon juice to your final rinse.

Foods to Avoid
- Cutting down on refined carbohydrates especially sweets, chocolates and soft drinks often helps. Reduce your intake of red meats, which take a long time to digest and can putrefy in the gut.
- Cut down on alcohol, caffeine and saturated fats, which place an extra burden on the liver. See *Liver Problems*.
- Avoid melted cheeses, which are difficult to digest.

Friendly Foods
- Eat more organic tofu, broccoli, cauliflower, Brussels sprouts, lentils and beans, which will help to regulate hormone levels.
- Drink at least 6 glasses of water every day.
- Eat more fish and especially oily fish, as well as more avocados, and sunflower, pumpkin and sesame seeds and linseeds (flax seeds). Also use their unrefined oils for your salad dressings.
- See also *General Health Hints*.

Useful Remedies

■ Vitamin A, 5000iu a day, helps balance oil production (only 3000iu if you are pregnant). Or eat liver once a week, which is high in Vitamin A.
■ Take an essential fatty acid formula – see *Fats You Need To Eat*.
■ Take a multi-vitamin and mineral plus 2–3mg biotin, the B-vitamin that is often deficient with this problem. (Good multis should contain biotin.)

Helpful Hints

■ Wash hair regularly with mild or very dilute shampoo (try a herbal shampoo, such as seaweed or rosemary).
■ Take plenty of exercise, which will help to reduce over-production of sebum.
■ Massage your scalp regularly.
■ Homeopathic Nat Mur 6x can be taken once daily for 7–10 days.
■ Dandruff, which sticks to the hair and scalp, can be loosened by rinsing the scalp with sour milk or a mild solution of lemon juice (2 tablespoons of lemon juice to a little under a pint/0.5 litre cooled boiled water).
■ Apply chickweed ointment to itchy areas.
■ Consult a qualified nutritionist, who can help you to rebalance your diet. For details of a good trichologist, see *Hair Loss*.
■ Avoid hair products containing sodium lauryl sulphate, which is used for cleaning concrete!

Head lice

This is a common problem especially in school-age children. The most obvious symptom is a constantly itching scalp and upon examination grey-coloured insects can be seen. These are the adult lice. The lice eggs (nits) are white and stick to the hair. As the eggs have a 7–14 day incubation period, patience and regular daily treatments are necessary. Many orthodox treatments contain organophosphates (pesticides), which are now linked to cancers. Head lice are attracted to clean and dirty hair alike.

Foods to Avoid

■ See *General Health Hints*.

Friendly Foods

■ See *General Health Hints*.

Useful Remedies

■ The spray Nice N Clear contains tea tree, lavender, citronella, nettle, thyme, orange and neem oil, which help to kill the lice. For details call 020 8875 9915.
■ Chinese Whispers is a herbal, non-chemical-based formula that has been shown in medical trials to kill the lice. For details of your nearest stockist call Tree of Life on 01782 567100. Website: www.treeoflifeuk.com
■ Bioforce make a tincture called Riddence, containing neem – a great insect repellent.

Helpful Hints

■ Comb the hair daily with a fine-toothed comb to remove the lice.
■ Check the head daily as close personal head-to-head contact with someone who is infested can spread the lice.
■ Wash all clothing in a really hot wash and then leave in the freezer for 2–3 days to kill any remaining lice.
■ Combine 1 part lavender oil and 1 part tea tree oil to 3 parts olive oil. Massage into the head and then rinse with vinegar.

SCIATICA

Sciatica is usually a symptom of a structural problem in the lower back, where the sciatic nerve becomes trapped or pinched. The pain tends to affect the buttocks and backs of the thighs, can travel down the back of the leg and in some cases as far as the feet. It may also cause numbness, pins and needles and/or weakness in those areas. The most common cause is a trapped nerve, but it can also be caused by a slipped or bulging disc in the lower back, which causes pressure on the sciatic nerve. Other causes include an abscess, an inflammation of the sciatic nerve, or the after-effect of minor injury to the back, for example resulting from lifting too heavy a weight in the gym, or sitting in an awkward position. If you suffer shingles in that area then you may experience post-herpetic neuralgia pain.

Foods to Avoid
- Avoid excessive consumption of foods that drain the body of thiamine and magnesium, such as coffee, tea, colas and fizzy drinks, chocolate and refined sugars, which reduce the body's ability to cope with pain. Sugar triggers inflammation in the body.
- Lack of magnesium and thiamine can also contribute muscular pain and spasms.
- Red meats, full-fat dairy and cheeses are high in arachidonic acids, which exacerbate inflammation.

Friendly Foods
- Cereals, wheat germ, meats, Bovril, fresh peanuts, Brewer's yeast and Brazil nuts are all rich in thiamine.
- Magnesium-rich foods are cereals, honey, wheat germ, almonds, Brazil nuts, mustard, and curry powder.
- Eat plenty of green leafy vegetables, yellow peppers and fresh fruits, which are all nutrient-rich, to support your nerves.
- Add more turmeric and cayenne pepper to foods, as they act like powerful anti-inflammatories.
- Ginger helps to reduce pain, so add to cooking or make fresh ginger tea.
- Eating porridge for breakfast helps support the nerves. Sweeten with a chopped apple and a few raisins (which are also rich in magnesium).

Useful Remedies
- Take NT188 containing B-vitamins and passiflora to help calm the nerves. **BC**
- Take magnesium malate – 500mg twice daily – to help relax the nerve endings.
- Calcium has anti-spasmodic properties; take 400–600mg daily.
- Take 100mg daily of thiamine (vitamin B1) to nourish the nervous system.
- Vitamin B12 injections may be helpful in some cases.
- As all B-vitamins work together, include a B-complex.
- Take 200iu of vitamin E, which helps to reduce any inflammation.
- Organic sulphur (MSM) plus the amino sugar glucosamine have shown great results in reducing this type of pain. Take 500mg twice daily until symptoms ease. If you are highly allergic to shellfish then ask for the Health Perception glucosamine, which is derived from corn.
- DLPA, an amino acid, encourages the production of the body's own pain-killing chemicals. 400mg can be taken 3 times daily until symptoms ease. Also helps to lift your mood. **FSC**
- Take 1–3 grams of vitamin C with bioflavonoids to aid tissue-healing.

Helpful Hints
- To reduce pain and discomfort, use an ice pack plus a hot-water bottle wrapped in towels. Place each alternately on the site of the pain for 10 minutes; try this twice daily.
- To relieve sciatica, lie down on your back with your knees bent, feet flat on the floor. Place your

hands underneath your buttocks (palms down) beside the base of your spine. Close your eyes, and taking long, deep breaths, rock your knees from side to side for two minutes. Reposition your hands every few minutes to enable different parts of the buttocks' muscles to be pressed. Gently move your legs from side to side with your knees pulled into your abdomen and your feet off the floor, and support your legs by holding them with your palms just behind your upper legs.

- Many alternative practitioners have found that regular deep-tissue massage gives enormous relief to sciatica sufferers, as muscular spasms in this area can be mistaken for sciatica.
- Essential oils of wintergreen and peppermint are nature's painkillers – for details of the best oils that I have ever found (from Young Living), contact Susie Anthony on 01749 679900. Website: www.psalifemastery.com (look for the Resources page).
- Homeopathic Lachesis is good for left-sided sciatica. Take 30c 3–4 times daily for up to 4 days. For right-sided – try Lycopodeum 30c.
- See a qualified osteopath or chiropractor as soon as possible and then try acupuncture, which is fantastic for pain relief. See *Useful Information*.
- Join a local yoga class to keep your spine and joints in great shape.
- When sleeping or resting, lie on your side with a pillow between your knees to minimize pelvic strain. If you sleep on your back put a soft pillow under your knees.

SHINGLES (HERPES ZOSTER) (see also *Immune Function*)

S

Shingles is caused by the same virus that causes chickenpox. The basic rule is that you cannot contract (or have a very low risk of contracting) shingles if you have not had chickenpox, as the virus lies dormant for many years in a nerve root in the spine. There is anecdotal evidence that a person suffering from shingles can pass the virus, especially to a young child, and give them chickenpox. Also, if a child who has chickenpox is in contact with an elderly relative who has once suffered chickenpox, the contact may reactivate the virus in the form of shingles. All people who have suffered chickenpox are at risk of contracting shingles. Someone who has never had chickenpox has a low risk of contracting shingles from someone else.

Shingles is common after the age of 60, but younger people are beginning to suffer from shingles. It is unusual to suffer more than one attack, but if you do then you need to boost your immune functioning. The virus can be activated by shock, stress, or lowered immune function. As the virus multiplies and attacks the nerve, it can cause searing pains along the nerve pathways. After a few days, the skin erupts in itchy blisters. These generally heal within a week, but nerve pains may last for several weeks. If the facial nerves are affected, there may be temporary paralysis. If the optic nerve is affected, the cornea may be damaged. It usually affects one side of the body or face. See also *Herpes* and *Cold Sores*, as shingles is caused by a form of herpes virus.

Foods to Avoid
- Foods that are rich in arginine, an amino acid found commonly in chocolate, carob, lentils, beans and nuts.
- Avoid sugar, refined foods made with white flour, and high-saturated-fat foods, which again have a negative effect on the immune system.

Friendly Foods
- Eat good-quality protein, such as lean meats including turkey, duck, and lean pork, plus fish, corn and tempeh, all of which are rich in lysine, an amino acid that has been shown to interfere

with replication of the virus.

- Most people feel very poorly indeed with shingles, therefore homemade vegetable soups that are easy to digest and rich in nutrients would be very beneficial.
- Add whey protein to smoothies to aid skin-healing. Solgar make Whey to Go. **SVHC**
- Live, low-fat yoghurts aid digestion and replenish the healthy bacteria in the bowel.
- Eat more garlic, which is highly anti-viral.
- See *General Health Hints*.

Useful Remedies

- At the onset of symptoms begin taking 500–1000mg of Lysine daily. If you are already suffering take up to 4 grams daily.
- Take up to 5 grams of vitamin C daily in an ascorbate form spread throughout the day with meals, whilst the situation is acute. This may trigger loose bowels, in which case reduce the dose by 1 gram at a time until this stops.
- Bee propolis, which bees make to sterilize their hives, is a powerful anti-viral agent and really boosts immune function. 3 grams daily for the duration of the attack.
- Try a cream containing St John's wort and lemon balm – both are anti-viral and regular applications will reduce pain and speed healing. **OP**
- Zinc in the form of a cream applied regularly can help fight the virus. Also take 30mg daily internally in the form of a multi-vitamin and mineral.
- Liquorice can also help to kill the virus.
- During an attack take 30,000iu of vitamin A daily for 2 weeks (only 3000iu if you are pregnant). This aids skin-healing and boosts immune function.
- Sold as Larreastat, an extract of the larrea bush has had a 97% success rate in treating all types of herpes. It is available in capsules or a lotion. Take 1 capsule up to 3 times daily and apply the lotion topically.
- Olive leaf extract acts as an anti-viral – see *Antibiotics* for details.

Helpful Hints

- Rest as much as possible when the attack starts.
- The herb St John's wort is very useful for relieving the depression and nerve pain associated with shingles. If you are not on blood-thinning drugs, take 500mg 3 times daily.
- Make sure you change your toothbrush and face towels regularly as these can harbour the virus.
- Calendula or melissa cream can be applied to the sores to help calm them down.
- Homeopathic Rhus Tox 6x, taken 3–4 times daily for 3 days, will help reduce the pain.
- Applying plain yoghurt mixed with a little zinc oxide cream along the path of the affected nerve 2–3 times daily can clear herpes zoster in 24–48 hours, if you start the regimen at the first sign of an outbreak.
- Hot and cold compresses help relieve nerve pain.
- Essential oils of wintergreen and peppermint are nature's painkillers. Dilute with a base oil and apply as close to the pain as possible but not on the sores – for details of Young Living oils contact Susie Anthony on 01749 679900. Website: www.psalifemastery.com (look for the Resources page).

SINUS PROBLEMS   (see also *Allergies, Allergic Rhinitis* and *Catarrh*)

Sinusitis is an inflammation of the mucous membranes in the sinuses. It usually occurs after a viral or bacterial infection, such as a cold or flu, which has affected another part of the respiratory system. It can also be caused by injury to the nose, dental treatment, or swimming. Common symptoms are a blocked nose and nasal-sounding speech, often accompanied by facial pain and headaches, which can be made worse by bending forward. If you suffer chronic sinus problems they may be linked to food intolerances and stress. Some people also have deviated septums or polyps in the nasal cavity, which can increase the likelihood of suffering chronic sinus problems.

Foods to Avoid

- At all costs avoid mucus-producing foods, such as full-fat milk, cheese, chocolate, white bread, croissants, pastries, cakes and anything else containing white flour and milk. Try the detox diet from Stephanie Lashford (see *Allergies*).
- At the onset of an acute sinusitis attack, try eating really lightly. This clears the body of toxins and gives the digestive system and liver a rest, which boosts immune function.
- Avoid sugar in any form for at least 6 days, as sugar greatly impairs your immune functioning and encourages bacterial growth.
- Basically avoid any foods to which you are intolerant – the most common being wheat and dairy, oranges or eggs. See *Allergies* for more information on being tested for intolerances.

Friendly Foods

- For 3 or 4 days live on really thick soups that are full of fresh vegetables and a little chicken, lentils, brown rice or barley.
- Eat more garlic and onions.
- Hot curries with cayenne pepper also help clear the sinuses as the spices dilate blood vessels and increase blood flow to the area and help clear any mucus.
- Drink plenty of freshly blended vegetable juices – especially cucumber, carrot, parsley, kale and apple, which are very cleansing.
- Snack on fenugreek seeds and add fresh root ginger to meals.
- Drink plenty of water and elderflower tea to help to reduce congestion.

Useful Remedies

- The amino acid N-acetylcysteine (NAC) really helps to support the liver and break down mucus – take 500mg before meals twice daily.
- The B-group vitamins are often lacking in this condition and while symptoms are acute take 250mg of pantothenic acid (B5) twice daily, 50mg daily of B6, and 1000mcg of B12. Or take a B-complex.
- Vitamin C – take up to 3 grams daily to boost immune function and reduce allergic responses to foods and external allergens. Vitamin C acts like a natural anti-histamine.
- Take a multi-mineral that contains 400mg of magnesium and 30mg zinc to boost immune function.
- The bioflavonoid quercetin, 400mg one to three times daily, acts as a natural anti-histamine.
- Echinacea and golden rod help reduce mucus – available in tincture. Ultimate Echinacea Complex contains these herbs. Available from the Nutri Centre or log on to www.holoshealth.com. **NC**
- Hyssop, elderflower or eyebright (if the eyes are affected) are good herbs to use for this condition. **SHS**
- Try the homeopathic remedy Kali Bich 6c three times a day in-between meals until symptoms are relieved.

Helpful Hints

- Inhaling steam is another useful treatment. Add a few drops of mint or eucalyptus oil to boiling water, place a towel over your head, and inhale for 5 minutes daily.

- Add some sea salt to tepid water and place a small amount in the palm of your hand, and inhale this mixture up each nostril. This really helps to clear the nasal passages. Otherwise ask at your health shop for Colloidal Silver or saline nose sprays.
- Avoid dry atmospheres; and when the central heating is on, make sure there is a bowl of water near the radiator to keep the air moist. Blow your nose very gently as some people can suffer nosebleeds when the nasal cavity becomes infected.

SLEEPING PILLS, ADDICTION   (see also *Insomnia*)

Sleeping pills are the most commonly prescribed drugs in the UK. They have their place for short-term relief of chronic insomnia, which is commonly associated with chronic stress, exhaustion, anxiety, an inability to shut down the mind at night, and so on. Once we begin taking sleeping pills, they alter brain chemistry and over time this situation gets worse until your brain can literally keep you awake most of the night if it does not receive its sleeping-pill 'hit'.

If you find that you cannot go to sleep without first taking a pill and if you believe that you are able to sleep only if you take a drug, then you are addicted. There are some newer generation sleeping pills available on prescription that are not as addictive as the older ones (like temazepam and valium). Nevertheless, if you take any sleeping pills in the long term, they can affect your memory and cause mood swings. If you decide to come off the sleeping pills, natural remedies may not work for the first couple of weeks due to the toxic residues left in your brain and liver from the drugs you have taken. It takes a month for the brain to register that it is no longer going to get its hit, and at this point you can then establish a healthier sleep pattern. Whatever happens – be patient with yourself. A good time to try to get off the pills would be when you are on holiday, when you are not as worried about sleeping. You would need to discuss a programme for coming off the pills with your doctor, as the withdrawal symptoms can be quite nasty if you have taken the pills for a long time.

Foods to Avoid
- Avoid eating late at night and eat at the same time every evening to establish a routine. Preferably before 8pm. Eat in a relaxed manner.
- Don't eat heavy, rich meals late at night, they are difficult to digest and can keep you awake.
- Greatly reduce your alcohol intake – drinking can make you drowsy initially, but can cause you to wake in the early hours feeling very dehydrated.
- Avoid all caffeine, cola, coffee, tea and cocoa. If you are really sensitive then even a few cups of coffee in the morning can interfere with the quality and quantity of your sleep at night.
- Generally avoid sugar, but if you find you cannot still your mind, then a small amount of sugar satisfies the hypothalamus area in the brain, which can help you to get off to sleep.

Friendly Foods
- Eat more pasta, wholemeal bread, bananas, wheat germ, avocados and cottage cheese at night. They are rich in a substance called tryptophan, which encourages natural sleep.
- Organic porridge made with rice milk makes a great breakfast cereal but it is also a calming food later in the day, packed with the B-vitamins that nourish your nerves. Make some before bed and add half a chopped banana and a little honey to sweeten; which really helps you relax.
- As a bedtime drink, try herbal teas such as camomile, valerian, passionflower or skullcap.
- To ease the load on your liver, eat more beetroot, artichokes, celeriac and celery – see *Liver Problems*.
- Drink decaffeinated green tea, which contains L-theanine, an amino acid that calms the brain.

Useful Remedies

- Niacinamide (vitamin B3) 500 mg before bed, acts as a natural sleeping pill, **but be certain to buy the no-flush variety**, as niacin can cause a dramatic skin-flushing effect that would keep you awake. This is particularly helpful for those who fall asleep readily, but can't return to sleep after waking up during the night.
- Vitamin B12; take 1000 mcg daily to aid natural sleep.
- As all the B-vitamins work together, also take a B-complex with breakfast.
- Take magnesium, nature's tranquillizer; 500mg before bed.
- 5-Hydroxy Tryptophan helps to raise serotonin levels and re-establish normal sleep patterns. Take 50–200mg before bed. **HN**
- Alpha Lipoic Acid is a great antioxidant. 100mg taken each day helps detoxify the liver from sleeping pills.
- The amino acid L-theanine extracted from green tea really helps to calm down the brain. You can take 100mg three times daily, with the last one before bed on an empty stomach.

Helpful Hints

- This may sound ridiculous, but if you can walk around in bare feet on grass for 5 minutes in the evenings, this discharges considerable amounts of pent up electro-magnetic pollution, which affects our brain, and this will help put you into a more relaxed Alpha-brainwave state. Then wear bed socks to keep your feet warm – especially in winter.
- There are many alternative remedies, such as Nytol, which you can find at your local health store.
- Stop working at least an hour before bedtime and read something light before going to bed.
- Generally try to take exercise throughout the day to relieve stress and reduce the amounts of stress hormones circulating in the body.
- Turn your bedside clock to the wall, stop worrying about the time.
- For more than 20 years I have had a problem sleeping, but find when I am on holiday I sleep like a log. Most of us today lead very stressful lives and have a lot on our minds, and at night our brains seem to wake up. If this is your problem, I strongly suggest you learn to meditate and include more regular exercise in your daily or weekly routine, which reduces stress (see *Meditation*).
- See also *Insomnia*.

SMOKING

(see also *Bronchitis*)

Smoking triggers 9 out of every 10 cases of cancer, and every 15 minutes someone dies thanks to smoking. Fifteen million people in the UK smoke and 450 children start smoking every day. Passive smoking also kills. Chronic Obstructive Pulmonary Disease (COPD) is an umbrella term for all chronic lung conditions – which is poised to overtake breast cancer to become the UK's fourth biggest killer of women. COPD can be fatal and is mainly caused by smoking. For more information on COPD log on to www.lunguk.org

If you smoke, the best favour you can do for yourself and those around you is to give it up. A pack a day equates to losing a month of life each year. One cigarette can increase your heart rate by 20 beats a minute and can also increase blood pressure. Smoking one packet of cigarettes a day depletes 500mg of vitamin C from your body – the average daily intake is 60–100mg. Cigarettes increase carbon-monoxide levels in the blood and it takes the circulatory system 6 hours to return to normal after you have smoked a cigarette. Perhaps now you understand why heart disease, cancer, and strokes, as well as high blood pressure and numerous other chronic diseases are linked to smoking. It's also worth noting that smoking ages your skin and tests have shown that the skin of a 40-year-old smoker is comparable to that of a 65-year-old non-smoker.

The more you can control your blood sugar, the easier it will be to give up smoking for good and avoid mood swings associated with withdrawal. You may also find it useful to also see the section on *Bronchitis*. People with A or AB blood types tend to have stickier blood – and therefore smoking would increase their risk for heart disease and strokes even more.

Foods to Avoid
- Cut down on the foods that you have just prior to enjoying a cigarette, such as wine, beer or a coffee.
- Cut down on saturated animal fats, which will harden your arteries over time.
- Cut down on caffeine, colas, sugar, tea and other stimulants.
- See also *Heart Disease*.

Friendly Foods
- As smoking makes your body more acid, eat plenty of foods that re-alkalise your body, such as fruits, vegetables, millet, buckwheat and wheat germ. See *Acid–Alkaline Balance*.
- Oats are a nerve tonic – and really help reduce addictions. Have organic porridge every morning.
- Begin using unrefined walnut, sunflower and olive oils for salad dressings, and use sunflower and pumpkin seeds and linseeds (flax seeds) over breakfast cereals and salads.
- Eating more leafy greens, such as cabbage, spring greens, spinach or kale, reduces your risk of lung cancer.
- Drink plenty of green tea, which is high in antioxidants. Some researchers believe that Japanese men who smoke suffer less incidence of cancer and other lung diseases thanks to the protective effects of green tea.
- Cantaloupe melons, pumpkin, apricots, carrots, French beans, mangoes, raw parsley, and watercress are all high in natural-source carotenes, which help to protect the delicate tissue in the lungs.
- Eat more oily fish, rich in vitamin A.
- Generally eat small meals regularly to control blood sugar (see *Friendly Foods* under *Low Blood Sugar*).
- Eat organic liver once a week as it is rich in lung-protective vitamin A.

Useful Supplements
- A high-strength multi-vitamin and mineral, in a formula that includes essential fats and antioxidants, helps to give some protection. See details of *Kudos 24* in *General Supplements* (p.160).
- Make sure any multi formula you take contains a full-spectrum of B-vitamins.
- Take 2 grams of vitamin C daily with meals.
- Take vitamin A – 10,000iu daily – to help protect lung tissue. If you are pregnant you should not be smoking, and the dose would need to be no more than 3000iu daily.
- Magnesium taken daily – 500mg – helps ease breathing.
- Take N-acetylcysteine, 500mg twice daily before meals. This amino acid helps bronchial conditions as it loosens mucus and strengthens tissue.
- The amino acid tyrosine – 500mg per day before meals – helps to reduce the craving for nicotine.
- 200mcg per day of the mineral chromium helps to keep your blood sugar on an even keel, thus reducing the cravings. Take between meals. (This is already in Kudos 24; see above.)
- MSM – an organic form of sulphur – helps the body to excrete the nicotine via the sweat. Take 1–2 grams daily before meals.

- A herbal extract tincture made from crushed lobelia leaves, ginger, oats, liquorice and thyme taken twice daily helps reduce the cravings and supports the lungs. Take with homeopathic Staphisagria, Tabacum and Nux Vomica – which really help reduce withdrawal symptoms and cravings. **OP**

Helpful Hints

- Soak in an Epsom-salt or sea-salt bath, which helps remove nicotine through the pores. Accompanying this with skin brushing would be even better.
- Scientists in Germany have developed a machine called Air Energy, which makes the oxygen we breathe easier to utilize. It has been shown to be very useful for people suffering COPD (see above). The air we breathe contains 21% oxygen – but our body can utilize only around a quarter of the available energy within this amount. Air Energy converts the oxygen into a form that the body can easily utilise. With regular use this machine is obtaining amazing results for all lung conditions. Clinical trials are ongoing in the UK and Europe. The machine is expensive, starting at £2100, but the results and research to date are very exciting. For more details call 01938 556800. Website: www.biolifesolutions.co.uk. These machines are also becoming available at many health clinics and doctors' surgeries – call the above number for your nearest clinic. Treatments start at around £35 an hour.
- For more help contact ASH – Action on Smoking and Health, 102 Clifton Street, London EC2A 4HW. Tel: 020 7739 5902. Website:www.ash.org.uk
- QUIT is a charity that helps people stop smoking. Tel: 0800 00 2200.

SORE THROATS   (see also *Colds and Flu* and *Immune Function*)

If you tend to suffer a persistent sore throat it usually denotes that your immune system is struggling to cope. When I become overtired and my throat becomes sore, I know that if I were to eat some foods high in sugar, this could send my immune system off the deep end and I would end up with a cold or infection. I now know my limits and listen to my body. If you are at this point, never underestimate how what you eat during the next 48 hours can be the deciding factor in whether you become ill or not; and get some sleep. Regular bouts of tonsillitis (see also *Tonsillitis*) mean that your lymphatic system is under stress and your body is telling you to detoxify. Regular sore throats are also associated with the yeast fungal overgrowth candida (see *Candida*).

Inflammation and pain in the throat can trigger symptoms such as pain upon swallowing or speaking, a dry tickling feeling, build-up of mucus in the nose and sinuses and occasionally a husky voice or loss of your voice. These types of infections are caused by bacteria or viruses. A sore throat caused by a streptococcal infection (often called strep throat) needs to be identified and treated, or it could trigger rheumatic fever in some cases. So if symptoms are severe, please see your doctor.

Foods to Avoid

- Eliminate sugar in any form for 4 days to give your immune system a chance to fight infection.
- Greatly cut down or avoid all white-flour-based products, snacks and burger-type meals. Avoid all 'white' foods.
- Coffee, sugary drinks and alcohol dehydrate the body and act as stimulants – if your adrenal glands are exhausted these foods will add to the problem.
- Cut down on all full-fat dairy produce.

Friendly Foods
- Increase fluid intake, include lots of filtered water, herbal teas especially green tea or rooibos tea, diluted fruit juices, and broths.
- Sip warm water mixed with powdered vitamin C, plus lemon, ginger and/or garlic with a little honey.
- See also *Friendly Foods* under *Colds and Flu*.

Useful Remedies
- Ask at your health shop for either a bee propolis or an echinacea throat spray and use as directed.
- Try Ultimate Echinacea Complex, which also contains astragalus (which boosts the immune system). **NC**; or log on to www.holoshealth.com
- While symptoms are acute take 10,000iu of vitamin A daily to boost your immune system (if pregnant only 3000iu), or eat organic liver once a week.
- Take at least 2–3 grams of vitamin C daily with meals.
- Take a B-complex to support your adrenal glands with an extra 500mg of B5.
- Low levels of selenium are linked to viral infections. Take a multi-vitamin and mineral that includes 200mcg of selenium and 30mg of zinc.
- Celloid Chloride compound, 200mg daily, helps to clear lymphatic congestion and relieve sore throats. **BLK**
- A natural source beta-carotene complex boosts immune function and fights infection.
- Zinc Gluconate lozenges really help reduce a sore throat – take 3–4 daily.
- If you end up taking antibiotics, make sure you replenish healthy bacteria by taking acidophilus/bifidus capsules twice daily for 6 weeks. See *Antibiotics*.

Helpful Hints
- Crush fresh sage, make into a tea, allow to cool, and gargle. Sage is antiseptic and eases the soreness. If the throat is really sore, soak a cloth in the sage mix and apply to the throat area.
- You can also crush an onion and wrap it in a cloth and place on the throat.
- Propolis tincture can be diluted in water and used as a gargle.
- Change your toothbrush regularly.
- At the onset of a sore throat use homeopathic Aconite or Belladonna 30c – if the throat is red and worse on the right hand side. For children's sore throats, a hacking cough and swollen tonsils, try Chamomila 30c – 3 times daily for 2 days.
- The herb thyme is also a natural antiseptic. It can be made into a solution and used as a gargle for sore throats or sipped as a tea mixture to help relieve sore throats and coughs. Or mix oregano, thyme and basil essential oils and massage onto the throat area.
- Tea tree oil is a natural antiseptic, use diluted with a little sea salt as a gargle, but do not swallow. Gargle with a mixture of warm water and a quarter teaspoonful of turmeric powder and a pinch of salt.

SPIRITUAL EMERGENCY
(see also Depression)

This title may appear out of place in a health book, but believe me spiritual emergency is a well-known phenomena in the East, and as our interest in spiritual subjects gains pace it is becoming far more common in the West. I have yet to meet an orthodox doctor (apart from a handful of GPs, including my own) who has heard of this condition, or recognises any of its specific symptoms, but it does exist.

Most psychiatrists tend to diagnose a spiritual emergency as psychosis, depression or schizophrenia – but if this subject could receive wider attention, many people could avoid being sent to mental homes and labelled as being mentally ill.

I experienced a huge spiritual emergency during 1998. I began affecting electrical equipment, could clearly see people's energy or auric fields, became super-psychic, telepathic, and could clearly hear people from the spirit world. I received huge amounts of information, which placed an enormous strain on my brain and nervous system. The full story is told in my book *Divine Intervention* (Cico Books).

People often experience various phenomena, such as seeing auras and hearing other realms, either spontaneously as in my case, or during spiritual development courses. We all have psychic abilities and are capable of miracles, but most of us don't truly comprehend this ultimate truth. When you undergo this type of experience you need to find professional help to determine the most appropriate course of action.

At this moment in our evolution the average human uses between 3 and 5% of their brain's *potential* capabilities. Certain highly evolved spiritual people use up to perhaps 50% and are capable of incredible feats, which need to be seen to be believed. In my book *The Evidence For the Sixth Sense* (Cico Books), I have included easy-to-read science on how miracles are possible and on enlightenment, and self-help during a spiritual crisis, both for the person and their family.

If during your spiritual growth, you begin to feel ultra-special and your ego comes into play – you need to ground yourself. Find your nearest spiritualist church, which will undoubtedly know of someone who can help you. Hands-on healing would definitely be of benefit during a spiritual emergency – see *Healing*. It's your choice whether to turn to an orthodox doctor, but you may end up on huge amounts of medication and be admitted to a psychiatric hospital. If I had not had tremendous support from my family and friends this could have easily happened to me.

Foods to Avoid
- Sometimes during this type of situation you don't want food, but it is imperative you eat to help ground yourself.
- The last thing you need is stimulants, so avoid caffeine, sugar (although see below) and alcohol.

Friendly Foods
- If your brain is in absolute overdrive and feels as though it's on fire, then eat some sugary food quickly. The brain uses pure glucose as a fuel, and as you may be processing huge amounts of information, your brain will need an energy supply. It is always preferable if you can eat small healthy meals regularly, but if the situation is acute then eat sugar or a banana. Controlling your blood sugar helps to control the events and your ability to cope with them – see *Low Blood Sugar*.
- Generally, eat what I term 'earthy' grounding foods, such as porridge made with organic rice milk, stews, and thick vegetable or grain-based soups.
- You may not want it, but you need protein, which helps balance your blood sugar levels for longer periods. Fish and animal products might repulse you, in which case eat some beans, pulses, cooked tofu and brown rice with plenty of fruits and vegetables. Otherwise make smoothies, with fruits, sunflower and pumpkin seeds and add a tablespoon of whey protein, which is easy for the body to utilise.
- Drink plenty of water, and as many calming herbal teas as you like.
- Your digestion may be upset, so include fresh ginger in soups and drink ginger teas.
- If you simply cannot eat whole food, at least make yourself some fresh vegetable juices with added aloe vera juice, a green food powder and some whey protein such as Solgar's Whey To

Go – which will help to keep you going. My favourite is apple, banana, blueberries, pineapple, whey, and sunflower and pumpkin seeds plus a couple of dried apricots. Try a few combinations to find one that you like.

Useful Remedies
- Begin taking Bach Rescue Remedy and Star of Bethlehem *and then* immediately every 2 or 3 hours.
- Also begin taking homeopathic Arnica 30c every few hours to help reduce feelings of shock.
- For anyone who is quite psychic, intuitive and has a very open personality, try homeopathic Phosphorous 30c, 3 times daily, which will help to balance the energies.
- Take 1 homeopathic Aconite 200c daily. Taken at the onset of any symptoms, this can help to relieve some of the stress and reduce fear.
- Take a high-strength B-complex to support your nerves. Try an extra 1000mg of pantothenic acid (vitamin B5) daily to support your adrenal glands, which are most probably working overtime.
- Take a multi-vitamin and mineral formula daily, such as Kudos 24 – for details see *General Supplements* (p.160).

Helpful Hints
- There is now a network called the Spiritual Crisis Network, which has been formed by clinical psychologist Isabel Clarke and her colleagues, plus Catherine Lucas, who went through a profound spiritual emergency. If you need help have a look at their website on www.SpiritualCrisisNetwork.org.uk; or email Catherine on clucas@spiritualcrisisnetwork.org.uk
- In London the College of Psychic Studies takes students from all over the world and helps them to integrate their newly found gifts and knowledge in a balanced and safe environment. Tel: 020 7589 3292. Website: www.psychic-studies.org.uk
- At this time you need all the support and patience friends and family can provide, as you may say and do many things – such as levitate or produce ash – that can initially be quite frightening. You may also experience periods of complete and utter bliss. I beg of you to write any insights or channelling down – don't try sharing them with everyone you know, which can have negative responses. At such times a person can also easily be persuaded to join cults. And if the person threatens to harm themselves or others, they made need a brief stay in hospital until things calm down.
- Avoid negative thoughts as much as you can. For every negative thought replace it with a positive one.
- Try not to panic – the experience will pass, it just takes time. See also *Panic Attacks*.
- Consult an expert, such as Susie Anthony based in Wells near Glastonbury, who has had great experience with acute spiritual awakenings. Contact her on 01749 679900 or log on to www.psalifemastery.com
- Read *Spiritual Emergency* by Stanislav and Christina Grof MD. To order in the UK call 020 7323 2382. This book really helps when personal transformation becomes a crisis. So would my book *The Evidence For The Sixth Sense* (Cico Books).

STITCH

This is a sudden, sharp pain in the side or abdomen, triggered by exercise, that wears off after a few minutes when we rest. The pain is almost certainly caused by a spasm in the gut wall. A stitch is the body's way of telling you that it needs more oxygen, so stand still and breathe deeply. It can also be triggered by too much exercise after a heavy meal. People who tend to be sedentary, eat insufficient fresh fruit and vegetables and too much sugar, caffeine and animal protein are often lacking in calcium and magnesium, which causes a build up of lactic acid, resulting in regular attacks of muscle cramps or stitch.

Foods to Avoid

- Avoid sugar and highly refined foods, such as croissants, biscuits, cakes, pizza and white-flour-based foods in general.
- Any foods that remove magnesium from the body, which is needed to alleviate stitch. Magnesium is particularly depleted by too much alcohol and caffeine.

Friendly Foods

- Magnesium-rich foods, such as green leafy vegetables, fruits plus brown rice, barley, lentils and whole grains rich in fibre will give you more protection in the long term. Black strap molasses is rich in magnesium and calcium.
- Honey and dried apricots are also high in magnesium.
- Include good-quality protein in the diet, such as fresh fish, cooked tofu and lean meats, at least once a day.

Useful Remedies

- Take a vitamin B-complex daily.
- Calcium 400mg and 600mg of magnesium to help reduce spasm and relax the muscles.
- Take Emergen C sachets – which are high in vitamin C and minerals. Take one sachet before exercising to help reduce any chance of stitch.

Helpful Hints

- Bend down and touch your toes to relieve a stitch. Or take a deep breath and have a good stretch.
- A stitch is more likely to occur if you exercise while food is still digesting in the gut. Avoid strenuous exercise for an hour after a substantial amount of food.
- Generally take regular exercise to avoid lactic acid accumulation in the body.
- A stitch generally occurs when you have not warmed up properly before exercise.
- Do not sit for long periods without going for a walk or a good stretch.
- Breathe deeply more often.

STOMACH AND DUODENAL ULCERS

(see also *Acid Stomach*)

Stomach ulcers are small raw areas on the walls of the stomach where the protective mucus coating has been worn away. This can be due to excessive stomach-acid production, insufficient mucus lining, and regurgitation of bile from the duodenum, which are linked to heavy smoking, alcohol, erratic eating habits, and a diet high in acid-forming foods.

Duodenal ulcers are small raw spots in the lining of the duodenum eroded by stomach acid. They usually trigger pain 3 hours or so after eating a meal. A bacterium called *Helicobacter pylori* has been found in over 90% of duodenal ulcers and 80% of gastric ulcers. This bacterium is also linked to stomach cancers, low energy levels, and skin conditions, such as rosacea and urticaria. Inflammatory conditions such as migraines are also linked with *Helicobacter pylori*. Treatment with high-dose antibiotics usually kills the bacterium – however it commonly re-occurs.

Stomach ulcers are more common in Type A blood types and tend to affect older people where the protective stomach lining has been eroded. There is a link between stomach ulcers and cancer. The pain of a stomach ulcer is often made worse after eating. Duodenal ulcers are more common in Type O blood types and tend to affect younger people. They generally do not progress to cancers and the pain of duodenal ulcers is usually relieved by food.

Stress is a major factor in any type of ulcer, as when you are stressed the body produces more stomach acid. Food intolerances to foods such as wheat, cow's milk and prescription drugs, plus long-term use of aspirin, steroids, and non-steroidal anti-inflammatory drugs, such as ibuprofen, are also linked to ulcers.

Foods to Avoid

- There is a proven link between over-consumption of caffeine and ulcers, so avoid all coffee, black tea and colas. Decaffeinated coffee is also a problem.
- Eliminate all dairy produce from cows for at least 1 month.
- Alcohol stimulates stomach-acid production.
- Don't eat too much sugar and too many rich fatty foods, which again tend to increase acid production.
- Avoid spicy foods, which can aggravate the gut lining.
- Avoid eating late at night, which places a great strain on your digestive system.
- Avoid citrus fruits, raw tomatoes, rhubarb, plums, and pineapple.
- Avoid all refined white-flour-based foods.
- Avoid thermally hot or cold foods and drinks.

Friendly Foods

- Eat lots more fresh cabbage, which is rich in L-glutamine, an amino acid that helps to heal the gut. Eat it raw, added to fresh vegetable juices. If you cook the cabbage, then use the cooking water for gravy or drink it once it has cooled.
- Replace cow's milk with soya light or organic rice milk. Sheep's or goat's milk is usually well tolerated.
- Eat plenty of vegetables and fruits, such as bananas, figs, lychees or pears.
- Include barley, brown rice and wholemeal bread, pastas and noodles plus lentils, millet, amaranth and couscous in your diet.
- Eat more jacket potatoes, peas, corn and apples, which are high in fibre.
- Add seaweed, such as kombu, to your bean dishes as it contains healing properties.
- Fish, nuts and seeds (linseeds/flax seeds, and sunflower, pumpkin and sesame seeds) are high in zinc, which aids tissue-healing.
- Eat more live, low-fat yoghurt, manuka honey, and liquorice, which all help to heal the gut.
- Add cinnamon to fruit dishes.
- Slippery elm – preferably in a tea – helps to soothe and heal the whole digestive tract including the stomach and duodenum. Sip throughout the day in-between meals. **SHS**

Useful Remedies

- Ulc-Dig capsules contain marsh mallow, barberry, pau d'arco, and poke root, which help to promote healing in the gut. **SHS**
- Chew 1 to 2 tablets of deglycyrrhized liquorice 20 minutes before food. This encourages healing of the stomach lining and helps to eradicate the *Helicobacter* if this is present.
- Vitamin A is vital for the stomach lining to be able to heal. If you are not pregnant take 20,000iu daily for the first month and then reduce to 10,000iu. If you are pregnant take no more than 3000iu of vitamin A.
- B-vitamins aid digestion and reduce the risk of ulcers. Take a B-complex daily.
- Take vitamin C as magnesium or potassium ascorbate, 500 mg before meals and at bedtime, as most ulcer patients are lacking this vital vitamin. **BC**
- Mastica is a resin from a plant found in the Greek Aegean sea. 500–1000mg per day for two weeks has been shown to rapidly heal gastric ulcers. It also helps to remove any *Helicobacter*.
- Take L-glutamine (500 mg 4 times daily) 30 minutes before meals to speed the healing process.

Helpful Hints

- Chew food thoroughly. Never rush a meal as digestion is made difficult when you are stressed or in a hurry.
- Don't drink too much liquid with meals as this dilutes digestive juices.
- Ulcers can be encouraged to heal by eating only small quantities of food at a time.
- Avoid stress and rushing as much as possible as stress over a prolonged period can cause great harm to our digestive system.
- Smoking greatly increases the risk of ulcers.
- Drinking 75ml of concentrated aloe vera juice 20 minutes before meals also helps to soothe the digestive tract.
- Homeopathic Merc cor or Arg nit 6c can be taken 3 times daily for a week.

STRESS
(see also Depression and Immune Function)

More than 7 million working days are lost in the UK every year through stress and it is a major contributing factor for a host of health problems. Not all stress is bad – it can help to keep you sharp and alert, but in the longer term how your body copes, depends on your *reaction* to the stress.

Aeons ago when our ancestors were faced with life-and-death situations, the hormones adrenaline and cortisol (see at the end of this section) would be released from the endocrine system (which is made up by the pancreas, thyroid, pituitary and the adrenal glands situated just above the kidneys), to make the heart pump faster; giving an instant energy boost to the body and brain. Muscles tensed, cholesterol increased and enzymes in the blood caused the blood to thicken, so that if the person was injured, then their blood clotted more easily. Blood vessels would constrict; endorphins, the body's own painkillers, would be released; and oxygen consumption increased. Known as 'fight or flight', these responses saved many lives back when our ancestors fought off marauding animals and invaders. However, today our automatic responses to stress remain the same, and unfortunately they trigger heart attacks, strokes, cancers, stomach ulcers and even Alzheimer's. Why? Because if we don't disperse stress hormones through regular exercise or relaxation, in the longer term they become highly toxic to every major organ, and set up inflammatory responses in the body. It's like putting rocket fuel in a scooter, you eventually burn out the engine.

But these days instead of going for a walk, breathing deeply and calming down – we tend to head for the coffee/cola machine or eat another sugary 'treat' to keep us going, which triggers even more adrenaline to be released, which exacerbates the situation. Make no mistake stress can kill you.

The first signs of stress usually show up in behavioural changes, such as feeling constantly irritable, a sense-of-humour failure, suppressed anger, you try to do more than one job at once, you begin to feel that you cannot cope, break down in tears, you are tired or wired.

Then come the physical symptoms, palpitations and headaches, lack of appetite/or cravings for sugary foods, insomnia, poor digestion, muscle cramps, frequent urination, constipation and/or diarrhoea, a dry mouth, constant thirst, feeling clammy or cold or too hot. Your brain doesn't work properly and you forget simple words or names. That's because stress creates more free radicals and research at Stanford University has shown that raised cortisol levels damage the connections between brain cells affecting brain functions. Luckily, if you stop the stress, the connections grow back. Long-term stress also makes the body more acid and vital minerals are then leached from the bones to re-alkalise the body (see *Acid–Alkaline Balance*).

If any or all of these symptoms sound familiar, you need to stop and rest, because the next stage could be total burn out, a heart attack or a stroke. Whether your stress comes from a bad relationship, work, children, illness, lack of money – whatever it is, if possible *make a space and time between what is stressing you and your reaction to it*. Talk to someone and tell them how you are feeling; ask your doctor to send you for counselling. If more people could do this, thousands of lives could be saved.

Research has shown that if you think negatively, tend to be angry a lot of the time, and are under long-term negative stress, especially after 50, then you are more likely to suffer heart and arterial disease. This is because so many of us hold in emotions that we should get off our chest. Remember, the more indirect you are – the more stressed you become. Emotions held in for long periods will eventually cause a fuse to blow.

There are also those infuriating (but wise) souls who are always positive, they love stress and positively thrive on it. However, we are all unique and you need to learn your limits and listen to your body. There are many things you can do to reduce the negative effects of stress on your body, which can help you to stay healthier.

Foods to Avoid
- Never underestimate just how much your diet can affect your stress levels and your ability to cope with it. Avoid any foods and drinks containing alcohol, caffeine, sugar and artificial sweeteners, especially aspartame, which are all stimulants that cause the adrenal glands to overwork .
- Reduce refined (white) and processed foods, they're high in additives/preservatives and sugar, and usually low in nutrients. The more refined and processed food you eat, the more stress you place on your liver, digestive system and ultimately your adrenal glands.
- Cut down on heavy meals, especially red meat which is hard to digest, and when you are stressed digestion is one of the first things to be affected.
- Don't eat in a rush.

Friendly Foods
- Stress breaks down protein in the body very quickly, this is why most people who are very stressed tend to lose weight. Make sure that you eat around 4–6oz (100–175g) of quality protein daily – preferably at breakfast and lunch, which helps to balance blood sugar levels.
- Whey is an easily absorbed form of protein. Solgar make an excellent formula called Whey To Go. **SVHC**
- Eat oily fish and unrefined sunflower, pumpkin and hemp seeds – all rich in essential fats that reduce inflammation triggered by stress hormones (see *Fats You Need To Eat*).
- Liquorice tea helps to support adrenal function and echinacea tea will help to support your immune system, which is greatly affected by stress. Valerian and camomile teas with a little honey help to calm you down.
- Green tea contains L-theanine – an amino acid that encourages production of Alpha waves, the brainwaves you produce during relaxation.
- Make sure you eat breakfast – a low-sugar muesli, eggs, or wholemeal toast would be fine. Try oats, especially porridge made with rice milk, as oats are a rich source of B-vitamins, which help you to stay calm.
- Wholewheat pasta, noodles and breads, couscous, quinoa, amaranth or oat crackers, lentils, brown rice and barley are all calming foods.
- Avocados, turkey, cottage cheese, bananas, potatoes, ginger, yoghurt, leafy green vegetables, lettuce and low-fat milks will also help to de-stress you.
- Generally increase your intake of easy-to-digest foods, such as homemade vegetable soups,

mashed sweet potatoes, poached fish, stewed fruits and so on, which helps take some of the burden off your digestive system.

- Eat smaller meals regularly – low blood sugar is common in people who are stressed (see *Low Blood Sugar*).
- See also *General Health Hints*.

Useful Remedies

- If the stress has been induced by shock or trauma, use homeopathic Aconite 30c – and take it every hour in-between meals for a few days. Give the shocked person some sweet tea, as at times of shock the brain uses more glucose.
- Jan De Vries has formulated Emergency Essence for Shock (use as directed). Available from all health stores, or visit www.avogel.co.uk.
- Take a high-strength multi-nutrient powder with vitamins, minerals, antioxidants and essential fats, such as Kudos 24. For more details see *General Supplements* (p.160).
- For general long-term stress try the herb Rhodiola root. In Siberia, where the root is made into a tea, many local people live healthy lives to well over 100. This could be because Rhodiola root has been proven to decrease the release of stress hormones and improve mood, and helps to lower blood pressure and aid memory. Take for 1 month, then stop for a month and then start again. Kudos make a high-strength (900mg), one-a-day capsule. **KVH**
- If you are *not* taking a high-strength multi-vitamin/mineral, then begin taking a B-complex to support your nerves. Even if you are taking a multi, for 2 weeks, in cases of severe stress, also take 500mg of vitamin B5 pantothenic acid 1–2 times a day, which really helps support adrenal function.
- You could also take pantethine – which is a more powerful version of B5. This helps regulate hormone production whilst the body is under stress. Take 300mg 1–3 times daily. Call the Society for Complementary Medicine for details on 020 7487 4334.
- Urinary excretion of vitamin C increases with stress, so take 1–2 grams of vitamin C plus 400iu of natural-source, full-spectrum vitamin E to thin your blood naturally, as stress also thickens the blood.
- BioCare's AD206 contains vitamins C and B5, and Siberian ginseng and other nutrients involved in the support of the adrenals in one convenient capsule to be taken 3 times per day. **BC**
- You need additional calming minerals, so take 600mg of calcium and 400mg of magnesium, which are known as nature's tranquillisers (they should be in any good multi).
- 5-Hydroxy Tryptophan (5-HTP), 50–200mg daily, helps to increase levels of the hormone serotonin in the brain, which helps to raise mood.
- Take a high-strength fish oil (1 gram) containing EPA and DHA essential fats that thin the blood naturally and help keep blood pressure down.
- To calm anxiety try a herbal formula called Advanced Stress Formula, containing the herbs ashwagandha, gotu kola, liquorice and Siberian ginseng. **NC**; or log on to www.holoshealth.com
- L-theanine is an amino acid found in green tea and in the mushroom *Xerocomus badius*. It is a natural relaxant that increases Alpha waves, which help you to feel more relaxed without inducing drowsiness. Take 100mg 3 times daily. **NC SL**

Helpful Hints

- Apply pure rosemary, nutmeg and clove oils directly to the adrenal area – around your waist area at the back – which will support adrenal function and help you to feel more positive. Excellent therapeutic healing oils are available from Young Living in the US. In the UK contact Susan Anthony at PSA Life Mastery on 01749 679900.
- If you tend to wake regularly between 3am and 5am, this is a sign that your adrenal glands are struggling.
- Take stock of your life. An important first step is to identify sources of stress. Keep a diary and

write down the things that are winding you up. After a month you will see it's most probably the same things over and over again. Take steps (if possible or practical) to remove what stresses you from your life.

- Laughter releases stress – learn to lighten up and don't take life too seriously.

- I know it's hard, but as much as you can stop worrying so much. Dale Carnegie once said that 85% of the things we worry about, never actually happen – trust that things will turn out for the best.

- Keep a pet. Studies with cat- and dog-owners have shown the considerable stress-reducing abilities of a furry companion. When cats purr they produce calming Alpha waves, so stroke your cat and de-stress!

- Concentrate on what you can change in your life and let go of the things you have no control over.

- Doctors agree that if we could all practice a pleasurable hobby that requires a fair amount of concentration, it would take our minds off what is stressing us and so reduce the release of stress hormones and help calm us down. At the very least watch a movie that makes you laugh.

- Make sure you get 8 hours sleep. Sleep deprivation is a major stress in itself and lowers your tolerance to other stresses.

- Avoid obvious pressures, such as taking on too many commitments and deadlines. Learn to see when a problem is somebody else's responsibility, and refuse to take it on.

- Learn to say no and mean it – stop feeling guilty.

- If you are in a very stressful situation, if possible walk away. Go for a walk, take some slow deep breaths, calm down and then go back. If you do this you will feel more able to cope.

- Get plenty of exercise, as relaxed muscles mean relaxed nerves, which reduces stress. A brisk walk or vigorous exercise session is good instant first aid for feelings of stress. If this is impossible you will still benefit from regular exercise.

- Take a deeper breath every 20 minutes, this helps to re-alkalise the body and slows the release of stress hormones.

- Learn how to relax. Try a simple progressive muscle relaxation exercise to free the body of physical tensions and distract the mind. Lying down flat on the floor with your palms up, breathe into your tummy. Then, beginning with your feet and calves, tense the muscles as hard as you can and then relax. Work your way up your body, tensing and releasing each muscle group in turn, finishing with your head and face. Then just relax and stay there for 5 minutes, imagining that you are simply empty space; and just let go.

- Learn to meditate – it's one of the best antidotes for stress (see *Meditation*).

- Have a regular massage using essential oils of lavender, valerian, frankincense, neroli, jasmine or ylang ylang, which will all help to calm you down. The oils are absorbed into the body, so leave them on overnight to increase their effectiveness.

- Hypnotherapy on a weekly basis will really help to calm you down (see *Useful Information*).

- If you have an emotional problem that you cannot solve or if you can't handle the stresses in your life, seek outside help and advice. Simply talking with a trusted friend can be very beneficial, although it is often better to find a professional counsellor, who can both help you to handle your problems and teach you effective stress-reduction techniques.

- For an excellent guide on how to lower the stress in your life read *Don't Sweat the Small Stuff…and it's all small stuff* by Richard Carlson PhD (Hyperion Books).

- For excellent stress-busting tips, try reading *10 Simple Ways to beat Stress Forever*, by Suzannah Olivier (Cico Books).

Cortisol and Stress

Cortisol is a steroid hormone made by the adrenal glands and is produced in response to any stressful 'fight-or-flight' situation. Aeons ago this perfectly normal and natural response gave us the extra energy boost and mental sharpness to either run from our attacker or stand and fight. Either way our bodies would utilise the cortisol and levels would then return to normal.

Cortisol is both good and bad. It is needed to help regulate blood pressure and cardiovascular function, as well as to regulate the body's use of proteins, carbohydrates and fats. It is also released during times of infections, trauma, fatigue, temperature extremes, and crucially when you worry too much. In the short term cortisol is a good guy, but if levels circulating in your body become, and remain, too high – that is, chronically elevated – then cortisol damages tissues and organs, and greatly affects memory and brain functioning. And stress hormones in the long-term deplete bone. Other common symptoms include palpitations, depression, sleep disorders, high blood pressure, anorexia, low blood sugar, insulin resistance, thyroid problems, menstrual disorders, osteoporosis and obesity (when combined with high insulin levels). You get the picture. Too much stress and cortisol can kill you. Think of Pacific salmon: after spawning it undergoes rapid cortisol-induced ageing, and death follows in a matter of days. You should also be aware that oestrogen replacement, from orthodox HRT, can increase cortisol levels.

One of the best methods for measuring cortisol levels is an adrenal stress index saliva test. This test measures cortisol levels from early morning to midnight. The results are plotted on a graph and compared with a normal daily output of cortisol. This test is available at the Individual Wellbeing Clinic. Tel: 020 7730 7010, or contact your health practitioner.

S

STROKE
(see also *Angina* and *Heart Disease*)

Strokes are the third most common cause of death in the West and account for the disability and dementia of approximately 130,000 people every year in the UK. Sixty thousand of these patients die as a result of a stroke. Children and young people can also suffer a stroke, but 9 out of every 10 cases occur in the over-55s – and the risk for stroke increases with age.

The good news is that most strokes can be avoided. A stroke occurs when there is a loss of blood supply to the brain that damages or destroys an area of brain tissue. Depending on the part of the brain affected, there may be sudden loss of speech or movement, heaviness in the limbs, numbness, blurred vision, confusion, dizziness, loss of consciousness, or coma. Stroke often causes weakness and paralysis on one side of the body, involving the arm and/or leg and face. Symptoms can last for several hours or the rest of one's life depending on the severity of the stroke. 'Mini' strokes may even go unnoticed and can contribute to subtle reductions in mental function. Many people who suffer a stroke go on to make a partial or even complete recovery.

Over time, arteries gradually narrow owing to a build of up of sticky cholesterol-like substances. Arterial blockages cause 9 out of 10 strokes (called ischemic strokes). The blockages may be the result of thickening of the arteries (atherosclerosis). Sometimes blood clots travel from another part of the body, such as the heart or neck, to the brain, causing a cerebral embolism. The other 10% of strokes (called haemorrhagic strokes) are caused by bleeding into the brain from a ruptured blood vessel, which is most commonly caused by high blood pressure.

The risk of having a stroke is higher among people with an unhealthy lifestyle – smoking, eating too much salt and too much saturated fat, high oestrogen levels, stress, high LDL (bad)-cholesterol levels, and being overweight. People who tend to be angry or aggressive a lot of the time are also at a higher risk – as stress and anger raise LDL-cholesterol levels, which thicken the blood. People with Type A or AB blood are also at a higher risk as they tend to have stickier blood.

The first step toward heart disease and stroke is damage to the delicate inner lining of your arteries, which leads to the development of plaque, which thickens the arteries and poses the eventual risk of a total blockage. But what causes the damage in the first place? We know that a lack of vitamin C weakens the matrix of the artery wall, making it more prone to damage. Free radicals, for example from smoking or eating fried foods, may lead to increased arterial damage, especially if the person is deficient in antioxidants, such as vitamins C and E. But there is another factor produced by the body that many doctors now believe to be more dangerous than having high cholesterol – it's called homocysteine.

High levels of homocysteine, a toxic by-product of the metabolism of proteins, are known to damage arteries, and the link to heart disease and strokes is now beyond question. Researchers have found that a high level of homocysteine in the blood is as great a risk factor for cardiovascular disease as smoking or having a high blood cholesterol level. However, if you have sufficient vitamin B6, B12 and folic acid, your body will convert homocysteine into less toxic substances, and studies have confirmed that the less vitamin B6 and folic acid in your blood, the higher your levels of homocysteine. This is why taking a B-complex daily could save your life. At times symptoms of stroke are not obvious. If you suspect that someone may have recently had a stroke, the American Stroke Association recommends asking these 3 simple questions – which could save the person's life;

* Ask the person to smile.
* Ask the person to raise both arms at the same time.
* Ask the person to speak a simple sentence, such as "It's sunny outside today."

If the person has trouble with any of these 3 tasks, take them to hospital or call for immediate medical assistance.

Foods to Avoid

■ Avoid white foods. Replace refined grains (white bread, pasta, rice, cakes and biscuits) with whole grains, such as brown rice, whole-grain breads and pastas, quinoa, and oats. Whole grains contain more vitamin B, which has often been removed in processed 'white' products.

■ Reduce your intake of saturated fats from red meats, full-fat dairy produce, cheese and chocolate.

■ Don't eat fried foods or hydrogenated margarines. Those most at risk of having high homocysteine levels are high-protein (meat) eaters with a poor dietary intake of vitamin B6, B12 and folic acid. See also *Fats You Need To Eat*.

■ Reduce your intake of dairy products – they're associated with an increase in cardiovascular disease, especially strokes. There are 2 possible reasons for this – first, while high in calcium (which is often poorly absorbed), dairy foods are relatively low in magnesium. Calcium requires adequate magnesium to be deposited in the bones, otherwise it is usually deposited in soft tissues including joints and arteries. Second, dairy foods are high in protein so raise homocysteine levels, but lack adequate levels of the B-vitamins needed to process it into less toxic substances.

■ Avoid all fizzy drinks because of the sugar content that causes damage to the circulatory system and leads to an increase risk of strokes.

■ Caffeine can drive up blood pressure. Cut down on coffee, tea, cola and other caffeine-based drinks and foods like chocolate cake! Good alternatives include green tea, peppermint tea, fruit teas, or diluted fruit juices.

- Eliminate sodium-based salts from your diet because of the effects on blood pressure. Replace them with magnesium or potassium-based salt, such as Solo salt, or sprinkle powdered kelp onto food. Ask at your local health food store.
- Avoid all highly preserved meats, salted nuts and smoked foods.

Friendly Foods

- Eat plenty of fresh fruits and vegetables and their freshly made juices for the vitamin C and the other protective antioxidants they contain. Especially good are brown rice, quinoa, barley and lentils, plus broccoli, sprouts, carrots, watercress, fresh and dried apricots, spinach, cabbage, spring greens, mangoes, cantaloupe melon, and tomato purée.
- Potassium-rich foods help prevent strokes and a recent study showed that a low potassium intake can increase the risk of stroke by 50% in the over-65s. Therefore, eat more potassium-rich foods. Bananas, low-fat yoghurt, baked potatoes with the skin, prune juice, tomato juice, Swiss chard, spinach and all leafy greens, squash, asparagus, dried apricots, oranges, kidney beans, and lentils are all rich in potassium. (Note: if you have kidney disease or take a diuretic medication to lower blood pressure, check with your doctor before taking any extra potassium.)
- Eat more beta-carotene-rich foods, such as carrots, sweet potatoes, watercress, mangoes, cabbage, broccoli, cantaloupe melon, pumpkin and tomatoes. In the Nurses' Health Study, which monitored 121,000 US female nurses ages 30–55, those who consumed more than 15–20mg of beta-carotene a day had a 40% lower risk of stroke than women who reported eating less than 6mg a day.
- Vitamin B6 and folic acid help prevent the build-up of artery-damaging homocysteine and can be found in oranges, lemons, bananas, tomatoes, green leafy vegetables, beans, nuts, seeds and whole-grain products. Many breakfast cereals are fortified with additional folic acid. Enjoy organic porridge oats for breakfast made with half skimmed milk and half water, add a chopped apple plus a few raisins for sweetness plus some wheat germ for its vitamin E.
- Make sure you eat a serving of greens, especially dark green leafy vegetables, every day. Spinach, cabbage, lettuce, spring greens, kale, chard, broccoli, peas and watercress are all good.
- Eat more foods rich in essential fats like oily fish and use unrefined olive, walnut and sunflower oil for salad dressings. Eat more raw, unsalted nuts and seeds – especially linseeds (flax seeds), and pumpkin and sunflower seeds. The easiest way to get seeds in your diet is to sprinkle them, whole or freshly ground, on your breakfast every morning (see *Fats You Need To Eat*).
- Garlic and onions help to thin the blood naturally.
- Magnesium-rich foods include honey, kelp, raw wheat germ, dates, almonds, Brazil nuts and curry powder.
- Sprinkle raw wheat germ over cereals and soups, as it is high in vitamin E.
- Cayenne pepper is a powerful heart and circulation tonic and has been known to reverse plaque formation on the arterial walls.

Useful Remedies

- Magnesium relaxes constricted arteries and reduces the risk of a blockage. Take 400–600mg per day. Many doctors have found that anyone who has suffered a stroke caused by a clot in the brain should be given intravenous magnesium as soon as possible after the stroke. Magnesium has a powerful dilatory action on the arteries and helps restore blood flow to the damaged tissue.
- Take a B-complex to help lower the level of the toxic amino acid homocysteine. Studies have shown that folic acid reduces levels of homocysteine in the blood and thus reduces its harmful effects on the arteries. Participants who consumed at least 300mcg of folate each day had a

20% lower risk of stroke. Recommended dose: folic acid 400–1,000mcg per day and vitamin B-complex 50mg per day.

- Take fish oils, 1–3 grams daily, to thin the blood naturally. If you are on blood-thinning medication consult with your doctor first.
- Take 1 gram of vitamin C, plus 400iu of natural-source vitamin E, which protect against clotting. Don't take vitamin E supplements if you are on blood-thinning medication without first consulting your doctor.
- Co-Enzyme Q10 x 30–60mg per day helps to strengthen the heart muscle. People high in CoQ10 are less prone to strokes.
- Bioflavonoids x 1000mg taken daily helps to strengthen capillaries.
- Ginkgo biloba helps to increase circulation to the brain. Ginkgo is known to inhibit platelets in blood from sticking together. Kudos make a high-strength capsule. Again, if you are on blood-thinning drugs, tell your doctor about taking any supplements, as over time and under guidance your medication may be reduced. **KVH**
- Take a good-quality antioxidant formula that contains at least 200mcg of selenium.
- Vinpocetine is an extract of the periwinkle plant that is used in more than 35 countries in the treatment of stroke and dementia triggered by poor blood-flow to the brain. It helps to increase oxygen levels in the brain by increasing blood-flow and in one study was shown to improve the transport of glucose (brain fuel) into the damaged brain tissue caused by the stroke. Try 10mg twice daily with food. Because this remedy can reduce the ability of blood to clot, never take vinpocetine if you are on blood -thinning drugs. For more information speak to the nutritionist at the Nutri Centre on 020 7436 5122.

Helpful Hints

- Research shows that people living in soft-water areas are more prone to high blood pressure, which can lead to strokes, as soft water is low in minerals including magnesium. Therefore, if you live in an area of soft water, supplement around 400–600mg of magnesium daily. Drink more bottled water.
- Stop smoking, which doubles your stroke risk.
- Certain types of combined oral contraceptives can make the blood stickier, which increases the risk of clotting. Orthodox HRT is also linked to an increased risk (see *Menopause*).
- Control your blood pressure (see *High Blood Pressure*).
- Take regular exercise, which makes the heart stronger and improves circulation. It also helps control weight. Being overweight increases the chance of high blood pressure, atherosclerosis, heart disease, and adult-onset (Type II) diabetes (see *Weight Problems*). Brisk walking, cycling, and swimming lower the risk of both stroke and heart disease. Remember to start gently if you've not exercised for some time and if you have heart or circulation problems consult your doctor before starting any new exercise regime.
- Untreated, diabetes can damage the blood vessels throughout the body and lead to atherosclerosis. See *Diabetes*.
- Homeopathic Aconite 30c – taken 3 times daily between meals for 3 weeks – helps to reduce the effects of shock on the body.
- Read *The Alternative Medicine Guide for Heart Disease, Stroke and High Blood Pressure* by Burton Goldberg (Future Medicine Publishing). To order call the Nutri Centre bookshop on 020 7323 2382.
- Or, read *Heart and Blood Circulatory Problems* by Jan de Vries (Mainstream Publishing).
- For more help contact the Stroke Association at www.stroke.org.uk

SUNBURN

(see also *Age Spots*)

Because the sun has had such a bad press over the years and skin cancer rates are rising, we are all supposed to have become more sensible in the sun. But most people haven't changed a bit. No matter where I am in the world, I see fair Europeans of all ages literally cooking their skin, as I once did. A few wise people stay out of the midday sun, but I still see so many young children with no hats or sunglasses or tee shirts out in the midday, tropical sun. Parents are often nearby doing the same thing. At the other extreme you have people like Nicole Kidman, who never sunbathe, so I hope she takes plenty of vitamin D!

Sunshine gives off a cocktail of frequencies, but principally ultra violet (UV) radiation. The UVA rays are the ageing rays; UVB are the burning; and UVC are the most dangerous. Both UVB and UVC are mostly absorbed by the ozone layer (what's left of it); UVA can penetrate deeper into the skin than UVB or C, and UVA causes damage down into the fat layer of your skin – 2.5mm into the dermis. To try to protect itself, your skin begins to thicken and of course it turns brown. We all know that too much sun accelerates ageing – in fact 80% of age-related skin damage comes from too much sun exposure. The slower you tan, the more you reduce the ageing effects on your skin. When the skin turns red in the sun, it is the red-blood-cells' response to the heat that is being generated on the skin. Your blood is basically trying to cool your skin.

Black and Asian skins contain more melanin, the thick treacle-like substance that resides in your epidermis. The darker the skin, the more melanin it contains and the more easily it can reflect UV rays. Also darker skin is able to resist the penetration of the sun's rays down to the dermis – 5 times more effectively than white skin. People with greasy skin make more sebum, which helps to block the UV rays, hence people with dark and oilier skins are able to tan better and suffer less wrinkling. Basically the fairer you are the more easily you will burn, the faster your skin will age, and the greater your risk of developing skin cancers.

But sunshine on your skin makes you *feel* so good. If you don't expose your skin to sufficient sunlight, then you can become depleted in vitamin D, which is vital for healthy bones and teeth. Too little sunshine can trigger SAD Syndrome as the body produces less serotonin – the feel good hormone. Full-spectrum light in natural daylight is vital for good health and your state of mind. Sunbathing helps to lower cholesterol and increases hair and nail growth, but too much will lower your immune function. People who live in colder climates and have little sun, tend to suffer a higher incidence of internal cancers. What we need to do, as always, is to find a healthier compromise. For example, if you expose your skin to just 15 minutes of sun a day, then you can produce several days supply of vitamin D.

Foods to Avoid
- Avoid foods and drinks that will trigger dehydration, such as alcohol, caffeine and too many fizzy drinks.

Friendly Foods
- Obviously if you are out in the hot sun, you will sweat more and you can quickly dehydrate, which can lead to low blood pressure, which in turn can make your faint. Drink plenty of water and if it's really hot, then add some extra sea salt to your food.
- The most important foods you need to eat more of to help protect your skin from the inside out are essential fats and carotenes.
- Eat lots more sunflower, pumpkin, sesame and hemp seeds and linseeds (flax seeds) and use their unrefined oils in salad dressings and drizzle over cooked foods (for more details see under *Fats You Need To Eat*).

S

- When you are in the sun, eat plenty of grilled oily fish and enjoy avocado and olive salads.
- For carotenes eat more organic or fresh locally grown carrots, tomatoes and tomato purée, asparagus, mustard and cress, raw parsley, red peppers, steamed spinach, apricots, pumpkin, spring greens, sweet potato, watercress, apricots, mangoes and cantaloupe melon.

Useful Remedies

- Take a high-strength multi-vitamin and mineral, and an antioxidant powdered supplement that is also high in carotenes and essential fats (for details see *Kudos 24* in *General Supplements*; p.160).
- Take 30mg of natural-source carotene complex for a month before and a month after your holiday in the sun.
- People who take 2 grams of vitamin C daily along with 400iu of vitamin E appear to have added protection. Obviously with a sun screen!
- Melanin is made up from the amino acid L-tyrosine, and taking 1000mg daily can help the body tan naturally. Start taking a week or so before you go away.
- Pine bark extract, known as pycnogenol, has been proven to reduce inflammation on the skin triggered by UV radiation.
- Try Urtica cream, which reduces the stinging and inflammation. From any homeopathic pharmacy; or call the Organic Parmacy. **OP**

Helpful Hints

- Skin cancers are on the increase, especially in countries and latitudes that enjoy hot sunshine all year round. And as the ozone holes become larger and more widespread, skin cancers are increasing proportionately, especially after the age of 50. The most dangerous type is malignant melanoma, which is a tumour of the melanocyte (the melanin-producing cells). They are usually pigmented either black or brown and can evolve from an existing mole, or simply appear. It begins to itch, grows larger, and the skin can break down around the 'mole'. The secret to surviving melanoma is to see a doctor, dermatologist or oncologist *as fast as you can.* If caught before the cancer spreads internally, it can be treated successfully. The good news is that if you have reached your 60s and have no skin cancer, the incidence of melanoma reduces.
- You may see small skin ulcers, tiny flaking patches, or small areas of skin that start to bleed, keep scaling and won't heal. This could be a squamous or basal cell carcinoma. These are not so dangerous, but again they need prompt checking and treatment.
- If you are using rejuvenating creams based upon Retin A, glycolic acids, AHAs etc, then wear a higher sunscreen factor and be really careful not to let your skin go red. I use these creams during the autumn and winter months and I stop using them 1 month before I go away.
- Don't allow your skin to go really red. This can trigger skin cancers and cause broken and unsightly capillaries on the face.
- If you suffer skin conditions such as eczema or psoriasis, moderate sunbathing and instead spend lots of time in the sea – the seawater will help your skin.
- No matter how much people tell you that sunbeds are safe, they are not, and continued use greatly increases the risk of skin and other cancers.
- If you carry the herpes simplex virus, too much sun can trigger an attack of cold sores, in which case begin taking 500mg of the amino acid lysine and 1 gram of vitamin C daily for 2 weeks before travel and keep away from chocolate as it contains arginine – another amino acid that makes cold sores more likely. See *Cold Sores.*
- Many scientists now believe that chemical-based sunscreens (containing ingredients such as sodium lauryl/laureth sulphate, octylmethoxycinnamate (OMC), benzophenones, sythetic fragrances and colourants) may do more harm than good. Certain preservatives in sunscreens, such as parabens, mimic the affect of oestrogens, which can disrupt hormones and are linked to

hormonal cancers. If you develop a rash after sun exposure, check out the ingredient list in the cream. PABA (a constituent of folic acid and a member of the B-vitamin family) is also a problem for many people.

- Try Green People's organic sunscreens. The UV protection comes from titanium dioxide and extract of cinnamon. Edelweiss, from the Alps, helps protect against skin cancers and is high in antioxidants. They also contain green tea extract, avocado oil, echinacea, myrrh and calendula that helps soothe the skin. They are available in an 8, 15 or 22 protection factor. Sold in good health shops and department stores, or order via www.greenpeople.co.uk. They also make wonderful shampoos, conditioners, and face and body creams.

- Another favourite is Dr Hauschka sun products. Again they use titanium dioxide, combined with rice germ oil (rich in vitamin E), chestnut bark extracts, quince seeds and jojoba oil. Sold at major department stores worldwide, or call 01386 792 622. Website: www.drhauschka.co.uk.

- The Life Extension Foundation in America make a sun cream called Total Sun Protection – containing green tea, grape seed, milk thistle, turmeric root, liquorice and rosemary, which all help reduce sun damage and inflammation. For details log on to www.lef.org. This one does contain some chemicals – which the majority of sun creams still do. It's a question of choice and reading labels.

- During tests it was found that the amount of suncream you put on your body can be crucial in protecting your skin. Most people only apply sufficient to achieve 20% of the sun protection factor on the bottle. Use plenty of cream regularly.

- To help avoid cataracts and ageing eyes, wear good wrap-around sunglasses that block 99–100% of the UVA rays.

- Wear a hat, which greatly reduces the UV radiation to the eyes.

- Avoid the sun between 11am and 3pm in an English summer – and make that 11am and 4pm in hotter climates.

- Please try to be sensible – wear a light wrap or tee shirt in the heat of the day and always re-apply the creams after swimming.

- Certain antibiotics, arthritis drugs, diuretic drugs and antihistamines (like Benadryl) can trigger extreme reactions. If you are taking any such drugs and you are going away to the sun, check with your doctor.

SUPERBUGS (see *MRSA*)

SWOLLEN FEET AND ANKLES (see *Foot Problems* and *Water Retention*)

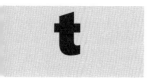

TACHYCARDIA (RAPID HEART BEAT)

(see also Palpitations)

Tachycardia is a sudden increase in heart rate to over 100 beats per minute in an adult. It occurs in healthy people during exercise, but if tachycardia occurs when you are resting, then you should consult a doctor as a matter of urgency. Symptoms may include palpitations, breathlessness and light headedness, and sweating and/or dizziness. These types of symptoms are common in people who suffer low blood sugar (see also *Low Blood Sugar*).

Foods to Avoid
- Avoid drinking too much alcohol, which can damage the heart muscle.
- Avoid caffeine which causes more adrenaline to be released into the bloodstream and can precipitate an attack.

Friendly Foods
- Eat potassium-rich foods. These include all leafy green vegetables, bananas, fresh and dried fruits, nuts, fish and sunflower seeds.
- See *Friendly Foods* under *Heart Disease*.
- Eat more garlic and onions, which are heart-healthy foods.

Useful Remedies
- Take a high-strength multi-vitamin and mineral that contains a full spectrum of B-vitamins. See details of *Kudos 24* in *General Supplements*; p.160.
- Co-enzyme Q10, 60mg daily, helps strengthen the heart muscle.
- Natural-source vitamin E helps the heart muscle get oxygen and naturally thins the blood. Take 400iu daily.
- The mineral magnesium is often deficient. Take 300–600 mg daily.
- All of these are in Kudos 24 (see above). Otherwise check at your health shop.
- Anything that helps you to relax usually helps reduce symptoms, speak to a nutritionist at any of the companies listed on pages 13–15 – and ask about L-theanine (extracted from green tea) or rhodiola root (which helps relaxation). **NC SL**

Helpful Hints
- As palpitations may be linked to an overactive thyroid, it may be worth asking your doctor to do a blood test.
- To combat worrying, which only exacerbates the condition, learn how to breathe properly by taking yoga or relaxation lessons.
- Practise meditation, which teaches you how to stay calm when stressed. If you feel an attack beginning, splash your face with cold water, then lie down, close your eyes, breathe deeply and slowly for a few minutes until the attack passes. See *Meditation*.
- Essential oil of lavender or ylang ylang has a calming effect, so add a few drops to your bath. Try regular aromatherapy massage, which is very calming.
- Go for leisurely walks, breathing deeply.

TASTE AND SMELL, LOSS OF

In young people this condition can occur after a cold or with blocked sinuses, but as we get older and our immune system weakens, loss of taste and smell is very common. If the nose becomes too dry and 'stuffed up' then the sense of smell can quickly be impaired. When you have a cold your ability to taste and smell can be reduced by up to 80%. Hayfever, allergic rhinitis, nasal polyps, and smoking can all interfere with taste and smell. Lack of zinc is associated with this condition, as many people do not absorb sufficient zinc from their diets. Certain heart drugs can also cause a loss of taste and smell. It is generally easier to smell and taste in warm, moist atmospheres rather than cold, dry ones.

Babies have many taste buds in their mouths – including the cheeks – and once we become adults the sensitivity of all our taste buds is diminished, and in old age it is greatly diminished. Your tongue is covered with tiny projections called papillae, inside which are the sensory nerves that enable you to taste. Saliva is needed for taste and without it our diet would be virtually tasteless.

The average nose can detect approximately 4,000 different odours, whilst an especially sensitive one can recognise around 10,000. Inside the nose we have 2 small receptor sites, which are yellow-brown patches of mucus-covered membrane found in the roof of the nasal cavities. They are covered in millions of hair-like antennae. As we age these antennae become less effective.

Foods to Avoid
- Generally you need to avoid mucus-forming foods, such as full-fat milk and dairy produce. Soya milk can be a problem for some people.
- Sugary, fatty foods will also make the situation worse.
- See *Foods to Avoid* under *Colds and Flu*.

Friendly Foods
- Keep your diet clean, with plenty of fresh fruits and vegetables.
- Eat more brown rice, barley, lentils, cereals, oats, and wholemeal bread and pastas.
- Zinc-rich foods include lean steak, lamb and beef, calves' liver, raw oysters, fresh peanuts, hazelnuts, Brazil nuts, ground ginger and dry mustard.
- Sunflower, pumpkin and sesame seeds and linseeds (flax seeds) all contain fair amounts of zinc.
- Try rice milk as a non-dairy substitute.

Useful Remedies
- Take 15–30 mg of chelated zinc or zinc picolinate, which can be useful in helping to restore the sense of smell. For best results take on its own at night before bed.
- If an infection triggers a loss of taste and smell, take 10,000iu of vitamin A for a month, which helps support the upper respiratory tract. If you are pregnant, take no more than 3000iu.
- Include a high-strength multi-vitamin and mineral, plus 1 gram of vitamin C daily.
- If the problem is linked to an infection, take echinacea, 500 mg twice daily, to boost your immune system. See also *Immune Function*.

Helpful Hints
- Tap water is often contaminated by chemicals, which can exacerbate this problem. Invest in a reverse-osmosis water-filter system, which is far more effective than over-the-counter carbon filters. For details contact The Pure H2O Company on 01784 221188; Email: info@purewater.co.uk Website: www.purewater.co.uk
- See a qualified nutritionist, who will help rebalance and detoxify your system.
- Homeopathic Nat Mur, Silica or Pulsatilla are also very useful for loss of taste, Belladonna or Hyos are useful for loss of smell.

TENNIS ELBOW

(see *Bursitis* and *Carpel Tunnel Syndrome*)

THROAT PROBLEMS

(see *Sore Throat*)

THRUSH

(see also *Candida* and *Cystitis*)

Vaginal thrush is caused by the same fungus, *Candida albicans*, that causes oral thrush. Infections develop when the bacteria in the vagina are destroyed. This happens if we take too many antibiotics, eat too much sugar and junk-type food, become very run down, use highly perfumed soaps and deodorants and so on. Symptoms can include itchiness or general soreness of the vagina, and sometimes the vulva swells and is accompanied by a thick, whitish discharge, which smells rather yeasty. You may feel the need to urinate more regularly and there could be some slight stinging when you pass urine. If the infection takes hold, the lymph glands in the groin can swell. If this happens you must see a doctor (see also *Candida*). If you suffer cystitis regularly, then you may be very run down – this can lead to thrush. Chronic thrush is also linked to diabetes – therefore see your doctor. If this is the case, then avoid sexual intercourse for at least a week to help ease symptoms.

Foods to Avoid
- See *Foods to Avoid* under *Candida*.
- As the body needs to be kept more alkaline, see the dietary advice in *Acid–Alkaline Balance*.

Friendly Foods
- Eating 250ml of plain, live yoghurt daily really helps to clear thrush.
- See *Friendly Foods* under *Acid–Alkaline Balance* and *Candida*.

Useful Remedies
- Take 1000mg twice daily of the herb pau d'arco – which has anti-fungal properties.
- Grapefruit seed extract, 800–1200mg, is anti-fungal. It also acts like a natural antibiotic.
- Take a course of acidophilus/bifidus – healthy bacteria, which really help to kill the yeast overgrowth. **BC**
- Thyme and rose essential oils – use a few drops diluted in a douche of lukewarm water twice daily to help kill the bacteria. For really powerful therapeutic grade oils have a look at the Young Living Products on the Resources page of www.psalifemastery.com
- Douche with yoghurt (1 pot natural live yoghurt to 3 pints/1.75 litres boiled cooled water); or with apple cider vinegar diluted into water (4 tbsp to 3/4 pint/1 litre of boiled cooled water). This helps to re-acidify the area, as the good bacteria prefer a slightly acid environment in the vaginal area.
- Include a high-strength multi-vitamin and mineral in your regimen.

Helpful Hints
- While an attack lasts avoid sexual intercourse, which could be extremely painful. Your partner will also need to be treated for any candida as you are more than likely passing the problem back and forth.
- Douche in lukewarm water with a few drops of tea tree oil, a crushed garlic clove and a little organic cider vinegar.
- Try lavender and tea tree pessaries until symptoms ease. **SHS**
- Wear cotton underwear and change it every day, and do not use vaginal deodorants, perfumed

bath salts, or talcum powder.
- Only use pH-balanced soaps.
- Vitamin E or calendula cream may relieve itching.
- Homeopathic Lycopodium 6c or Kali Mur 6c – take 2–3 times daily for up to a week to help to reduce symptoms.
- For oral thrush use Borax 6c twice daily for up to a week.

THYROID, UNDERACTIVE AND OVERACTIVE

Undiagnosed thyroid problems are now reaching epidemic proportions – as symptoms can vary so hugely. Your thyroid is often the most ignored gland in your body. It is situated in your neck, just below the Adam's apple, and produces hormones that affect every major organ and the metabolism and repair of every single cell, and it has a major influence on hormonal function. Every drop of our 8–10 pints (4.5–5.5 litres) or so of blood circulates through our thyroid every hour, bringing with it the substances the thyroid needs to do its work. The most important thyroid hormone is thyroxine (also known as T4), which outside the thyroid is converted to T3 (tri-iodothyronine), which is the active form of the hormone. Basically, the more T3 you produce, the faster your metabolism. If you don't produce sufficient thyroid (T3) hormones, many systems in your body begin to slow down – heartbeat, circulation, blood pressure, energy levels, metabolism and temperature. Slower metabolism will mean that you don't burn calories as efficiently as you could, so you gain weight more easily. Also when the body slows down, the body's ability to detox is greatly impaired.

Up to 20% of the population are probably suffering from some degree of hypothyroidism (underactive thyroid), and the older you get, the more prone you are to the condition. But it needn't be that way. Symptoms that should make you investigate whether your thyroid may be underactive include low energy, mental 'fogginess', depression, cold hands and feet, weight gain even with a poor appetite, high cholesterol, even when you eat sensibly, a slow pulse, low blood sugar (see *Low Blood Sugar*), headaches, infertility, dry and sometimes puffy skin, brittle nails, poor vision and memory, constipation, sore throat, nasal congestion, thinning hair, low libido and heavy periods. Phew!

An underactive thyroid is 7 times more common in women than in men. Unfortunately because some of the symptoms associated with an underactive thyroid are so often attributed to the menopause, thousands of women go undiagnosed or are offered orthodox HRT as a one-stop cure-all. But there is so much you can do to help yourself.

If you have your thyroid tested by a doctor it's very likely they'll report that everything is fine. Unfortunately the tests are rather crude and your thyroid would have to be very underactive indeed before it would show up as altered blood levels. The quoted 'normal' range is so wide it is relatively meaningless – you could be 50% down on 'average' and still said to be within normal limits.

To test your own thyroid, there's a simple temperature test developed by Broda Barnes that's now widely used by nutritionists. Here's how it works. Shake out a thermometer and keep it by your bed. When you wake up in the morning, and **before getting up**, put the thermometer under your arm and lie there for 10 minutes. Your temperature should be 36.5–36.7°C (97.7–98°F). Do this for at least 2 days. (Women should do this test on days 2 and 3 of their period as body temperature fluctuates during the cycle.) If either of your temperature readings are below 36.5°C (97.7°F), take it again over a longer period, say a week, to see if it is low on a fairly regular basis. If it is, you're probably hypothyroid – your thyroid gland is under-functioning. For more help log on to www.brodabarnes.org

In many cases a low temperature will not necessarily indicate a condition that would be medically diagnosed as an underactive thyroid (and treated with synthetic thyroid hormones), but nevertheless you could benefit from the following guidelines.

If you take steps to improve your thyroid efficiency, take your early-morning temperature again for a couple of mornings every month or so. As it starts to increase, you should find that some of your symptoms also start to improve.

An overactive thyroid (excess T3 production) is known as hyperthyroidism and is relatively rare. In this condition the thyroid produces too many hormones, which can trigger symptoms such as goitre – when the thyroid becomes more prominent and the eyes bulge. Other common symptoms are anxiety, insomnia, an inability to relax, shakiness, excessive sweating, feeling warm even on cold days, rapid heartbeat, palpitations, breathlessness, and weight loss even with a hearty appetite. If you are diagnosed with an overactive thyroid, you need the help of a competent physician or nutritional practitioner.

Foods to Avoid – for an underactive thyroid

- Certain foods are known to inhibit thyroid function, these includes soya (soya milk, tofu, and so on), apples, cruciferous vegetables (such as cabbage, broccoli, mustard and kale), spinach, peaches, pears and turnips. Also avoid walnuts and peanuts. These foods are generally good for you, but avoid them just until the thyroid has stabilised.
- Avoid all foods and drinks containing caffeine, which stimulate the release of adrenaline, which can affect the thyroid.

Friendly Foods – for an underactive thyroid

- Iodine (an element) and the amino acid tyrosine are the 2 nutrients the body uses to make thyroid hormones. Iodine can be found in seafood and seaweed (for example kelp, nori and arame), mushrooms, Swiss chard, butter beans, pumpkin seeds, and sesame seeds (tahini), egg yolk, lecithin, minced beef, artichokes, onions, and garlic.
- Use organic sea salt or sprinkle powdered kelp over meals.
- Tyrosine is in all protein-rich foods, especially fish, butter beans, pumpkin seeds, bananas and avocados. If you have adequate protein in your diet you should be getting enough tyrosine.
- Essential fatty acids are essential for proper thyroid function, so include oily fish, seeds and cold-pressed oils in your regular diet. See *Fats You Need To Eat.*
- Eat more radishes, watercress, wheat germ, brewer's yeast, mushrooms, tropical fruits, watermelon, seeds and sprouted foods such as alfalfa. Make your own watermelon juice and add aloe vera juice, a great thyroid blend.
- Use coconut oil for cooking and for flapjacks – it helps to stimulate the thyroid.
- The trace mineral manganese is important for thyroid function – therefore eat more pecans, almonds, Brazil nuts, rye, barley and buckwheat.

Useful Remedies – for an underactive thyroid

- A high-strength multi-vitamin and mineral complex taken every day provides a baseline of nutrients for the body to work with. Try Kudos 24 – for details see *General Supplements*; p.160.
- Kelp tablets contain iodine, follow the directions on the label, aiming for around 150mcg of iodine a day. But don't take more than 500mcg of iodine a day, unless under your doctor's instruction, as too much iodine can upset thyroid balance.
- The body makes thyroxine from the amino acid L-tyrosine, so take 500mg twice daily on an empty stomach (plus 50mg of B6 and 100mg of vitamin C to aid absorption).

- Take Siberian ginseng – 1–3 grams (or 2–6ml of tincture) daily for a month, then leave off and start again a month later. This can help reduce the effects of stress on your adrenals, your thyroid and your health in general. Avoid Korean ginseng if you suffer from high blood pressure.
- 1 gram of vitamin C, as well as 100mg of CoQ10, can help raise energy levels within the body .
- Thyro Complex is a formulation by naturopath Martin Budd, an established authority on thyroid health. He has spent 15 years researching the nutritional support required for healthy thyroid function, and his formula contains all the nutrients needed to help support the thyroid. Take 1–3 tablets daily 30 minutes before food. **NC SL**

Helpful Hints

- Stop smoking – smoking is known to make an underactive thyroid worse. Cigarettes aren't an easy addiction to give up, but worth the effort. For smokers, the number-one thing they can do to improve their health and healthy lifespan is to quit smoking.
- Avoid stress. Stress stimulates the adrenal glands to produce the hormone cortisol, which is known to hinder the conversion of the thyroid hormone T4 to the more potent T3. Avoiding stress is easier said than done, so managing stress is often the key – learn to relax, ensure you have 'down time' regularly, try yoga, Tai Chi, massage or meditation, and exercise regularly (see *Stress*).
- Support your digestion. It is well established that our enzymatic function and digestive capacity decline with age, and when you are under stress at any age. Tyrosine, needed to make thyroid hormones is a component of protein. Protein is relatively difficult to digest, so less digestion means less tyrosine and therefore less thyroid hormones. The answer is to chew well, relax over meals, and ensure you have an optimum level of nutrients in your diet to support digestion. If you have low stomach acid (needed to digest protein), you'll find that beetroots give you pink urine, which can be used as a simple test at home. Both digestive enzymes and HCl capsules may be needed in the short term till your digestion becomes more efficient.
- Consider food intolerances. Dr James Braly has reported in his book *Dangerous Grains* (Avery Publishing) a surprising correlation between wheat intolerances or allergies and thyroid problems. You can test for food intolerances with a kinesiologist or a simple at-home blood test from York Laboratories (call 01904 410410, or find it through a nutrition consultant; see *Useful Information* for further details).
- Exercise regularly. Exercise stimulates thyroid function – 30 minutes of aerobic exercise at least 3 times per week. If you are just starting an exercise program, start gently and build up.
- Avoid fluoride (in toothpaste) and chlorine (in tap water) as they are both chemically similar to iodine and block the iodine receptors in the thyroid. Consider putting in a pure water filter.
- If an underactive thyroid is diagnosed early enough and the patient is otherwise vigorous, homeopathic thyroid treatment can be very useful. One such product called Thyroidea Compositum, made by the German company HEEL, is one of the most powerful and useful non-drug substances in the holistic physician's repertoire. Available from homeopathic pharmacies.
- Try reading *Hypothyroidism, the Unsuspected Illness* by Borda O'Barnes and Lawrence Galton (Harper and Row); or *Why Am I So Tired – Is Your Thyroid Making You Ill*, by Martin Budd (Thorsons).
- For further help log on to www.brodabarnes.org

TINNITUS

Tinnitus is a chronic and distressing condition in which the patient suffers a ringing, buzzing or humming in one or both ears. This condition can have a variety of causes, which include high blood pressure, exposure to loud noise or an explosion, long-term use of aspirin, use of beta blockers and antibiotics, compacted ear wax, spinal or cranial misalignment (which can reduce circulation to the ears), or food intolerances. Tinnitus is more common in older people, but is appearing in younger people who are exposed to excessively loud music. In Chinese medicine adrenal and kidney function are linked to ear problems – therefore if you are totally exhausted and/or stressed, this could also trigger tinnitus or make any existing problem worse. Ageing rock stars, who are exposed to loud music over many years often suffer from tinnitus. This condition can also be linked to a congested liver. See *Liver Problems*.

Foods to Avoid
- Avoid alcohol, smoking and caffeine, all of which may aggravate the condition.
- Cut down on salt, which may increase blood pressure.
- Avoid all full-fat cow's milk and products for 2 weeks as they are mucus-forming, which can block the ears and sinuses.
- Generally cut down on saturated fats, such as red meat, cheese, chocolate, highly refined white-flour-based foods, pies, pastries, biscuits and so on.
- Yeast-based foods such as Marmite, Bovril and yeasty breads can also make this problem worse.
- Don't use hard margarines or highly refined cooking oils and eliminate fried foods.
- Read labels carefully and avoid any foods containing hydrogenated or trans fats. See *Fats You Need To Eat*.

Friendly Foods
- Eat plenty of garlic and onions, which are very cleansing.
- Choose low-fat dairy options, such as fully skimmed milk or cottage cheeses.
- Use organic rice milk for making porridge and with cereals, and try live, low-fat yoghurts in desserts instead of creams.
- Generally increase fruits and fresh vegetables, and include more nutritious foods such as lentils, barley and corn, rice and spelt-based pastas in your diet.
- Jacket potatoes are a wonderful food, but add yoghurt instead of lots of butter or use a non-hydrogenated spread such as Vitaquell, Biona or Benecol.
- Add more cayenne pepper to foods to help increase circulation.

Useful Remedies
- For 1 month take 25,000iu of vitamin A to nourish the inner ear nerve cells. (If you are pregnant or eat lots of liver, which is high in vitamin A, then limit your intake to 3000iu a day.)
- Take 30mg of zinc in a multi-vitamin and mineral, as lack of zinc is associated with tinnitus. For the first month take an extra 30mg of zinc daily before bed to aid absorption until symptoms ease.
- Taking vitamin B12 – 1000 mcg a day – helps noise-induced tinnitus.
- As all the B-vitamins work together, also take a B-complex.
- Taking ginkgo biloba, 120–240mg of standardised extract daily, increases circulation to the ear.
- Try garlic and horseradish tablets or tincture, which act as decongestants.
- Herbs such as gotu kola, cayenne pepper and prickly ash will all help to increase circulation to the head. Have a word with the herbalist at Specialist Herbal Supplies and find out which herb might help you most effectively. **SHS**

Helpful Hints
- Recordings of soothing music or sounds help mask the unwanted noise, especially when you are trying to get to sleep.
- Regular exercise may provide relief by increasing blood circulation to the head.
- Practise relaxation techniques.
- Cranial osteopathy or chiropractic can release built-up tensions in the head and neck, which can trigger tinnitus.
- Acupuncture has proved very beneficial for some sufferers (see *Useful Information*).
- You can call the Tinnitus Helpline, for up-to-date research. Freephone 0808 808 6666 (Monday–Friday).
- Impacted wisdom teeth and tooth decay can cause this problem. When we grind our teeth over many years, the jaw can be misaligned, this is known as TMJ (Temporo-mandibular Joint Syndrome). Dentists who specialise in treating TMJ problems can make a small brace to be worn at night that holds the jaw in its correct position, which often alleviates tinnitus. There is now a craniofacial pain clinic in Surrey, which is dedicated to the treatment of head, neck and facial pain; call 01737 767100. I go to dentist Richard Dean in London on 020 7580 2644 who specializes in facial pain treatments – he is wonderful.

TONGUE PROBLEMS

The tongue is a great indicator of your overall health and mirrors the levels of toxicity in the body. A healthy tongue should be pink, moist and clean, with little or no coating. A white coating usually denotes the digestive system is not working as it should; liver and bowels are sluggish; and you are eating too many mucus-forming foods – such as full-fat dairy food, sugar and red meat. Smokers are more likely to have a coated tongue. Candida can cause a thick white coating on the tongue (see also *Candida*). If you have a heavily coated tongue, this can also contribute to bad breath, so buy a tongue scraper from large chemists and use daily.

A swollen tongue can denote dehydration, so drink at least 6 glasses of water every day, and it can also denote iron deficiency (in which case have a blood test). If your tongue swells suddenly, this is an acute allergic reaction (can be triggered by nuts, shellfish or anything to which you have a severe allergy) and you would need to seek immediate medical attention.

Foods to Avoid
- Red meat, full-fat dairy produce and most foods made with white bread can add to the mucus load in the body and slow digestion.
- Reduce alcohol, caffeine, fried foods and junk-type take-aways, which place a strain on the liver. See *Liver Problems*.
- See also *General Health Hints*.

Friendly Foods
- To clear the coating you would need to keep your diet really clean for 7 days. Try the Lashford Technique detox diet (see *Allergies*).
- Drink plenty of fresh vegetable juices made with garlic, ginger and any fresh vegetables you have to hand. Celery, artichoke, chicory, celeriac, kale and beetroot are great liver cleansers.
- See *Friendly Foods* under *Constipation*.

Useful Remedies
- Take acidophilus/bifidus for at least 6 weeks to replenish healthy bacteria in the bowel.
- Take a digestive enzyme with main meals.

- The herb milk thistle – 500mg 3 times daily – will help to improve liver function.
- The celloid mineral sodium phosphate – 600mg daily – helps to reduce a creamy coating. **BLK**

Geographical tongue

This is so named because the tongue often resembles a map, when discolouration forms irregular shapes on the surface. Usually it disappears of its own accord, but sensitivity to certain foods can make it worse (see *Allergies*). I have had letters from pregnant women whose geographical tongue disappeared once the baby was born. It is also linked to iron and/or vitamin-B deficiency. The patches can also be caused by infection or irritants, such as vinegar.

Foods to Avoid.
- Cut down on caffeine, highly spiced foods, vinegar, pickles, pineapple and plums.
- Alcohol will also irritate the delicate tissues in the mouth.

Friendly Foods
- Include more ginger and live, low-fat yoghurt in your diet, which is very soothing.
- Garlic and onions are very cleansing.
- Drink plenty of water.
- See the cleansing Lashford Technique under *Allergies*.
- Eat more foods containing B-vitamins, such as wholegrains, wheat and rice bran, wheat germ, brown rice, organic muesli, oats, lecithin granules and brewer's yeast. Liver is also high in B-vitamins and vitamin A.

Useful Remedies
- CT 241 is a formula of herbs, such as horsetail, and silica, kelp, vitamin C, boron and digestive enzymes, which improve absorption of nutrients from food and encourage soft tissue healing. **BC**
- Take a B-complex.
- Ask your doctor to check if you are low in iron, in which case take a liquid formula, such as Spatone, which will not cause constipation.
- Take New Era calcium fluoride tissue salts 4 times a day.

Helpful Hints
- Tea tree oil can be diluted in warm water and used as a mouthwash as well as 1% hydrogen peroxide in water.
- Some sufferers report an improvement after taking a garlic capsule daily.

TONSILLITIS
(see also *Sore Throat*)

Sore throat, accompanied by difficulty swallowing and ear pain are the most common symptoms of tonsillitis. It makes you feel dreadfully low and symptoms may also include fever, nausea and headache. Tonsillitis is especially common among children. Antibiotics are not necessarily needed as more often that not tonsillitis is caused by a virus, which is not killed off by antibiotics – and it is only if a secondary bacterial infection occurs that antibiotics are warranted. Recurrent infections indicate that the immune system is struggling or that food intolerance, especially to dairy, is involved (see *Immune Function*).

Foods to Avoid
- Whilst an infection is present anything that increases mucus needs to be avoided. This includes

dairy produce (most especially from cows) – cheese, milk, chocolates, cream and butter – along with eggs, soya milk and nut butters.

- Foods like toast, crisps and spicy foods, which will cause discomfort to an inflamed throat.
- Fizzy pop, and other sugary foods and drinks, contain lots of sugar, which greatly lowers immune function.
- Caffeine, found in tea, coffee, chocolate and colas adds stress to the immune system and is best avoided.
- Once the infection is over and if you suspect that dairy foods are causing a problem continue to keep them out of the diet. Keep calcium levels high by eating lots of sesame seeds or tahini (ground sesame seeds), almonds and Brazil nuts, bony fish like sardines and tinned salmon, and dark green leafy vegetables, including kelp, broccoli, cabbage and watercress.
- Reduce packaged and processed foods high in hydrogenated and trans fats, artificial flavourings, colourings, preservatives and sweeteners.

Friendly Foods

- Freezing low-sugar, diluted fruit juices by making them into ice lollies is a great way to help soothe a sore throat whilst an infection is present – blackcurrant and apple is particularly good.
- Vegetable soups and chicken broths are full of healing nutrients that will boost the immune system and are easier to swallow than regular food. Use plenty of sweet potatoes, cabbage, squash, pumpkin, carrots, plus lentils or brown rice – with a little chicken.
- To tempt a child with a low appetite, put lots of different colours on the plate – oranges, reds, purples, blues, yellows and greens. Colourful foods contain bioflavonoids, which have many immune-boosting and protective properties. A bowl full of blueberries, cherries, plums, apricots kiwi and oranges will give any child lots of nutrients. Or blend these fruits with a small amount of rice milk to make a nutritious smoothie.
- When your child is ready to go back to solid foods, begin with light, easily digested meals, as the digestive system is taxed during an infection. Go for lightly steamed vegetables with chicken or fish.
- Increase all fresh fruits and vegetables and wholegrains as these will help to supply the immune system with the raw ingredients it needs in order to function well.
- Include more vitamin-C-rich foods, such as strawberries, kiwi, sweet potato, red and yellow peppers, broccoli and peas.

Useful Remedies

- Try Sambucol, an extract of elderberries, which has proven anti-viral action and tastes great too. Children can have 2 tsp twice a day and adults a dessertspoon 4 times a day. It also comes as a lozenge – adults should have 1 lozenge 4 times a day.
- Vitamin A is known to help heal inflamed mucous membranes and boost immune function. During an infection children over the age of 5 can have 10,000iu for 2 days then reduce to 2,500iu daily; and for 7–10-year-olds – 10,000iu for just 2 days and then 3,500iu daily until symptoms ease.
- Applying a little neat tea tree oil externally to the painful area on the throat should help ease the pain.
- Suck zinc lozenges 3 times a day as zinc aids the immune system, and has been shown to reduce the duration of a sore throat.
- During an infection add 4 grams of powdered vitamin C to water and sip throughout the day. This will keep levels boosted and help the immune system to fight the infection. BioCare makes a good non-acidic one called magnesium ascorbate. **BC**
- Bee propolis helps to boost immune function and fight infection. It has proven anti-viral properties. Take 500mg every 3 to 4 hours for several days when you start to feel a sore throat coming on. For general immune support take 1 capsule daily especially in winter.
- Bioforce make a formula for kids combining the herb echinacea with the herb plantago, which

helps boost immunity, has anti-inflammatory properties and is anti-bacterial. A child of age 2–5 needs 4 drops in water 2 or 3 times a day; aged 6–12, 8 drops; and aged over 12, 15 drops. Add to a low-sugar fruit juice.

Helpful Hints

- Add Manuka honey and root ginger to hot water for a soothing drink. The ginger is full of zinc, which is healing, and the Manuka honey has strong anti-bacterial action.
- Gargling with salty water, or red sage and echinacea – used 4 times daily – really helps. **SHS**
- Slice an onion, wrap it in an old cloth, and wrap around the throat. Replenish every 3 hours. This can really help to clear congestion from the lymph glands in the neck.
- Get lots of rest and maintain a high fluid intake.
- Humidifiers can help to keep a dry throat moist and ease discomfort.
- If the tonsils become infected and antibiotics are necessary, then follow them up with a probiotic. These are healthy bacteria needed by the gut, which are killed along with the infection by the antibiotics. BioCare's Replete is an excellent way to replenish healthy bacteria.

TRAVEL SICKNESS

This is extremely common especially in children and older people. Just worrying about a journey can be sufficient to trigger symptoms in a sensitive individual. Eating a large meal prior to travelling, and stuffy atmospheres, can also make symptoms worse. Some people can read while moving, but for others trying to focus on something stationary while in a moving vehicle can disturb the balance in the inner ear, resulting in nausea. Also, if anyone who suffers from travel sickness notices the scenery flashing by – such as on a train – often this makes symptoms worse, because the balance of the inner ears is linked to the receptors in the eyes. Symptoms include looking pale, feeling clammy and sometimes nausea, vomiting and, in extreme cases, fainting.

Food to Avoid

- On short trips avoid eating and drinking anything.

Friendly Foods

- On the day prior to travel, eat light foods, salads, and fresh fruit compotes; or grilled fruits, soups and low-fat yoghurt.
- If you are on a long trip and can face food, eat really light, low-fat foods such as a rice or oat cakes. Otherwise try dry toast or a cheese biscuit.
- Sip small amounts of fresh lemon or lime juice in warm water.
- Peppermint and ginger herbal teas can also be sipped to calm the digestive tract and stomach.
- Recently on a cruise I suffered sea-sickness and was told that if I ate a green apple very slowly it would help – and it did.

Useful Remedies

- Magnesium is nature's tranquillizer. If you tend to get nervous the day before your trip, begin taking 200mg of magnesium 3 times a day for a couple of days prior to travelling.
- Ginger is really successful at reducing the feelings of nausea and you can take 4 ginger capsules 2 hours prior to travel – but it is often more effective when you can taste the ginger.
- Make tea with a small piece of fresh root ginger and a little honey and take in a flask to sip during your journey; or take 1–2ml of the tincture in a little water.
- Take a B-complex daily to support your nerves.

Helpful Hints

- Stay fairly still and breathe calmly. Look ahead to the horizon and not downwards to help keep

the fluid in the ears balanced.
- Try to sit at the front of any vehicle.
- If possible, open a window.
- Avoid the company of people eating strong-smelling foods.
- A drop of peppermint oil on the tongue helps reduce feelings of nausea.
- Acupressure can help control motion sickness. Press the point that is approximately 2 inches (5cm) up from the centre of your wrist on the underside of your arm – it's the point between 2 tendons. Press for 20 seconds every half or so to reduce symptoms; or wear Sea Bands, which work on a similar principle. Available from most large chemists.
- Try homeopathic Cocculus 30c – take 1 before travelling and 1 every few hours during the journey.

TREMORS

This problem can be triggered by a huge variety of causes, such as extreme nervousness, excessive consumption of caffeine or alcohol, and an overactive thyroid gland. Recovering alcoholics and drug addicts often suffer tremors. If the tremors occur when resting or you suffer involuntary jerking, this may be associated with conditions such as Parkinson's Disease and rheumatic fever. On rare occasions tremors can be inherited. Mercury and heavy-metal toxicity are linked to tremors (if you have mercury amalgam fillings – see *Mercury Fillings*); cigarettes are high in cadmium and nickel, so stop smoking. If you suffer blood-sugar problems this could make symptoms worse (see *Low Blood Sugar*).

Foods to Avoid
- Any foods or drinks containing aluminium (see *Alzheimer's Disease*).
- Greatly reduce any foods or drinks containing caffeine, this includes chocolate, fizzy canned drinks, guarana, coffee and strong tea.
- Avoid alcohol and spicy foods, which are stimulants.
- Don't eat too many highly sugary foods, which can make you feel more nervous.
- Avoid preservatives and additives.

Friendly Foods
- Generally you need calming foods, such as potatoes, pasta, wholemeal bread, brown rice, lentils, barley, cereals and oats.
- Porridge made with organic rice milk, and a chopped raw apple or banana plus a little Manuka honey to sweeten, makes a very calming breakfast or supper.
- Turkey, chicken, cooked tofu, bananas, wheat germ, avocados, sunflower seeds, pumpkin seeds, linseeds (flax seeds) and oily fish are all calming foods – and the oily fish and seeds help to nourish your nerves.
- Almonds, dates, Brazil nuts, mustard, curry powder and all green leafy vegetables are a good source of magnesium, which calms the muscles.
- Drink more water.
- Drink more green or white tea, which contains L-theanine, an amino acid that helps to calm you down. Avoid at night as these teas contain some caffeine, or ask for decaff versions. Otherwise you can take 100mg of L-theanine twice daily in-between meals.

Useful Remedies
- Include a multi-vitamin and mineral that contains a full spectrum of B-vitamins to nourish your nerves and also contains at least 20mg of zinc. Have a look at details of *Kudos 24* in *General*

Supplements (p.160). (Often when we are falling off to sleep our bodies jerk, this is often due to lack of zinc.)

■ Calcium and magnesium help to reduce muscle spasms. Most vitamin companies supply them in one formula. Take 600mg of calcium with 400mg of magnesium.

■ Either take 4 evening primrose oil capsules daily or 400mg of GLA (a fatty acid found in evening primrose oil that helps to reduce tremors). **BC**

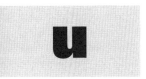

ULCERS, DUODENAL AND STOMACH   (see *Stomach Ulcers*)

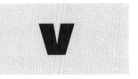

VARICOSE VEINS (see also *Circulation, Constipation* and *Raynaud's Disease)*

Varicose veins are caused by long-term poor circulation and weakened valves in the veins, which allow blood to accumulate thus stretching the vein walls. The most commonly affected areas are the legs, where eventually the veins can be clearly seen on the skin's surface. Over time they bulge, become bluish and lumpy looking, and can become painful. If they are not treated, they can also ulcerate, especially in older people. Anything that slows the return of the blood from the legs to the heart will aggravate varicose veins.

This condition is closely linked to constipation and if you strain when you go to the toilet, then blood is forced into your lower body, which makes the problem worse. Vein problems are also linked to standing or sitting for long hours, being overweight, pregnancy and crossing your legs too much. Perhaps most frightening of all, vascular surgeons are now seeing children as young as 11, who are 'couch potatoes' and sit at computers or watch TV all day.

Another common condition, known as thread or spider veins, involves chronically dilated and overly permeable capillaries near the surface of the skin. Whilst they are harmless and rarely cause any problems, they can be distressing for cosmetic reasons. You can prevent them developing or worsening with much of the same advice below (see also *Helpful Hints*).

When I became pregnant at 18, after working long hours standing in a supermarket, I developed bad varicose veins. In my 20s these were made worse when I worked for 9 years as an air stewardess and often had to be on my feet for 15 hours at a stretch. Today I tend to sit at a desk for 8 hours at a time, which greatly restricts circulation. My mother and father both had vein problems. Yes, you can inherit a tendency for veins, but if I had known then what I know now, I could definitely have prevented their onset. In my 40s I had some veins stripped, but the problem has returned. However, today, thanks to more efficient diagnostic techniques and improved surgical procedures, you can in many cases eliminate varicose veins – but much better to prevent them in the first place.

Foods to Avoid

■ Cut down on heavy meals, red meat and cheeses, as they're low in fibre and take a long time to pass through the bowel, potentially contributing to constipation. Furthermore, saturated, fried and hydrogenated fats thicken the blood, which make it travel more slowly through your veins and arteries, increasing the risk of vascular problems.

■ Foods made with flour from any source tend to block the bowels; therefore reduce your intake of flour-based foods especially croissants, meat pies, pizzas, cakes, biscuits and so on. Choose whole grains instead where possible. For example, try rye or spelt breads, brown rice, rolled oats, quinoa and barley grains.

■ Coffee, tea, colas and especially alcohol will dehydrate the bowel.

■ See also *Constipation* and *Circulation*.

Friendly Foods

■ Bilberries, blueberries, blackberries, sweet potatoes, pumpkin, squash, cherries, apricots, spinach, spring greens and cabbage. In addition eat more citrus fruits, broccoli, red grapes, papaya, tomatoes, tea and red wine, which are all rich sources of flavonoids and vitamin C – powerful antioxidants that help to strengthen capillaries and reduce the risk of haemorrhoids, thrombosis and bruises.

■ Rose hips (try rose hip tea), buckwheat and apple peel contain the bioflavonoid rutin, which also helps to strengthen your veins. Buckwheat makes great pancakes and can also be added to breads and biscuits.

■ Avocados, sprouted seeds such as alfalfa, plus eggs, raw wheat germ and unprocessed nuts are rich in vitamin E, which reduces stickiness in the blood.

■ Garlic, onions, ginger and cayenne pepper all aid circulation.

■ Eat plenty of fish, especially oily fish. The essential fatty acids (EFAs) they contain reduce pain and keep blood vessels soft and pliable. Aim for 2–3 portions per week. Eat more unrefined, preferably organic sunflower, pumpkin and sesame seeds and linseeds (flax seeds), which are all high in essential fats and fibre (see *Fats You Need To Eat*).

■ Drink more water – 6–8 glasses a day of bottled or filtered water. Water maintains blood pressure and helps reduce constipation.

■ Make sure that your diet contains plenty of fibre to prevent constipation. Fruits, vegetables, whole grains, such as brown rice and quinoa, beans and lentils are your best sources. If you feel you need more than you're getting in your diet, skip the bran – a harsh, insoluble fibre – and use instead soluble fibre-rich (cracked) linseeds (flax seeds), such as Linusit Gold or psyllium husks, both available in your local health food store.

■ If constipation is a real problem for you, in addition to the fibre, water and exercise recommended above and below, eat 4 prunes prior to each meal.

Useful Remedies

■ For centuries plant extracts, such as butcher's broom and horse chestnut seeds (commonly known as conkers), have been used to reduce inflammation and swelling associated with leg problems, and science has now validated these age-old remedies. Dr John Wilkinson, a scientist who specialises in plant research says, "We have found that saponins, a group of active agents found in the roots and seeds of these plants, constrict and strengthen veins, have anti-inflammatory properties, and reduce swelling, thus making venous return to the heart more efficient. The compounds in these plants are safe and can be taken internally in capsule form daily (but not during the first 3 months of pregnancy, or by people on blood-thinning drugs). Plant extracts can also be used topically in a cream or gel. We have found that butcher's broom is highly effective when taken in isolation, but its effects appear to be amplified when combined with horse chestnut, vitamin C, and the flavonoid rutin."

- Most health shops sell butcher's broom, which also reduces heaviness, tingling and cramping associated with varicose veins. Take 100–300mg standardised extract 2–3 times daily, or try V-Nal combination capsules made by Bional, available at most chemists and health shops worldwide.

- Horse chestnut seed extract can also be taken either as a combination or on its own. Clinical trials have confirmed its ability to aid vein contraction, reduce vein fragility and permeability and significantly reduce lower-limb swelling. You need 50–75mg of aescin twice daily (aescin is the active ingredient in horse chestnut). If you prefer a tincture, take 1–4ml twice a day.

- Another herb, gotu kola, has also shown impressive clinical results in treating both varicose veins and varicose ulcers by improving circulation in the lower limbs and stimulating connective tissue repair. Try 500mg twice daily.

- Bioflavonoids help reduce swelling and strengthen the vein walls. Take 1000mg of the bioflavonoid rutin daily.

- Silica is an excellent mineral for toughening up veins. Take 200mg of silica compound daily. **BLK**

- An antioxidant complex containing vitamins A, C and E, selenium and Co-enzyme Q10 helps prevent free-radical damage to the blood vessels as well as aiding in connective tissue repair. Take 1–2 grams of vitamin C daily with meals and 400iu of natural-source vitamin E, which also enhances circulation through its anti-clotting effects.

- If veins are sore and swollen, buy some witch hazel in tincture or cream form and apply directly to the veins. Witch hazel in capsules and tincture can also be taken internally to reduce the swelling. **OP**

- Apply a little vitamin-E cream mixed with 2 drops of juniper oil topically where the skin is sore.

- If you have facial thread veins, try Jason Vitamin K Cream for the face, which contains bioflavonoids, ginkgo biloba, and calendula. It is available from most good health and department stores worldwide. For your nearest stockists call Kinetics on 0845 0725825.

Helpful Hints

- For those on their feet all day, physiotherapist Geraldine Watkins recommends lying on the floor, bending the knees and placing the lower legs on a chair or bed for 15 minutes daily to give the leg valves a rest and encourage excess fluid to be absorbed back into the system. If the legs are swollen then a cold compress should be applied.

- It's vital for your overall health that you stay active. Even brisk walking for 45mins to an hour a day will help. Otherwise rebounding, skipping, playing tennis, jogging and dancing are all wonderful exercises for supporting veins. And if your legs ache, no matter what your job, swimming is the best all round exercise for keeping legs healthy.

- Also, if you stand a lot all day, wear insoles to support your arches from John Bell and Croydon in London on 020 7935 5555, or any good chemists or back shop. Avoid heels over 2 inches (5cm), and at the first sign of vein problems wear support tights or socks.

- If you are at a desk for much of the day, take regular breaks, look for some stairs and climb them! Make sure you move for at least 30 minutes a day. But whilst seated use a D-shaped foot rest, available from chemists such as John, Bell and Croydon in London, as bending and circling the feet keeps circulation moving. When at your desk make sure your knees are lower than your hips, which reduces compression in the arteries and veins in the groin area. Also avoid wearing tight-fitting trousers, which adds to compression in the groin and the back-of-knee areas when seated for long periods.

- Avoid crossing your legs, doing heavy lifting, or putting any unnecessary pressure on your legs.

- Reflexology, acupuncture and a firm massage can all help to increase circulation (see *Useful Information*).

- If the veins are sore and throbbing make a warm-water compress with added cypress and geranium essential oils. Use cold compresses to reduce any swelling.

- Avoiding constipation and/or straining to pass stools is essential for avoiding varicose veins. Straining to go to the toilet forces blood into your lower body, which makes the problem worse. Haemorrhoids are actually varicose veins of the anus – follow the dietary guidelines above to avoid constipation, and see also *Piles*.

- Facial thread veins can be treated using a fine needle, often called Red Vein. The needle is quickly inserted into each end of the vein and a current passes through the needle, which cauterizes the tiny capillary, then the needle is quickly injected down the length of the vein, which makes the vein disappear. Available at most beauty salons. Costs around £35 for 15 minutes. You then need to keep the treated areas dry for several days.

- You can also have thread veins lasered, which I found more effective. The laser literally 'smashes' the thread vein and although you may have some bruising for a few days, it works very well. For details contact Lasercare, who have several clinics around the UK. Tel: 020 7224 0988; or visit www.lasercareskinandbody.com

- To avoid facial thread veins in the first place, don't use very hot or very cold water on your face, as any extremes can cause delicate veins to rupture.

- Avoid strong winds, and if you are out on a boat or skiing, wear really thick protective creams.

- Avoid too much sunbathing.

- Finally get a proper diagnosis, says Mr John Scurr, a consultant vascular surgeon based at the Middlesex Hospital in London. "Many people believe there is little point in having veins, haemorrhoids and so on treated, thinking they will return. But these days newer diagnostic and treatment techniques are giving good long-term, and in many cases permanent, relief." For any further queries on all aspects of vein problems, Dr Scurr's website is excellent: www.jscurr.com

VEGETARIANISM

This subject is obviously not a health condition, but I do receive numerous letters from parents who are concerned that their children are not getting sufficient nutrients from their diet. After the BSE and CJD crises in the UK and Europe, more and more people are turning to a vegetarian diet, which basically means not eating any foods or products derived from the slaughter of animals. Generally, a vegetarian diet is a healthy diet and vegetarians tend to suffer less arthritis and inflammatory conditions than meat eaters. But many people, especially teenagers who call themselves vegetarians, often have a pretty unhealthy diet that includes lots of dairy foods, especially melted cheese, plus sugar- and white-flour-based foods. These people are at a higher risk for increased homocysteine levels because they are more likely to have fewer B-vitamins and zinc in their diet. For full details of homocysteine – see *High Blood Pressure*.

Vegetarians generally suffer less ill health, heart disease and cancer than meat-eaters, mainly because vegetarian diets tend to be higher in fibre and lower in saturated fats than carnivorous ones. Many parents worry that their children will become deficient in nutrients, especially vitamin B12, iron, zinc and vitamin D, but this tends to be more of a problem for vegans. Simply make sure you or your children eat as great a variety of foods as possible.

Foods to Avoid
- Don't go overboard on full-fat cheeses, which are high in saturated fats.
- Products that are high in processed palm oil should be kept to a minimum as they are also very high in saturated fats.

- Avoid too many foods high in white flour, sugar and unsaturated fats (see *Fats You Need To Eat*).

Friendly Foods

- Green leafy vegetables, sesame seeds, low-fat yoghurts and Parmesan cheese are all high in calcium.
- For protein, eat lentils, quinoa, beans (especially soya beans), tempeh, miso, brown rice, cereals, corn, almonds, Brazil nuts, peanuts, sunflower seeds and sesame seeds, which also contain good levels of zinc.
- Mozzarella, goat's or sheep's cheese (such as feta) are better absorbed by the body than cow's products.
- Eggs and dried skimmed milk are rich sources of vitamin B12. Alfalfa sprouts, spirulina also contain small amounts.
- For carbohydrates, eat low-sugar cereals, oats, wholemeal bread, brown rice and pasta, barley, amaranth, millet, buckwheat and rye. Quinoa is an excellent source of protein.
- Potatoes, parsnips, pumpkin, turnips and swedes are also good sources of carbohydrates.
- Red or yellow vegetables, carrots, tomatoes, pumpkin, sweet potatoes, dried apricots, and leafy green vegetables are all rich in vitamin A, so is liver.
- Nuts and seeds are high in essential fats.
- Wheat germ can be sprinkled onto cereals and desserts as a rich source of B-vitamins.
- Mushrooms and peas also contain the B-group vitamins.
- Use unrefined walnut, sunflower and olive oils for salad dressings.

- Iron is found in leafy green vegetables, wholemeal bread, black strap molasses, eggs, dried fruits (especially apricots), beans, seeds, pulses (peas and chickpeas), nuts, chocolate and cocoa.
- Eat plenty of fruits rich in vitamin C, such as kiwi and cherries, as vitamin C aids absorption of iron from foods.

Useful Remedies

- Take a high-strength B-complex.
- Take a multi-vitamin and mineral that contains a full spectrum of B-vitamins, plus zinc and selenium, and is suitable for vegetarians, such as Kudos 24 (see *General Supplements* for details; p.160).
- If you have been found to be low in iron, take a formula such as Spatone – available worldwide from health stores.

Helpful Hints

- Most bookshops now sell a huge range of healthy vegetarian cookbooks. Treat yourself to a couple, and remember that the greater the variety of foods you eat, the more nutrients you will be ingesting.

VERRUCAS

(see also *Immune Function*)

Verrucas are 'plantar warts' that occur on the soles of the feet. They are extremely common, highly contagious and can be very painful. Verrucas are essentially a viral infection and you are more likely to contract them if you are really run down.

Foods to Avoid

- Reduce your intake of all foods and drinks containing sugar, which lowers immune function.
- Reduce caffeine, alcohol and all highly processed white-flour-based foods.
- See also dietary advice in *Immune Function*.

Friendly Foods
■ Eat lots of garlic, asparagus, parsley, avocados, sea vegetables, such as kelp, plus whey protein, apples, cucumbers, millet, rice bran and sprouts.
■ See also *Immune Function* and *General Health Hints*.

Useful Remedies
■ If you suffer with verrucas regularly, start taking a high-strength bee propolis tincture or capsules, which are highly anti-viral and greatly help to boost your immune system.
■ To fight the virus take 20,000iu of vitamin A daily for 1 month and then reduce to 5,000iu daily in a multi-vitamin and mineral complex. (If you are pregnant take no more than 3,000iu of vitamin A daily.) Or eat organic liver once a week.
■ Take a garlic capsule daily.
■ Vitamin C is vital for boosting your immune system; take 2 grams daily with food.
■ Take 30mg of zinc daily for its anti-viral properties – this is found in most multi-vitamin/mineral complexes.
■ See this section under *Immune Function*.

Helpful Hints
■ Apply a tiny amount of crushed garlic or tea tree oil onto the affected area twice a day. Garlic oil can burn, so make sure it is placed only directly on the verruca for several minutes at a time.
■ There is an enzyme in banana skin that can attack the verruca. Many people have written to say that, although somewhat bizarre, this remedy really does work! Apply the inside of the banana skin to the verruca and tape on. Change every 2 days until the verruca disappears.
■ Homeopathic Thuja 6C can be helpful as well as Thuja Mother tincture applied directly onto the warts and covered with a plaster.
■ Place a tiny amount of fresh urine on a small cotton-wool ball and attach it over the verruca with a plaster. Change the dressing twice daily. Urine is a sterile liquid that contains anti-viral and anti-bacterial components.

VERTIGO
(see also Ménière's Syndrome)

Vertigo is a very unpleasant sensation of moving or spinning, a feeling that you are losing your balance even when you are standing or sitting still. It can be accompanied by nausea. Vertigo usually lasts for a few minutes, but can continue for hours and even days. It can be caused by impacted ear wax, blockage of the Eustachian tube, or by a viral infection of the balancing mechanism of the inner ear (see also *Catarrh* and *Sinus Problems*). Vertigo can also be triggered by high blood pressure and iron deficiency (see *Anaemia*). It is also linked to blood sugar problems (see *Low* and *High Blood Sugar*) and poor circulation. Vertigo is also a symptom of Ménière's Syndrome. Beta blockers and some prescription drugs can trigger an attack – make sure you carefully note any contraindications on drugs. Extreme exhaustion and an overgrowth of the fungus candida can also trigger vertigo (see also *Candida*). A misalignment of the neck and skull can also trigger symptoms. If you suspect this is the cause, consult a cranial osteopath or a chiropractor.

Foods to Avoid
■ Generally, you need to cut down on saturated fats found in full-fat milk and dairy produce, cheeses, meat, chocolates, cakes, biscuits, pies, sausages and so on.
■ Avoid caffeine, especially cappuccinos and chocolates, fizzy drinks, fried foods, alcohol and aspartame.

- Cut down your intake of sodium-based salts; there are now plenty of magnesium and potassium-based salts available from health stores.

Friendly Foods

- Vitamin A and carotene-rich foods are needed for sensory cells in the inner ear to function normally. Eat more oily fish and fish oils, sweet potatoes, pumpkin, apricots and sweet potatoes. Liver is very high in vitamin A.
- Eat more garlic, onions and ginger.
- Calves' or lambs' liver, eggs and leafy green vegetables are a rich source of iron and vitamin A.
- Use organic rice, oat or almond milk instead of cow's milk.
- Eat more sunflower or pumpkin seeds and linseeds (flax seeds), which are rich in essential fats and zinc, and use their unrefined oils for salad dressings.
- Eat more bananas, dried fruit, fish and sunflower seeds, which are rich in potassium.
- See *General Health Hints*.

Useful Remedies

- Vitamin A, 25,000iu per day for one week. The inner ear needs a high concentration of vitamin A and sensory cells are dependent upon vitamin A. If you are pregnant only take 3000iu daily.
- A full-spectrum B-complex helps nourish the nerve endings in the inner ear.
- Take a multi-mineral that contains at least 100mg of calcium and 99mg of potassium. The potassium reduces the sodium (salt) levels in the body – high levels of sodium in the blood can make symptoms worse.
- The herb ginkgo biloba helps to improve circulation to the inner ear. Take 120–150mg of standardised extract twice daily until symptoms ease.
- Take a vitamin C and bioflavonoid complex – up to 2000mg daily.
- Ginger capsules can be taken 4–6 times daily during an attack to help reduce feelings of nausea.
- Co-enzyme Q10, a vitamin-like substance, helps to improve cellular function in the brain and may help to alleviate the vertigo. Take 60–100mg daily.

Helpful Hints

- If you smoke, stop as it thickens your blood and slows circulation to the head.
- Avoid rapid body movements, especially of the head. Avoid standing up quickly after lying down, especially first thing in the morning.
- Generally reduce stress and make sure you are getting sufficient sleep.
- See a chiropractor or cranial osteopath to make sure your neck and spine are not misaligned, which can trigger problems in the ear. Hypnotherapy and acupuncture have helped in some cases (see *Useful Information*).
- High blood pressure and beta-blockers have been known to trigger vertigo in some people. If you have been taking prescription drugs for a long period of time, check with your GP.
- Ask your doctor to check if you have impacted ear wax, which can trigger vertigo-like symptoms, or use Hopi ear candles. (See *Glue Ear*.)

VIRAL INFECTIONS   *(see Immune Function)*

VITILIGO

This is a difficult multi-factorial condition that causes white patches to appear on the skin when the natural pigment production stops. The darker the skin colour, the more obvious and distressing the appearance of the skin. This condition has been linked to low stomach-acid levels, stress, low levels of the B-group of vitamins, pernicious anaemia, and an overactive thyroid gland. It could also be triggered by nutritional deficiencies or a fungal overgrowth.

Foods to Avoid
- Alcohol, caffeine, processed foods, and sugar all deplete the body of B-vitamins.
- See *General Health Hints*.

Friendly Foods
- Papaya and pineapple contain enzymes that aid digestion and absorption of nutrients.
- Foods rich in B-vitamins include wheat germ, brewer's yeast, Bovril, calves' liver, eggs, whole grains (such as brown rice), nuts, fish, chicken, turkey, dates, oats, cereals, mushrooms, green vegetables (especially kale, broccoli and spinach), black strap molasses, dried skimmed milk, fruits and apricots.
- As low zinc levels are linked to vitiligo, eat more fish, shellfish, and sunflower and pumpkin seeds.
- Live, low-fat yoghurt also aids digestion.
- Drink plenty of water – at least 6 glasses daily.
- Eat more foods high in natural carotenes – apricots, cantaloupe melon, pumpkin, carrots, tomatoes, sweet potatoes, papaya, red and yellow peppers and mangoes.

Useful Remedies
- As lack of stomach acid is linked to this problem, take Betaine (HCl) for up to 2 years with main meals. If you have active stomach ulcers just take a digestive enzyme with main meals instead of the Betaine.
- Take a high-strength B-complex, plus 400mcg of folic acid and 500mcg of vitamin B12.
- PABA is a B-vitamin – take 100mg, 3 times daily, to help to re-pigment the skin.
- Include 1–2 grams of vitamin C daily – which is vital for collagen production.
- Copper 2mg per day. Copper is needed for certain enzymes that are required for skin pigmentation. Take 30–40mg of zinc at the same time. Both of these are usually found in most multivitamin and mineral formulas.
- The amino acid phenylalanine – 50mg per kilo of body weight – taken on an empty stomach with careful sun bathing should help to re-pigment the skin. Use a high-factor sunscreen and don't sit in the midday sun. Just take 15 minutes twice daily for a few days and gradually the skin should re-pigment.
- Natural-source carotenes are great for the skin. **HN**
- There is a herb from India called *khella* – extracted from khellin seeds, which acts like a natural steroid. The tincture can be taken by mouth, or applied topically on the affected areas. For more help contact Herbs of Grace on 01638 712123, or log on to www.herbsofgrace.co.uk

Helpful Hints
- Some people believe that small amounts of sun are beneficial for vitiligo. However, I believe that you should keep areas of vitiligo out of the sun, or at the very least use a strong sunscreen (see *Sunburn*). Never allow these areas to burn as your skin has no natural protection.

VOMITING
(see also *Food Poisoning*)

Vomiting can have many causes, the most obvious being food poisoning, food intolerances, and binge drinking, but it could also be prescription drugs that disagree with you – certain antibiotics have this affect on me. Morning sickness, migraines, bulimia, drinking too much alcohol and eating a really high-fat, rich meal can all trigger nausea. If an infant vomits violently within a few minutes of being fed, you would need to seek medical attention. If a child drinks a poison, such as bleach, or swallows an object and begins to vomit, urgent medical attention is needed.

Dehydration is the biggest concern with vomiting. If the person is small, also has diarrhoea, and cannot keep down any fluids, obviously the rate of dehydration will be much faster than in a tall, weighty person. If a baby or small child suffers frequent vomiting and diarrhoea, they are at a greater risk of dehydration and need immediate medical attention.

If I start to vomit, low blood pressure kicks in and if I vomit regularly, I pass out and need a saline drip to bring me round very quickly. If you suffer low blood pressure and begin vomiting frequently, call a doctor. If you have severe abdominal pain or begin vomiting any blood, have a fever and the vomiting has continued for more than 24 hours, seek urgent medical help. Nausea after fatty foods can be related to liver congestion, in which case you need to greatly reduce your intake of fats, coffee and alcohol. See *Liver Problems*.

Foods to Avoid
- See also all dietary advice in *Food Poisoning*.

Friendly Foods

- Sip clear fluids, such as boiled water, fruit juices, or an electrolyte powdered drink, such as Re-hydrate, available from all chemists.
- If you can tolerate it, sip a little ginger ale or ginger tea.
- Don't drink more than a couple of tablespoonfuls of liquid at any one time until the nausea has stopped.
- Once vomiting has stopped gently increase your fluid intake. No coffee or black tea for 24 hours.
- Sip apple cider vinegar while feeling nauseous or vomiting. Put one teaspoon of apple cider vinegar in a glass of water and sip. This helps settle your stomach and flushes out the toxins from the digestive system.
- Slowly begin eating again: dry toast, dry crackers, arrowroot, tapioca or semolina, fresh soups, a little poached fish with mashed potato, low-fat yoghurts or brown rice should be fine.

Useful Remedies
- Don't take these supplements until at least 24 hours after the vomiting has stopped.
- Take a vitamin B-complex to calm down the digestive system – but take with food.
- Deglycerrhized liquorice – 15 drops twice daily – helps to soothe the digestive tract.
- Acidophilus/bifidus – take 2 capsules daily for a couple of weeks – to replenish healthy bacteria in the bowel.

Helpful Hints
- Place some essential oils of ginger and peppermint under your nose, this helps to reduce the dreadful feeling of nausea.
- Homeopathic Nux Vomica 6x or Arsenicum Album 6x – take 1 dose every 30 minutes up to 10 doses daily until symptoms ease.

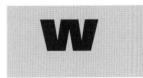

WARTS

Warts are caused by a varied assortment of viruses, which invade the skin, causing cells to multiply rapidly forming raised lumps. When your immune system is at a low ebb, you are more likely to pick up the virus. Warts are contagious, and touching warts can transfer viruses to new sites, and encourage new warts to develop. They are commonly found on the soles of the feet (see *Verrucas*) and on the hands or arms.

Foods to Avoid
- See *Foods to Avoid* under *Immune Function*.

Friendly Foods
- As vitamin A and carotenes are vital for healing the skin, eat more leafy greens (especially spinach and kale), pumpkin, apricots, sweet potato, tomatoes, cantaloupe melon, oily fish, and liver.
- Eat more sulphur-containing foods, such as onions, garlic, Brussels sprouts, cabbage, and broccoli.
- Eat more low-fat, live yoghurt.
- See *Friendly Foods* under *Immune Function*.

Useful Remedies
- If you are not pregnant take 20,000iu of vitamin A daily for 1 month to help fight the virus. If pregnant only take 3000iu daily.
- Take 400iu of natural-source vitamin E daily.
- Take 1 gram of vitamin C twice daily with food to boost your immune system.
- Take a high-strength multi-vitamin and mineral that contains 200mcg of selenium and 20mg of zinc – see details of *Kudos 24* in *General Supplements* (p.160).
- The herb echinacea is anti-viral, as is bee propolis.

Helpful Hints
- Oregano oil or thyme therapeutic grade essential oils are very powerful – dab a little neat oil onto the wart twice daily until it disappears. It will take about 2–3 weeks. For more details of Young Living oils, which are some of the most potent oils I have ever come across, call Susie Anthony on 01749 679900, or look at the Resources page at www.psalifemastery.com
- Soak a small cotton-wool ball with a little apple cider vinegar and hold it in place over the wart with a plaster. Or crush half an aspirin, place this on the plaster and immediately place it over the wart. Change the plaster regularly and keep adding more vinegar. If you use an aspirin – it's the salicylic acid that helps to break the wart. The wart should disappear within 2 weeks.
- Dandelion tincture can be added to the wart through a small piece of card in which you have cut a small hole. Dab on the tincture for 3 days.
- Apply the following mixture twice daily for up to 10 days: add a little freshly crushed garlic to the contents of 1 vitamin E and 1 vitamin A capsule and mix with some zinc cream. Add only to the site of the wart and cover with a dressing. If the skin surrounding the wart becomes inflamed then eliminate the garlic.
- Homeopathic Thuja 6c or Causticum 6c can be taken twice daily – but you must stop this remedy as soon as you see an improvement.

WATER ON THE KNEE
(see also *Water Retention*)

This condition is triggered when the little fluid-filled sacks that surround the knee joint become inflamed. The problem is usually triggered by a knock or a fall, or by a chronic condition such as arthritis.

Foods to Avoid
- Avoid meat, salt, caffeine, black tea and all highly processed foods. Any foods like crisps, olives, preserved meats and foods high in salt will make the body retain more water.
- Avoid foods from the nightshade family – tomatoes, potatoes, eggplant and sweet peppers.
- See *Foods to Avoid* under *Bursitis*.

Friendly Foods
- Eat foods high in magnesium, dark leafy greens (especially kale, spinach and cabbage), plus squash, fruits, vegetables and organic honey. These are all foods that help to alkalise the body, as an overacid system can make this condition worse. For more help see *Acid–Alkaline Balance*.
- Add a teaspoon of apple cider vinegar and a touch of honey to cooled, boiled water and sip throughout the day. This also helps to re-alkalise the body.
- Eat plenty of potassium-rich foods: bananas, linseeds (flax seeds), sunflower and pumpkin seeds, and nuts.
- Eat more avocado and raw wheat germ, which are rich in vitamin E.
- Pineapple is a rich source of bromelain, which has anti-inflammatory properties.
- Eat oily fish, such as mackerel, salmon and sardines, twice a week.
- Drink plenty of water – for details as to why, see *Water Retention*.

Useful Remedies
- Celloid Chloride compound helps to lessen the inflammation – 200mg daily. BLK
- Silica helps to strengthen the tissues in the knees. Take 200mg daily, or drink more Fiji water, which is high in silica.
- Take 1 gram of vitamin C twice daily with bioflavonoids to help reduce the swelling.
- Take 400–600iu of natural source vitamin E to help reduce the inflammation.
- Take zinc 30mg per day – zinc helps the body fight inflammation.
- The amino acid DL-Phenylalanine, 1000–2000mg per day, will help to reduce the pain.
- Take a 1 gram of omega-3 fish oils daily – which are highly anti-inflammatory.
- MSM is an organic form of sulphur that counteracts inflammation and pain. Start on 1 gram a day and then increase to 2 grams daily. Great for your skin too.
- Celery seed extract acts as mild diuretic, which helps to flush the excess fluid from the body. Take 200mg twice daily with food.

Helpful Hints
- At the onset of inflammation rest the affected area and avoid putting pressure on the joint for a few days. Keep your leg raised as much as possible.
- Alternating hot and cold compresses can help to disperse the swelling.
- Homeopathic Ruta 6c, taken twice daily for 3–5 days, really helps reduce knee problems. Also Apis 6c taken 3 times daily between meals helps to reduce the swelling.
- Perseverance with this regime is important as knee problems can take some time to heal.
- Regular acupuncture can not only greatly reduce the pain but also the swelling (see *Useful Information*).
- Ask at your local health or sports shop for a knee support that contains magnets, as magnets help increase blood flow and therefore bring more oxygenated blood to the area, which speeds healing.

■ Drink strong camomile tea, particularly at bedtime, to help relieve pain.

WATER RETENTION (OEDEMA)

Water retention can be seen throughout the body and, unlike water on the knee, general water retention is not caused by an injury. It can usually be seen in the hands, legs, ankles or feet, or around the eyes. The most common cause is excess salt in the body, but it can also be triggered by food intolerances (the usual culprits being wheat and dairy from cows). It can also occur during pregnancy, when taking the pill or HRT, and is very common in women, especially those over 60.

Another trigger can be standing for too long in hot weather. Occasionally, fluid retention can denote more serious problems that affect the heart, kidneys or liver. Therefore, if my suggestions do not work after 2–3 weeks please have a thorough check up with your doctor. Some people mistakenly think that if they cut back on their fluid intake their water retention will disappear, but in fact the opposite is true. The problem is that, as we get older, water finds it harder to penetrate your cells, and therefore a person can be suffering from water retention, but technically be dehydrated. The secret is getting the water into the cells that need them.

Foods to Avoid
■ Cut down on high-salt foods and pre-packaged meals – and don't add salt to meals.
■ Meat pies, cheese, sauces, pizza, olives, crisps, preserved meats and pickles can all be high in sodium.
■ Some breakfast cereals contain more salt than an average bag of crisps.
■ Don't add salt to cooking unless it's a potassium and magnesium-based salt, such as powdered kelp.
■ Even some chocolate drinks can be very high in salt.
■ Alcoholic and caffeinated foods and drinks act as diuretics, but they cause water to be leached out of the cells where it is needed, which increases dehydration.

Friendly Foods
■ Eat lots of fresh fruit and vegetables, as they are very rich in potassium.
■ Include more spinach, celery, kale, cabbage, bananas, almonds, sunflower seeds, apricots, potatoes, raisins, bilberries and blueberries.
■ Add the spice curcumin (turmeric) to your meals, which helps strengthen the kidneys.
■ Drink at least 6–8 glasses of pure filtered water daily.
■ Eat good-quality protein, such as fish, chicken, turkey or tempeh, at least once a day.
■ Ask at your health shop for various seaweeds, such as kombu, arame, nori or kelp. Soak them for 5 minutes and chop over meals. These are high in potassium and really help to remove excess fluid from the body. They are also high in organic sodium, but this does not hold water like normal table salt.

Useful Remedies
■ Dandelion leaf tea or tincture – 1ml can be taken 3 times a day – is a gentle diuretic, which puts more potassium into the body than it takes out. **FSC**
■ Take 1–2 grams of vitamin C as potassium ascorbate, which can help lymph drainage. **BC**
■ Take a B-complex that contains 100mg of B6, which is a natural diuretic.
■ Take celery seed extract – 1 x 200mg capsule twice daily. Celery is a natural liver and kidney cleanser and helps to neutralise excess acid in the tissues.
■ The herb gotu kola stimulates circulation in the lower limbs and improves lymph drainage. Take

up to 500mg twice daily when symptoms are acute.

- Celloid sodium sulphate is known as the problem-fluid remover. Take 200mg 3 times daily. **BLK**; or ask at your local pharmacy for the tissue salts.

Helpful Hints

- Try to elevate your feet for at least 15 minutes every day. Lie on the floor and place your lower limbs higher than your waist. This really helps the excess fluids to drain via the lymphatic system.
- Rebounding on a mini-trampoline is particularly good for enhancing lymph drainage. Have regular lymph-drainage massage (see under *Useful Information*).
- Take regular exercise, such as swimming, walking, skipping or jogging.
- If you are overweight, try to lose weight.
- It may be well worthwhile fitting a pure water filter – as purer water can more easily penetrate the cells. Contact The Pure Water Company on 01784 221188; or log on to www.purewater.co.uk

WEIGHT PROBLEMS

(see also *Allergies, Candida, Insulin Resistance, Low Blood Sugar* and *Thyroid Problems*)

More than 8 million men and women in the UK are now obese – that's 1 in 5 adults. 62% of men and 53% of women are now overweight and the problem is escalating. Among 6–15-year-olds obesity has trebled from 5% in 1990 to 16% in 2004. One in 5 adults is clinically obese, which causes more than 30,000 premature deaths a year in the UK alone. Research shows that women who gain more than 44 pounds after the age of 18 (above the weight they should be for their height and age) are 2.5 times more likely eventually to suffer a stroke. People who are significantly overweight are 5 times more likely to develop late-onset diabetes. More than 85% of people with type II diabetes are overweight when first diagnosed. Obese men are 33% more likely to die of cancer and this rises to 55% in women.

The basics of finding your perfect weight and then maintaining it are: controlling your blood sugar levels, eating a varied diet that contains plenty of fibre, and taking sufficient exercise. If you feel that you have truly tried every diet and you are still finding it hard to lose weight, then you may have an underactive thyroid, a chronic food intolerance that is causing water retention, or an overloaded liver that's allowing toxins to accumulate, which your body then stores away in fat cells. Steroids are well known to trigger weight gain.

The human body contains 30–40 million fat cells and any extra calories we eat are stored as fat. A lot of people now take regular exercise, but the majority still do not. This slows our metabolic rate and toxins begin to accumulate. The net result is 'middle-age spread' – which is now happening to teenagers.

How many overweight people do you know who say "I really cannot imagine why I'm overweight, I hardly ever touch bread, cakes, Mars Bars" and so on, and when they think no-one is looking they eat a chocolate croissant followed by a full-fat hot chocolate drink. I realise that weight gain can have a multitude of causes – but 98% of people who are overweight are simply eating too much and taking insufficient exercise. After all, if we are truly honest about obesity, I have yet to see anyone leave a prison-type camp looking overweight. This book is about living consciously – you can choose. Choose what you put in your mouth and you can choose your weight. And if you choose to lose weight, then do it for yourself, and if you are happy being 'overweight' then so be it.

Meanwhile, I believe it is important to stop thinking about the word 'diet' and start thinking 'eating more healthily for the rest of our lives'. There are cabbage diets, zone diets, protein-only diets, carbohydrate-free diets, eat-a-twinkie-only-at-night diets – and so on. And almost half of women between 25 and 35 are on a diet, but in the long term they don't work. For example, if you go on a diet trying to survive on only 1,000 calories a day, your brain will begin craving more glucose, which is the only form of fuel it utilises, and the more sugar you eat, the more this disrupts blood sugar levels and the more you will go on craving sugary foods. When you suddenly restrict your calories to fewer than you need, your body thinks there's a famine on, and your metabolic rate slows down to protect your energy reserves to help you survive the shortage. When you come off your diet, and start eating as you did before, your slowed metabolism means that you put anything you lost straight back on, and it's now harder than ever to lose it. This yo-yo dieting experience is all too common. Yet many studies show that 90% of dieters regain every ounce lost and 30% of these people actually become heavier than before their diet. Rather than going 'on a diet', I recommend simply changing the one you are already eating.

If you are 20% or more over your ideal weight, you are technically obese. This extra weight puts undue stress on your back, legs, joints, circulation and internal organs. Obesity increases the body's susceptibility to infection, the risk of heart disease, high blood pressure, arthritis, diabetes, stroke, and other serious health problems that can result in premature death. So how do you know if, for your height, build, age and sex, you're 'normal', overweight or obese? There have been numerous charts produced, but the most recognised method, that's easy to do, is the Body Mass Index (BMI). Simply the ratio of your weight in kilograms to your height in metres squared, it's a good rough guide and is widely used. The 'normal' range is 20–25, over 25 is considered overweight, over 30 is moderately obese and over 40 is very obese. As an example, a 6-foot man weighing 80kg has a BMI of 24 (80 divided by (1.83x1.83)) and is a normal weight, but a 5-foot man weighing 80kg has a BMI of 34 and is regarded as obese – his 'normal' weight would be no more than 58kg. Calculate your BMI and use it to determine what your target weight should be.

Also, research from America, Japan and France has confirmed that a tendency to overeat and to store fat is largely controlled by biochemical signals emitted by a part of the brain called the hypothalamus. As well as governing many important processes, such as temperature and hormone balance, the hypothalamus controls the feeling of being satisfied. It also interprets emotional upset, stress or low blood sugar as hunger, and sends a message to the body to eat. Snacking on sugary foods gives the brain a quick energy boost for a short time, but then triggers a further drop in blood sugar levels, which causes the hypothalamus to demand more fuel. This vicious cycle can trigger numerous symptoms ranging from chronic exhaustion, mood swings and brain 'fog' to black outs. The answer is to keep the hypothalamus happy by controlling blood sugar levels (see *Low Blood Sugar* for more details).

Don't omit all your favourite foods at once, as this can cause you to become despondent and go on a binge. The slower you do this, the easier it will be for your body to adjust. Sugar is highly addictive and it takes a good month to educate your body to a new way of eating.

The high-protein/low-carbohydrate diet has attracted a lot of attention in recent years (often called the Atkins diet). The theory is that carbohydrates are bad for weight control, being turned into sugars and then fat. But it's mostly the refined 'white' carbohydrates that cause the weight gain, not the unrefined ones like brown rice.

Many of the 'new' diets suggest lots of protein and no carbs at all, but protein can be harder to digest and metabolise, releasing energy more slowly and not being stored as fat. This diet isn't a good long-term weight loss strategy. Excessive protein is very acidic in the body and a major risk factor for osteoporosis in later life. Excess protein also places a great burden on the kidneys, metabolism becomes imbalanced, and the saturated fat that accompanies animal protein can increase the risk of heart disease. People do experience initial weight loss on this diet, perhaps due in large part to the exclusion of wheat and sugar (most people's main carbohydrate). A far better approach is to eat as great a variety of foods as possible and to make a life-long change to your diet, whilst cutting down on wheat-based foods.

Many people find that on a trial 'exclusion diet' for food intolerances they lose weight easily, while eating heartily. The most common food intolerances are usually starchy or sugary in nature (wheat, corn, milk from cows, sugar and potatoes) and this is not unlike the low-carbohydrate diet mentioned above. But avoiding any food that is badly tolerated, whether it be 'fattening' or not, usually enables rapid weight loss. Also, naturopath Stephen Langley says "If people can eat according to their blood type, they will naturally lose weight. For example, people with Type A blood will tend to put on weight if they eat meat and dairy; whereas those with Type O will increase their weight by eating gluten and corn." Therefore I suggest that people read Peter J. D'Adamo's books such as *Fatigue, Fight It With The Blood Type Diet* or *Eat Right For Your Blood Type*.

Finally, don't be tempted to cut corners and use weight-loss pills claiming to be fat blockers or fat magnets. These products encourage you to eat a cheeseburger, then take a pill so you won't gain weight. This is definitely not the way to try to improve your health, and like low-fat diets, they can stop you absorbing essential fats (the good ones), plus other fat-soluble nutrients that depend on fats to be transported into the body, such as vitamins A, D, E and K. Weight loss is best done slowly and for the long haul if you want to improve not just your weight, but your health too.

Foods to Avoid

- Cut down on the refined carbohydrates, white breads and rice, croissants, Danish pastries, meat pies, desserts, anything with pastry, burgers, pizzas and melted-cheese-type snacks. By all means have a treat, once a week or so, but once you start losing weight and stop eating these foods all the time, your need for them will gradually disappear.
- Artificial sweeteners, found in more than 3,000 foods and low-calorie drinks, place a strain on the liver and can slow weight loss. The worst offender is aspartame.
- Cut down on fried, fast foods and high-fat take-aways and processed foods – Indian foods in sauces are among the worst offenders.
- Keep in mind that most low-fat foods are high in sugar or sweeteners; check labels. Reduce foods high in sugar – sugar converts to fat inside the body if it is not used up during exercise. We all need a certain amount of fat and fat-free diets are dangerous (see *Fats You Need To Eat*).
- Chocolates are highly acid-forming, and although dark chocolate is high in antioxidants and can often contain fewer calories than crisps, please remember it is still high in saturated fats and sugar. The occasional piece of dark chocolate is fine, but keep in mind the word 'occasional'.
- Avoid salted nuts and highly preserved meats.
- Reduce sodium-based table salt.
- Avoid all hard margarines, full-fat milk and full-fat cheeses.
- Stop ordering desserts when you eat out – or try the fruit salad.
- It is the foods that you eat **every** day, and crave the most, that trigger the majority of your problems. Keep a food diary and note what you eat and when – you will soon know the culprits!

Friendly Foods

- Eat more organic foods, which contain fewer pesticides – pesticides live in your fat tissue and are really hard to eliminate.

- In summer, eat nothing but fruit before midday – this is a great way to kick start a sluggish metabolism. In winter have porridge with a grated raw apple and a few raisins for breakfast, which helps reduce cravings mid-morning.
- Instead of white-flour-based foods, use wholemeal bread and experiment with various pastas and meals made from corn, rice, spelt, quinoa, buckwheat, millet, lentil, amaranth and potato flour.
- Instead of wheat-based breads try amaranth crackers, rice or oatcakes, spread with a little hummus or cottage cheese; add a tomato and cucumber for a quick healthy snack.
- Eat more brown rice, lentils, chickpeas, barley and dried (or tinned) beans.
- Eat plenty of fresh fruits and vegetables – the more fibre the better. Cabbage, broccoli and cauliflower are great healthy foods, but avoid them if you have an underactive thyroid or have Type O blood. (See *Thyroid*.)
- Onions, ginger, spring greens, spinach, pak choy, celery, pineapple and apples are all great foods for assisting weight loss. Radicchio, chicory, fennel, celeriac and bitter foods help to cleanse the liver, which aids weight loss (see *Liver Problems*).
- Use organic rice milk, or skimmed milk (or skimmed goat's milk) instead of full-fat milk.
- Eat 1 portion of quality protein a day, such as fish, eggs, chicken or cooked tofu, as protein balances blood sugar for a longer period. Try to eat the protein at breakfast and/or lunchtime.
- A small jacket potato is fine, but fill it with low-fat yoghurt and chives instead of butter. Or use a spread like Benecol.
- Always eat breakfast – there are dozens of organic low-sugar cereals now available and a great breakfast is organic porridge made with half water and half rice milk. Use a few raisins and a chopped apple to sweeten.

- If you are desperate for sugar, use a little fructose, which is many times sweeter than ordinary sugar, so you use far less and it has a lower glycaemic index. See *Low Blood Sugar* and *Insulin Resistance*.
- Drink lots of herbal teas and at least 6–8 glasses of water a day. Water suppresses appetite and helps prevent fat depositing in the body; it reduces water retention and encourages toxins to be flushed through the body.
- Essential fats are vital if you want to lose weight (see *Fats You Need To Eat*).
- Use rice or oat bran for extra fibre.
- Ask at your health shop for a magnesium- and potassium-based salt such as Himalayan Crystal Salt (sold at most health stores), or use powdered kelp.
- Vegetarians tend to suffer less obesity, less heart disease and significantly less cancer. See *Vegetarianism*.
- Caffeine is an appetite suppressant, although a fairly toxic one.

Useful Remedies

- Junk foods deplete many vital minerals from the body and virtually everyone who eats too many refined foods is lacking in the mineral chromium. Begin taking 200mcg daily to help reduce your chance of developing late onset diabetes and to reduce cravings for sweet and refined foods. Take 200mcg twice daily in between meals. It takes a while to kick in, but it really does help to reduce sugar cravings. Furthermore, scientific investigations show that during exercise it can help reduce body fat and increase muscle concentration.
- Take a high-strength B-complex to support your nerves and aid digestion.
- Include a good-quality multi-vitamin and mineral in your regimen, such as Kudos 24 – for details see *General Supplements* (p.160).
- The essential fatty acid conjugated linoleic acid (CLA) helps to burn fat while increasing muscle mass. This seems to be most effective during the first year of taking this supplement. **BC**

- Co-enzyme Q10 is needed for the conversion of fat into energy within the cells. Research shows that as many as half of all obese people are deficient in CoQ10. Take 30–150mg per day.
- Soluble fibre, such as ready cracked linseeds (flax seeds) or psyllium husks taken prior to meals has been shown to induce the feeling of fullness. This type of fibre also aids fat elimination from the intestines and helps prevent the re-absorption of toxins by keeping you regular. Try taking a heaped teaspoon of psyllium husks in a full glass of water 30 minutes before meals. They taste awful, but do the job! It is imperative that you drink sufficient water when taking psyllium, and it can take a few days to start working. In some people these husks can trigger bloating. If the bloating were severe, you would need to stop taking them.
- The amino acid tyrosine helps you to maintain your chosen weight once you have reached it. Take 500mg twice daily before meals.
- Try Freecarb, made from white kidney bean extract, which helps prevent the digestion and absorption of approximately 60% of starches (such as pasta, rice, cereals, potatoes, bread) that you may consume. If you continue to eat lots of white-based cakes, biscuits and desserts this supplement will be less effective. **HN**

Helpful Hints

- Some people find it easier to lose weight by 'grazing' all day on healthy snacks, to balance their blood sugar. So regular nibbling is one of the simplest but most effective ways to start losing weight. Others says that if they eat 3 sensible meals a day – which includes a porridge-type breakfast, a good lunch (without dessert) and a light supper, with no snacks in-between – they also lose weight. Listen to your body.
- Many people now consider food combining as being out of date – but naturopath Stephen Langley adds "There is no doubt that food combining aids better digestion and encourages weight loss. The basic rule is, if you are eating a protein such as meat, eggs, cheese, fish or chicken – then avoid the major starches such as bread, pasta, rice or potatoes in the same meal. And if you are eating starches – then eat them without any of the major proteins." Ask at any bookshop for Kathryn Marsden's *Complete Book of Food Combining*.
- Two-time Nobel Prize-winner and pioneer of optimum nutrition, Linus Pauling, advised avoiding fad diets you can't stick to, and to reduce your calorie intake from all sources; eat a diet you like and can continue.
- Regular exercise increases your metabolic rate, decreases fat deposits, reduces food cravings and suppresses appetite. Regular exercise also increases muscle mass, which burns more energy just to keep the muscles functioning properly. The most important part of regular exercise is that it needs to be **regular**, and burning yourself out in the first week is the surest way to not continue. Aim for 30 minutes of exercise at least 5 times per week. The best way is simply to walk for 30 minutes or more every single day. I have a girlfriend who was 16 stone, and would not diet at all, but she agreed to start walking daily. At first she hated it, but as the pounds and then stones fell away over several months, she was delighted, and now feels irritable if she does not get her daily walk. She is 67. It's never too late to start!
- Gradually build the intensity, and vary the style of exercise. Consider joining a local dance, aerobic exercise or swimming club. It really helps if you work with people who have the same goal in mind. For this reason join Weight Watchers. Call 08457 123000 to find your nearest club, or log on to www.weightwatchers.co.uk
- Eat the majority of your food before 7.30pm if possible and try to make breakfast and lunch your larger meals of the day.
- An excess of oestrogen can cause weight gain and water retention if your body is low in progesterone (for details of natural progesterone cream see *Menopause*).
- An interesting book is *The Detox Diet* by Dr Paula Baillie-Hamilton. She argues that our natural

weight regulation system is being poisoned by the toxic chemicals we encounter in our everyday lives, and that this damage makes it increasingly difficult to control our weight.

- As Dr Dean Ornish likes to point out, his complex carbohydrate diet is the only one scientifically proven to work against ageing. Try reading his book *Eat More, Weigh Less* (Quill Press).
- If you suffer from an eating disorder, get professional help. Contact The Eating Disorders Association via their Helpline on 01603 621414 (Monday to Friday). Website: www.edauk.com

* *

Well, I thought this update would take me only two months – but after almost six months, I am delighted to have reached the end of the Hints Section. I have learned a lot and I hope you have too. I have added several new headings, but if your specific condition is not mentioned I apologise. If we had tried to feature every illness, this book would be thousands of pages thick, but we have endeavoured to give you a good basis to enable you to become your own health detective.

Due to my work schedule I can no longer answer individual letters, but there are plenty of names and addresses to turn to for more help. Or find me via my website www.hazelcourteney.com

Remember, you can still enjoy treats, but simply balance them out with plenty of healthy foods. It's never too late. Your body is perfectly capable of healing itself, when given the right tools for the job. Above all, reduce the stress in your life, exercise regularly, and as much as possible enjoy your journey.

Good luck and good health.

Hazel Courteney, Stephen Langley and Gareth Zeal

USEFUL INFORMATION

ACUPUNCTURE

This practice goes back over 3,000 years. Basically an acupuncturist inserts fine sterile needles into specific points in the body, which encourages energy and blood to flow more freely in the body. Specialist scanners can now clearly see blocked energies within the human body (see *Electrical Pollution* and *Healing*). And when these blockages are released the body's self-healing mechanism becomes more effective. Acupuncture is great for reducing pain, inflammation, water retention, balancing hormones and emotions, infertility and pregnancy problems, nausea, sciatica, back and neck pain, migraines, and so on.

To find your nearest practitioner, send an SAE to British Acupuncture Council, 63, Jeddo Road, London W12 9HQ.
Tel: 020 8735 0400
Fax: 020 8735 0404
Website: www.acupuncture.org.uk
E-mail: info@acupuncture.org.uk
Stephen Langley, my co-author, specialises in facial acupuncture at the Hale Clinic in London.
Tel. 020 7631 0156

ADVANCED REFLEXOLOGY

Anthony Porter has been a reflexologist since 1972. During the 80s he went to China and the Far East to teach reflexology and found that their methods, when combined with his own, gave even better results. He has taught his advanced techniques to thousands of reflexologists internationally and says "With ART we can not only balance various parts of the body (which is what happens with normal reflexology), but we can also feel more subtle changes within the 7000 nerve endings or reflex areas of the feet, and after working on them – this has a profound therapeutic affect." Medical research with a leading gynecologist has shown huge success with easing the pain and distress of many gynecological conditions that might otherwise need surgery. He also has had great success with infertility, stress, and a host of health problems. A lovely man. To find details of Anthony's practice in Central London or for an ART therapist in your area log on to www.artreflex.com or call 020 8920 9555

ALEXANDER TECHNIQUE

Teaches you how to use your body more efficiently and how to have balance and poise with minimum tension in order to avoid pain, strain and injury. To find your nearest practitioner, or list of affiliated societies worldwide, contact:

Society of Teachers of the Alexander Technique, 1st Floor, Linton House, 39-51 Highgate Road, London NW5 1RS
Tel: 0845 230 7828
Website: www.stat.org.uk
E-mail: office@stat.org.uk

AROMATHERAPY

The use of essential oils to improve health and well-being, by massage, inhalation, compresses and baths. Excellent for reducing muscle spasm, stress, and anxiety.

For a register of practitioners, contact the International Federation of Aromatherapists (IFA), 61-63 Churchfield Road, London W3 6AY.
Tel: 0208 992 9605
Fax: 0208 992 7983
Website: www.ifaroma.org
E-mail: office@ifaaroma-org
Or, contact The International Society of Professional Aromatherapists, 82 Ashby Road, Hinckley, Leicestershire, LE10 1SN.
Tel: 01455 637987.
Fax: 01455 890956.
Website: www.ifparoma.org
E-mail: admin@ifparoma.org

BACH FLOWER REMEDIES

A healing system used to treat emotional problems such as fear and hopelessness. The liquid remedies are made from the flowers of wild plants, bushes and trees.

For further information contact The Bach Centre, Mount Vernon, Bakers Lane, Sotwell, Oxfordshire, OX10 0PZ.
Tel: 01491 834678 (Monday to Friday, 9.30am–4.30pm)
Fax: 01491 825022
Website: www.bachcentre.com
E-mail: mail@bachcentre.com

BOOKS

If you have difficulty finding any of the recommended books, or simply want to find a book on your condition, the Nutri Centre bookshop in London has an extensive library of self-help books and would be happy to order for you, or give assistance on specific subjects.
Tel: 020 7323 2382 or 0800 587 2290
Website: www.nutricentre.com

CHELATION

Chelation, an intravenous treatment using the synthetic amino acid EDTA, has been proven to improve blood-flow in blocked arteries in heart, diabetic and stroke patients, by removing toxic metals from the body. When combined with antioxidants and other substances, the healing and anti-ageing effects are amplified. It is very useful if you have any of the above conditions, plus senile dementia, Alzheimer's, Parkinson's, ME, Chronic Fatigue, arthritis or multiple sclerosis, or you want to prevent cancers. It is now being called IVAT – Intravenous Antioxidant Therapy. For further details read *Forty-Something Forever* by Harold and Arline Brecher (Healthsavers Press). To order, tel: 020 7323 2382. In the UK there are several chelation clinics. Call 01942 886644 for details, or log on to www.chelationuk.com In London I go to Dr Robert Trossell at 4 Duke Street, London W1U 3EL. Tel 020 7486 1095. Or Dr Wendy Denning on 020 7224 2423.

CHIROPRACTIC

Manipulation to treat disorders of the joints and muscles and their effects on the nervous system. Chiropractors treat the entire body to bring it back into balance and restore health. Once a month I visit my chiropractor, who keeps my spine and neck mobile after an injury several years ago. To find a practitioner in your local area, contact:
The British Chiropractic Association, 59 Castle Street, Reading, Berkshire RG1 7SN. Tel: 0118 950 5950
Fax: 0118 958 8946
Website: www.chiropractic-uk.co.uk
E-mail: enquiries@chiropractic-uk.co.uk
McTimoney Chiropractic Association, Wallingford, Oxfordshire OX10 8DJ
Tel: 01491 829211
Website: www.mctimoney-chiropractic.org
E-mail: admin@mctimoney-chiropractic.org

COLONIC HYDROTHERAPY

A method of cleansing the colon to gently flush away toxic waste, gas, accumulated faeces and mucus deposits. Very safe treatment when given by a qualified professional. Check with your GP before undertaking this therapy. Colonics are very useful if you are chronically constipated or have taken antibiotics or painkillers, which can cause constipation.
I go to Margie Finchell, who is brilliant, at 58B Crawford Street, London W1H 4JW
Tel: 020 7724 1291.
A list of practitioners is available online:

Association and Register of Colon Hydratherapists,
Tel: 01271 871 177
Website: www.colonic-association.org

COUNSELLING

If you, or a member of your family, are in need of professional counselling, send an SAE to
British Association for Counselling and Psychotherapy (BACP), BACP House, 15 St John's Business Park, Lutterworth LE17 4HB
Tel: 0870 4435252
Website: www.bacp.co.uk
E-mail: bacp@bacp.co.uk

CRANIAL OSTEOPATHY

A gentle method of osteopathy concentrating on nerves and bones in the head, neck and shoulders. Many readers have reported relief from ME (Chronic Fatigue Syndrome), facial pain, jaw pain and arthritis from this therapy.
A list of practitioners can be found on the website of
The Bio-Cranial Institute (Europe), 41–43 Castle Street, Comber, Co. Down, BT23 5DY
Tel: 028 9146 0680
Fax: 078 7578 7164
Website: www.biocranial.com
E-mail: bcranial@aol.com

GENERAL ORGANISATIONS

If you want to know more about specific alternative therapies, the following organisation will be happy to give you advice and put you in touch with the practitioners and societies that now meet with their high standards of practice and therapy.
Institute for Complementary Medicine (ICM), PO Box 194, London SE16 7QZ.
Tel: 020 7237 5855
Fax: 020 7237 5175
Website: www.icmedicine.co.uk
E-mail: info@i-c-m.org.uk

HALE CLINIC

This clinic is the largest alternative treatment centre in Europe with more than 100 practitioners, many of whom are also qualified medical doctors. Some of the best people working in alternative medicine in the UK are based at the Hale. The Hale Clinic, 7 Park Crescent, London W1B 1PF
Tel: 020 7631 0156
Fax: 020 7580 5771
Website: www.haleclinic.com
E-mail: admin@haleclinic.com

HEALING

A healer channels healing energies through their bodies and out through their hands into the patient's energy field, which encourages the body to heal itself. It is especially good for chronic fatigue and for raising energy levels when you are under the weather or suffering any illness. There is now a wealth of scientific research to show how healing works. See *Healing*.

To find your nearest practitioner, send a SAE to:

National Federation of Spiritual Healers,
Old Manor Farm Studio, Church Street, Sunbury-on-Thames, Middlesex TW16 6RG
Tel: 01932 783164
Fax: 01932 779648
Website: www.nfsh.org.uk

HEALING, REIKI

A very popular form of hands-on healing.
For general enquiries, contact

Sonia Thornton, The Reiki Association,
Westgate Court, Spittal, Haverfordwest SA62 5QP
Tel: 07704 270727 (As this is a mobile number, Sonia will be happy to call you back)
E-mail: enquiries@reikiassociation.org.uk
Website: www.reikiassociation.org.uk

HERBALISM

The practice of using plants to treat disease. Treatment may be given in the form of fluid extracts, tinctures, tablets or teas.
For further details and a register of qualified members, send a SAE to:

The National Institute of Medical Herbalists,
Elm House, 54 Mary Arches, Street, Exeter
EX4 3BA
Tel: 01392 426022
Fax: 01392 498963
Website: www.nimh.org.uk
E-mail: nimh@ukexeter.freeserve.co.uk

HOMEOPATHY

Works in harmony with the body to stimulate the body's natural healing mechanisms. Some researchers state that homeopathy is in the mind, but having used many remedies very successfully during the past 15 years homeopathy has proven very useful to me and thousands of people.
For a register of professionally qualified homeopaths and general information about homeopathy contact

The Society of Homeopaths, 11 Brookfield, Duncan Close, Moulton Park, Northampton NN3 6WL
Tel: 0845 450 6611
Fax: 0845 450 6622
Website: www.homeopathy-soh.org

E-mail: info@homeopathy-soh.org
Homeopathic Medical Association (HMA),
7 Darnley Road, Gravesend, Kent DA11 0RU.
Tel: 01474 560336
Website: www.the-hma.org
E-mail: info@the-hma.org
British Homeopathic Association (BHA),
Hahnemann House, 29 Park Street West, Luton LU1 3BE
Tel: 0870 444 3950
Fax: 0870 444 3960
Website: www.trusthomeopathy.org

HYPNOTHERAPY

By allowing external distractions to fade, the therapy allows you to fully relax and understand the root cause of many of your problems, phobias and addictions.
To find your nearest practitioner, telephone:

The National Council for Hypnotherapists on 0800 952 0545.
Website: www.hypnotherapists.org.uk
I visit Leila Hart in central London – a highly qualified accredited clinical hypnotherapist. She works with emotional and physical problems, phobias, weight loss and stress and can be contacted from 10am to 6pm on 020 7402 4311.

INSTITUTE FOR OPTIMUM NUTRITION

The Institute for Optimum Nutrition prints a wonderful quarterly magazine that is packed with up-to-date health news and the latest research in alternative medicine. The Institute also holds seminars on health and it has in-house nutritionists. For details contact:

Institute for Optimum Nutrition (ION),
Avalon House, 72 Lower Mortlake Road, Richmond, Surrey TW9 2JY
Tel: 020 8614 7800
Fax: 0870 979 1133
E-mail: reception@ion.ac.uk
Website: www.ion.ac.uk

IRIDOLOGY

A method of analysis rather than treatment, based on the theory that the whole body is reflected in the eyes. Using a magnifier, the practitioner examines the visible parts of the eyes to pinpoint physical weaknesses or potential areas that might cause you problems in the years to come.
Send an SAE for a list of qualified practitioners to:

Guild of Naturopathic Iridologists Int.,
94 Grosvenor Road, London SW1V 3LF
Tel: 020 7821 0255
Website: www.gni-international.org

KINESIOLOGY

The science of testing muscle response to discover areas of impaired energy and function in the body. Kinesiology is especially useful if you think you have a sensitivity or negative reaction either to a food or an external allergen.

To find your nearest practitioner, send 4 loose first-class stamps to the **Association for Systematic Kinesiology,** 16 Iris Road, West Ewell, Epsom, Surrey KT19 9NH
Tel: 0208 391 5988
Website: www.kinesiology.co.uk
E-mail: info@kinesiology.co.uk

MANUAL LYMPHATIC DRAINAGE

A very gentle pulsing massage, which helps to drain the lymph nodes, thereby reducing swelling and pain related to the lymph glands. A very useful treatment for ladies who have had breast and/or lymph surgery. Also great for reducing water retention anywhere in the body.

To find your nearest practitioner, send an SAE to: **Manual Lympatic Drainage UK**, PO Box 14491, Glenrothes, Fife, KY6 3YE
Tel: 01592 748008
Website: www.mlduk.org.uk
E-mail: admin@mlduk.org.uk

NATUROPATHY

Naturopaths are keen to treat the whole person, on a spiritual, physical and emotional level, to discover any underlying dysfunctions in a patient's life. They then offer advice on dietary changes, supplements and herbs to help your condition. Many naturopaths are also qualified homeopaths and/or acupuncturists. They help provide the right tools for the body to heal itself naturally. They are especially keen on detoxification and correcting any deficiencies in the body.

For more help contact:
The College of Naturopathic Medicine
Tel: 01342 410 505
Website: www.naturopathy-uk.com
They run college courses in London, Bristol, Manchester, Edinburgh, Dublin, Belfast and Cork. In central London I visit Bob Jacobs, who is a brilliant naturopath and homeopath – and a great friend.

Bob Jacobs, The Society of Complementary Medicine, 3 Spanish Place, London W1U 3HX
Tel: 020 7487 4334
Website: www.scmhealth.com
E-mail: admin@scmhealth.com

NEURO-LINGUISTIC PROGRAMMING

This is a profound and yet simple way to re-programme any negative thoughts or habits to more positive ones. Great for phobias and panic attacks, and for attaining your goals in life.
British Board of Neuro-Linguistic Programming (BBNLP), 46 Alexander Gate, Stevenage, Hertfordshire SG1 5RG
Tel: 07795 976 458
Website: www.bbnlp.co.uk
E-mail: nlp@bbnlp.com

NUTRI CENTRE, THE

The Nutri Centre, located on the lower ground floor of the Hale Clinic at 7 Park Crescent, London, is unique in being able to supply almost every alternative product currently available from any country, including specialised practitioner products. The Nutri Centre offers an excellent and reliable mail-order service worldwide for all its products.
For supplements:
Tel: 020 7436 5122
Fax 020 7436 5171
For books:
Tel: 020 7323 2382
Website: www.nutricentre.com
E-mail: customerservices@nutricentre.com

NUTRITIONAL THERAPY

To find your nearest qualified nutritionist who can help you to balance your diet and suggest the correct vitamins and minerals, and so on. Send £2 plus an A4 SAE to:
The British Association of Nutritional Therapists, 27 Old Gloucester Street, London WC1N 3XX
Tel: 0870 606 1284
Website: www.bant.org.uk
E-mail: the administrator@bant.org.uk
Contact **The Institute for Optimum Nutrition** (see above). For a directory of nutritionists send £5.00 to ION, Avalon House, 72 Lower Mortlake Road, Richmond, Surrey TW9 2JY
Tel: 0870 979 1122
Website: www.ion.ac.uk
E-mail: info@ion.ac.uk
The directory is also available on-line.

NUTRITIONIST WHO IS ALSO A MEDICAL DOCTOR

You will need to be referred by your own GP who will be able to find the address of your nearest practitioner by contacting:
British Society for Allergy Environmental and Nutritional Medicine (BSAENM), PO Box 7, Knighton, Powys, LD7 2WF
Tel: 01547 550380
Website: www.jnem.demon.co.uk

ORGANIC PRODUCE

The Soil Association has published an Organic Directory, which is packed with information on where to buy organic produce throughout the country.
This is available on-line for free at www.whyorganic.org
Soil Association, South Plaza, Marlborough Street, Bristol BS1 3NX
Tel: 0117 314 5000
Fax: 0117 314 5001
Website: www.soilassociation.org.uk
E-mail: info@soilassociation.org.uk
Soil Association Scotland, 18 Liberton Brae, Tower Mains, Edinburgh, EH16 6AE
Tel: 0131 666 2474
Fax: 0131 666 1684
E-mail: contact@sascotland.org

OSTEOPATHY

A system of healing that works on the physical structure of the body. Practitioners use manipulation, massage and stretching techniques. If you suffer chronic or sudden back, hip, neck or shoulder displacement or injury, go to see an osteopath.
To find your nearest practitioner, contact the
General Osteopathic Council, 176 Tower Bridge Road, London SE1 3LU
Tel: 020 7357 6655
Website: www.osteopathy.org.uk
E-mail: info@osteopathy.org.uk

PILATES

This is a highly effective, low-impact, isometric form of exercise, which you can practice even if you have suffered some kind of injury. Very powerful but gentle.
Pilates Foundation UK Ltd, PO Box 58235, London N1 5UY
Tel: 07071 781859
Website: www.pilatesfoundation.com
E-mail: admin@pilatesfoundation.com

QIGONG

An extremely gentle form of exercise (like T'ai Chi), which helps people with impaired mobility like severe arthritis. Anyone can practice qigong and no special clothes are needed. For further information contact:
TSE Qigong Centre, PO Box 59, Altringham, Cheshire WA15 8FS
Tel: 0161 929 4485
Fax: 0161 929 4489
Website: www.qimagazine.com.
E-mail: tse@qimagazine.com

REFLEXOLOGY

Gentle stimulation of the reflex/nerve-ending points on the hands and feet correspond to every part of the body. By working with pressure on these points, blockages in the energy pathways are released, which encourages the body to heal itself. This is a great way to boost circulation and really relaxing.
To find your nearest practitioner, contact
Association of Reflexologists, 5 Fore Street, Taunton, Somerset TA1 1HX
Tel: 0870 567 3320
Web: www.aor.org.uk
E-mail: info@aor.org.uk
AOR is a member of Reflexology in Europe Network and International Council of Reflexology.
The British Reflexology Association, Monks Orchard, Whitbourne, Worcester WR6 5RB
Tel: 01886 821207
Fax: 01886 822017
Website: www.britreflex.co.uk
E-mail: bra@britreflex.co.uk
See also details of Advance Refloxology on p.360.

YOGA

The ancient principles of yoga are beneficial for staying healthy and supple well into one's 80s and beyond. Yoga teaches relaxation and breathing techniques, together with gentle stretching exercises, which help keep the 'whole' self fit for life. Especially useful for keeping the spine strong. There is also now a monthly YOGA magazine, especially for yoga enthusiasts.
To find your nearest class click on-line
The British Wheel of Yoga, 25 Jermyn Street, Sleaford, Lincolnshire, NG34 7RU
Website: www.bwy.org.uk
E-mail: office@bwy.org.uk Tel: 01529 306851

INDEX

Other Books by Hazel Courteney

500 of The Most Important Ways to Stay Younger Longer
(Cico Books, £10.99)
Packed with cutting edge information on all aspects of ageing from the Brain and Blood Type in Ageing to Genes, Hormones and even Teeth in Ageing. More than 150 headings in another easy-to-read, A–Z book, covering all you need to know to help slow your ageing process.

* *

Divine Intervention
(Cico Books, £8.99)
Tells the true story of Hazel's amazing near-death experience during 1998, when she began levitating, giving intense healing, became super psychic and much more.

Robin Morgan – Editor of *The Sunday Times Magazine* – says, "*A provocative and compelling page turner – even the skeptics will be riveted.*"

* *

The Evidence For The Sixth Sense
(Cico Books, £9.99)
This is the sequel to *Divine Intervention*. Hazel continues her journey by taking part in the landmark Afterlife experiments in Arizona, which offer amazing evidence into the survival of human consciousness. She also interviews several world-class scientists who explain how miracles are possible in a language that anyone can understand. In addition she writes about what proves if a spiritual man or woman is truly enlightened.

Psychology Professor Gary Schwartz from the University of Arizona says,
"*This is an Important and inspiring book.*"

For more information on Hazel's work log on to www.hazelcourteney.com